Doctor Guilt?

Doctor Guilt?

Benefits of Medical Treatment
Compared with Hazards — A tradeoff

Everett Winslow Lovrien, M.D.

Brent died at age seventeen from AIDS after he became infected with HIV from medicine he used to treat hemophilia. Was the doctor that prescribed the contaminated medicine guilty of causing harm? Or were the drug companies that produced the medicine guilty of sacrificing safety for profitability?

iUniverse, Inc.
New York   Bloomington

Doctor Guilt?
Benefits of Medical Treatment Compared with Hazards — A tradeoff

iUniverse books may be ordered through booksellers or by contacting:

iUniverse
1663 Liberty Drive
Bloomington, IN 47403
www.iuniverse.com
1-800-Authors (1-800-288-4677)

Because of the dynamic nature of the Internet, any Web addresses or links contained in this book may have changed since publication and may no longer be valid. The views expressed in this work are solely those of the author and do not necessarily reflect the views of the publisher, and the publisher hereby disclaims any responsibility for them.

ISBN: 978-1-4502-1682-1 (sc)
ISBN: 978-1-4502-1684-5 (dj)
ISBN: 978-1-4502-1683-8 (ebk)

Library of Congress Control Number: 2010906298

Printed in the United States of America

iUniverse rev. date: 08/23/2010

Contents

Part I
Brent's Early Years

Part II
The Appearance of a New Disease

Part III

HIV and Hepatitis in Persons Attending the Clinic

Part IV
Differing Effects of HIV and Hepatitis

Part V
Origin of Hepatitis and HIV

Part VI
Onset of AIDS

Part VII
HIV in the School

Part VIII
Conclusion

List of Tables, Figures, and Photographic Plates

Tables

Figures

Plates

Acknowledgments

Many persons helped with this story. The assistance from families who were saddened by the loss of their son—or sons—or their father, their husband, or friend brought this tale together. Jim and Esther McAlpine provided information and photographs. Jim and Marjorie McAllister provided useful comments and a valuable perspective. Dave and Sharon Gibson graciously recounted events for this book. Nora Warren helped bring the events together. Carmelita Witbeck Perez supplied details of the school life of the two sons she lost. Wayne and Louise Cobb provided encouragement and a photograph. Linda Charles encouraged this writing and furnished information for the text. The Roseburg newspaper, the *News-Review*, was the source of a great amount of information. Jan Crider provided significant information and encouragement. Support is gratefully acknowledged from the Child Development and Rehabilitation Center. Help from the Oregon Hemophilia Treatment Center is acknowledged, especially from Patti Adams, Dave Oleson, Tammy Vogel, Robi Ingram, Monica Kraus, Jan Goldman, Alice Sprague, and Thallia. I also received inspiration from Dr. Lawrence Wolff, Dr. Scott Goodnight, Dr. David Noall, Dr. Robert Pittenger, Dr. Fred Ey, Dr. Dick Zimmerman, and Dr. Chuck Fagan. I appreciate the encouragement from Fred Adams and Dr. Vic Menashe as well as the support from Jerry Elder and Chuck Carter. The support from Dr. Art Thompson was important. Mary Jane Webb provided welcome assistance in Idaho. I acknowledge with appreciation the help and advice received from Dr. Dave Spence and Dr. Dale Webb in Alaska. I am grateful for approaches to judicial issues arising from the dilemma of HIV and hemophilia offered by John McCulloch and Rod Norton.

Every life has a story. All the persons who were part of the treatment center—patients, their families, and staff, as well as the Hemophilia Foundation of Oregon—though their names may not appear in this writing, are gratefully acknowledged and will not be forgotten.

The encouragement, patience, support, and professionalism from the editors at iUniverse have been inspirational for me as a first-time author.

I am grateful to Vicki Menard, editor of the Roseburg newspaper, for permission to quote and cite articles discussing HIV in the school.

Steven Paul Taylor inspired completion of this writing. Without his example and the encouragement from the supportive book discussion group he assembled, including Marci Taylor, Stacy Thomas, Nick Thomas, Seth Irish, and Pierrette Lovrien, I would not have achieved the finishing stroke.

The love received from my family, especially from my wife and children, has sustained me during the time this project came to life.

E. W. Lovrien

To those persons who had hemophilia and were infected with HIV or hepatitis while attending the Oregon Hemophilia Treatment Center, became ill, and died

Preface

Persons affected by medical disorders are confronted with the risks of their treatment. To weigh risks compared to expected benefits, they rely on their doctors' recommendations. Doctors make recommendations based upon accepted standards of medical care. When new therapy becomes available for a medical condition that previously had no satisfactory treatment, doctors often prescribe the medicine, hoping to relieve suffering, prevent complications and deformity, and to prevent fatalities. Rarely, but sometimes, the effectiveness of the medical recommendations from the doctors is nullified by unanticipated events that diminish the benefits and increase the harm caused by the treatment. The doctors and their patients are forced to choose between accepting the hazards without treatment and accepting the harmful aspects of a new medicine. They do not always accept the new medicine.

A medicine became available in the 1970s for the treatment of recurrent bleeding episodes in persons affected by hemophilia. The new medicine was regarded as miraculous for its potential to end suffering and prolong life. After the new miracle medicine was introduced, it was discovered that the medicine was polluted with hepatitis viruses and HIV, the virus that causes AIDS. The medical professionals working at the Oregon Hemophilia Treatment Center, which provided care and prescribed the new medicine, were devastated when they discovered the harmful side effects of their treatment.

This book includes the story of a young person named Brent, who died of AIDS when he was seventeen years of age. Brent was born with a medical condition that never went away during his short life, requiring repeated medical treatment. Brent received contaminated medicine at a hemophilia treatment center.

The events in this story do not take place in the "dark old days." The setting is during the times of modern medicine in the 1980s and 1990s. Events in Brent's life are set down as he would have described them if he had lived a few more years. Experiences related are real, although exact conversations, Brent's intimate thoughts, dates, places and details of events are not completely factual. Some names of places and living persons have been changed.

Through his treatment, Brent met other youths and men, not exactly like him, but who had the same medical disorder and required similar medical care. He met men and boys in the clinic where he was cared for—as well as at summer camp. Some of the events in their lives are also described in this story. He also met medical doctors, nurses, physical therapists, social workers, and a list of persons who served him in the clinic. Brent had a close family and loving relatives.

The medical condition Brent lived with, hemophilia, was treatable but not curable, and it required frequent infusions of medicine into his veins. Modern treatment with a revolutionary medicine brightened his life. But the medicine he received for treatment also led to his early death. By the time of the discovery of HIV tainting the medicine, Brent was already infected. Even though the doctors and the manufacturers of the medicine suspected a threatening virus, use of the medicine continued. The decision to continue using polluted medicine was made by the family as well as the doctor.

The families and doctors faced a dilemma—the threat of a life-endangering bleed if the medicine was withheld … or infection with a mysterious lethal virus if the medicine was infused into their veins.

Although he didn't live to see manhood, Brent matured from infancy and childhood constantly challenged by his medical disorder. Despite the heavy burden of medical complications from his treatment, he was always a cheerful, positive youth; however, he was skeptical and questioned decisions and procedures that affected him. Brent died at a young age, which is sad, but his life was not filled with sadness even though he consciously faced death. There were agonizing, painful days of suffering in Brent's life, from recurrent bleeds and the misery of the complications of AIDS, but the joyous moments dwarfed them. He chose a bright path to recognize the meaning of his life.

Brent wondered why the medicine he required led him to disaster rather than the longevity he had been promised. It came down to using a medicine that relieved suffering, helping him get through each day, but was polluted with deadly viruses that would overcome him and possibly result in death, or being safe and suffering from his medical condition, accepting the risks of not getting treatment.

Toward the end of his life, Brent became ill after using the medicine. The other persons he had met with hemophilia also became ill. By the time he questioned the merits of the medicine, he was already poisoned. It was too late once the harm of the medicine was discovered.

Brent was aware that he would die by his sixteenth birthday. Before he and all the others he knew died, they wondered why the doctors gave them medicine that led to suffering and an agonizing death rather than to good health and wellness. Following the discovery of HIV contamination of the medicine used to treat hemophilia in 1983, nearly one-half of males affected with hemophilia in the USA died of hepatitis or AIDS. How did this happen?

Families who lost a person to hepatitis or AIDS have been revisited to obtain their impressions, which are recorded in this book. They were asked whether the doctors who treated their sons were guilty of giving them medicine that led to their deaths. The survivors who related their impressions of the dynamics that resulted in the pollution of the hemophilia medicine with the virus that causes AIDS were nearly unanimous. They wanted their voices heard. Although the families acknowledged that the drug companies had produced a miraculous medicine, they maintained that the disaster was the result of the practices of the pharmaceutical manufacturers of the hemophilia medicine. Parents, wives, and daughters of hemophilia persons who died of AIDS or liver failure want their opinions to be known—that the deaths of their loved ones could have been prevented.

Doctors are the responsible directors of their patients' medical care. Although the doctors were unaware that the medicine was contaminated, shouldn't they have known? Rather than accept the word of the pharmaceutical manufacturers, wasn't a demand for greater safety in order? Were the doctors guilty of allowing harm to befall their patients, or were they only wrong because of their lack of knowledge?

Most readers of this book will never meet anyone who has hemophilia. Yet readers should care what happened when hepatitis and HIV claimed the lives of thousands of boys and men all over the world. Modern medicine is not without risks. Because of human nature, regulations and safeguards are necessary to control actions of a few who affect the lives of many.

Introduction

This book was written to commemorate the many young boys and men who died from AIDS after being treated for hemophilia. The purpose of writing this book is to stimulate discussion of the circumstances and events that doomed hemophilia patients to death from hepatitis and AIDS. It explores the intricacies of life, human nature, and medicine. This book is intended for the general reader, to make him aware of the difficulties in balancing new treatments against the possibilities of future serious or fatal complications.

It is about boys and men, but it is also about women—the mothers, spouses, sisters, and daughters of those men and boys. Some males inherited a medical disorder from their mothers. Although the origin of their medical disorder is from their mothers, their mothers are not to blame. Humans are part of nature. Nature's way of altering living things sometimes appears unreasonable. Things happen.

In the past, children born with hemophilia usually died during childhood or as young adults. And while they were alive, they suffered from pain and became disabled from recurrent bleeding into their joints.

During the last quarter of the previous century, a treatment was developed to relieve pain and suffering and prevent deformity in persons born with hemophilia. With this new method of treatment, it was hoped that the young boys would not die early in their lives—instead, by using the medicine, they would grow to adulthood to become men with near-normal life spans ... with lives free from pain and disability. During the 1970s and 1980s, the new medicine for treatment of hemophilia, AHF[1] concentrate, became available in the Western world, North America, Australia, parts of Europe, and some countries in South America. The new concentrate to treat hemophilia dramatically changed the lives of affected males living within advantaged countries, for the better.

In the beginning of this new era in hemophilia treatment, concentrate was produced as a derivative of blood obtained from paid donors. In recent years, medicine for treating hemophilia has been manufactured by genetic methods, without blood as its source. Before the methods to produce the medicine without using blood were developed, over a period of twenty years, thousands of males who had hemophilia were infused with the blood derivative. The blood-derived AHF concentrate had a great impact, relieving suffering and preventing premature deaths. Lives in the world of hemophilia were sailing along smoothly in the 1970s and beginning of the 1980s.

But nature changed all that with the discovery that the concentrate was contaminated with viruses. The hepatitis virus and HIV,[2] the virus that causes AIDS, were lurking in the concentrate derived from blood. Regarding the hepatitis virus, doctors were aware of its presence in the concentrate made from blood. They assumed that all persons infused with concentrate would become infected with the hepatitis virus. But they also assumed that the fate of a person affected with hemophilia was doomed without the medicine. The risks of the medicine were overshadowed by the benefits of the treatment. Doctors believed that illness caused by hepatitis was less serious than the risk of a bleed into the brain if treatment was avoided. Aware that the medicine was contaminated with live hepatitis virus, patients and doctors agreed that the best action to relieve pain and prevent disability and premature death was to treat bleeding episodes with infusions of concentrate.

---

1   antihemophilia factor
2   human immunodeficiency virus

In the case of hepatitis, doctors knowingly gave the virus to males with hemophilia when infusing them with concentrate. In the case of HIV, the doctors were unaware of its existence. By the time the virus was detected in concentrate, it was too late to prevent its devastating effect. Many males who were infused with concentrate, some over a period of ten or twenty years, were doomed to die of AIDS, a fate worse than hemophilia. The years of a miracle treatment for hemophilia had ended.

After the passage of years, time has revealed that the doctors were mistaken about the harmless presence of hepatitis. The hepatitis virus is not harmless. Doctors believed that the trade-off between hepatitis and untreated hemophilia was acceptable. Many of those men who were infused with polluted concentrate during the 1970s and 1980s, who did not die from AIDS, subsequently died from liver disease, including cancer of the liver and liver failure, an outcome of hepatitis.

The doctors were unaware of the virus that causes AIDS, a new illness, until it was too late. They did not knowingly give HIV virus to persons with hemophilia.

The world for persons born with hemophilia seemed so bright with the advent of the new concentrate to treat their recurrent bleeding episodes in the 1970s. A dark curtain unexpectedly descended upon their lives, at first from AIDS and subsequently liver failure and liver cancer, in the 1980s and 1990s. In the era of modern medicine, when treatment for a medical disorder was well established and accepted, if the treatment leads to disaster rather than the expected relief, shouldn't there be some accountability? Were the doctors justified when they knowingly gave the hepatitis virus to their patients? Were they correct when they assumed the risks without treatment exceeded the hazards from their prescribed treatment utilizing hepatitis-contaminated medicine? Although the doctors did not know about AIDS and HIV contamination of the concentrate, should they have known? Doctors are not malicious. Doctors are supposed to prevent suffering and save lives. They did not knowingly infuse their patients with HIV; nevertheless, they did give them the virus that causes AIDS. Should the doctors be held accountable? Are they to blame for the hepatitis and AIDS that snuffed out the lives of thousands of persons who had hemophilia? The doctors knowingly gave their patients an old disease, hepatitis, and unknowingly a new disease, AIDS.

Prescribing the new miracle medicine for the treatment of recurrent bleeds of hemophilia by the doctors is only half the AIDS story. The other half of the story originates from the producers of the medicine, the pharmaceutical manufacturers. Revisiting families whose son or husband became a victim of AIDS or liver failure from hepatitis reveals a nearly unanimous sentiment that they wish to be expressed in this account. The wives and parents of those who died profess that the drug companies sacrificed safety for profitability. How could this happen, they wonder? Why wasn't more regulation applied to assure the safety of the blood supply?

Why didn't the drug companies who produced the medicine eliminate hepatitis viruses? If they would have purified concentrate to eliminate hepatitis, HIV would have also been eliminated. AIDS in hemophilia could have been prevented.

Were the doctors too complacent, the sharpness of their judgment blunted by financial support from the drug companies in the form of research funds, travel expenses, and discounts?

Another purpose of writing this book is to acknowledge all those who suffered from hemophilia and died from hepatitis or AIDS. Of those who received care where Brent did, nearly ninety persons who had hemophilia died from HIV or hepatitis-related illness.[3] Some of their names are included in table 5. More than 10,000 persons who infused concentrate to treat hemophilia became infected with HIV in the United States. In one report (Chorba et al. 2001), 4,781 deaths occurred in those affected by hemophilia during a ten-year period. The cause of deaths was HIV related in 2,254 persons (47 percent).

---

3   Oregon Hemophilia Treatment Center 2008

Many persons believe those losses were avoidable and could have been prevented.

Those whose lives were ended after using concentrate are entitled to the dignity and respect that all humans deserve. They suffered and died not because of their own doing; they were innocent. They were grand people. Let us love them rather than forget them.

E. W. Lovricn
Fairview, Oregon

Part I

Brent's Early Years

In the Beginning

Brent was born in Spokane, a town nestled within the most eastern part of northeastern Washington, over in a corner, distant from most of Washington, as well as away from the main part of the United States. Spokane is larger than a town; it is a small city.

Gwyn Margaret McCann, Brent's mother, born August 18, 1946, was an attractive twenty-nine-year-old woman. She was not a native of Spokane. She was the second oldest of four beautiful sisters, preacher's kids, no brothers, born to a Canadian Protestant minister and his attractive Detroit wife. The family moved from Detroit to San Diego, California, where Gwyn's father served his church.

Brent's lovely mother became a college student at San Diego State College where her handsome professor turned her pretty head. They fell in love, which culminated in a trip to the altar. After they married, Gwyn and her husband moved to Spokane, where he accepted a faculty position in the Modern Language Department of Gonzaga College. Brent's oldest sister, Paula, was born in Spokane on Thanksgiving Day in 1969, before Brent's mother discovered that her husband no longer wished to be married to her. She and her first husband divorced, although they continued to remain amicable.

Gwyn married another man, a dynamic twenty-nine-year-old Spokanite: Leland Hubert Perry. With Lee, Brent's mom had a second child, Colette, who was born in 1971. His mom and dad and two sisters lived in a cute little one-story brick house at West 2905 32nd Street in Spokane. Not far away from the house, in the early morning hours, Brent came into this world at 10:24 AM on October 4, 1975, in Sacred

Heart Hospital, Spokane, Washington. His first view of the world outside his mother's womb was in the hospital where his life began. Like many of us, his life did not end in the same hospital, or the same city, or even in the same state where he was born.

Preceding Brent's birth, Gwyn's older sister, Louise McCann Carson, gave birth to an infant son who was born with hydrocephalus, a birth defect presenting with an abnormally large head. Hemophilia was not suspected at the time of his birth, and no tests were completed. However, it is possible that the cause for the child's large head was an undiagnosed bleed inside his skull. In 1962, he died at six months. A second son was born to Gwyn's sister, a normal child. Eight years before Brent's birth, a third child was born to the same sister, Louise, in 1967, a baby boy, Brent's cousin, Bill Carson, who was circumcised and almost bled to death a few days later. Tests completed in California, where the family lived, revealed that the baby boy had hemophilia. There had been no ancestors with bleeding tendencies in the family. He was the first case of the bleeding disorder in the McCann sisters' family. Everyone in the family was tested to identify carriers of hemophilia—who would be at risk of giving birth to another male infant—by obtaining blood samples that were sent to Johns Hopkins Medical Center for analysis. The 1967 test results were normal for the mother of the infant born with hemophilia, her three sisters, her mother, and her grandmother.

They were informed that they were not carriers of hemophilia. If they had sons, they were told, none would be affected with hemophilia. The family assumed the birth of an infant male with hemophilia to one of the sisters was an instance of a new mutation, and hemophilia was not inherited in the family. Gwyn thought she was off the hook if she were to have a son—he would not have hemophilia. Even though Gwyn was informed that she was not a carrier of hemophilia, she wasn't completely confident of the test results.[4] When Gwyn and her husband

---

4   Gwyn's friend Pierrette recalls hearing Gwyn proclaim after the birth of her first
     child, Paula that she was glad it was a girl, implying that she harbored worry
     about the possibility of having a son with hemophilia.

moved away from her family in Santa Barbara, she did not know that she was a carrier of hemophilia. Gwyn became pregnant for the third time. Again, she was told she was not a carrier and not at risk for having a son with hemophilia, as her sister had before her. At six months of gestation, Johns Hopkins Hospital notified her, reporting that the tests previously completed were not reliable. A new method of testing for carriers of hemophilia, which was more accurate, had become available. However, she was already far along in her pregnancy.

Brent, the third child, her first son, was born headfirst. "And it was fast," his mother proclaimed. There were no abnormal signs of bleeding at birth, no scalp hematomas, and no bruises.

Birth is a rough trip. During birth, the infant's head is squished against the inside of the hard bones of the mother's pelvis. The arms and legs, shoulders, and hips are twisted and squeezed, and yet the slippery baby usually emerges unscathed, a miracle of nature.

Why don't all infant boys who have severe hemophilia bleed during their birth? Some mothers believe their blood protects their babies from bleeding, and some doctors let the mothers continue to harbor their maternal protective beneficial beliefs because it makes them feel better, even if the mother's impression is incorrect.

Brent did not bleed excessively after a heel stick to collect newborn blood samples. This test is accomplished by jabbing the point of a sharp blade into the soft skin of a newborn's heel, followed by squeezing the baby's foot until blood flows from the wound.

Before Brent went home from the hospital, the doctor examined him. He proclaimed that Brent was a healthy, normal little boy. Brent opened his eyes. He moved his arms, legs, fingers, and toes; he had a robust cry. His testicles were descended. Gwyn remembered that she had a nephew, her sister's son, Bill Carson, who was a bleeder. He had hemophilia. He was Brent's maternal cousin. She decided not to have her son circumcised.

One way to find out if Brent would manifest signs of abnormal bleeding, to discover if he had hemophilia similar to his maternal cousin, would be a simple test: snip off the foreskin of his little penis and see if he bled afterward, the test of circumcision. But such a test is not without hazard. There is risk of uncontrollable bleeding afterward. Circumcision is not an accurate procedure to establish the diagnosis of hemophilia. Nearly one-third of the infant males who have hemophilia and have been circumcised, their unsuspecting parents unaware of hemophilia[5] at their son's birth, have not bled following circumcision.[6] A preferable test to establish whether Brent would develop signs of abnormal bleeding from hemophilia would be to complete a test after obtaining a sample of blood from one of his veins. However, obtaining a blood sample from the tiny vein of a newborn is not an easy task. To diagnose hemophilia, by measuring the clotting activity of blood to determine the amount of antihemophilia factor (AHF), special care must be exercised when obtaining the sample. A free-flowing blood sample must be collected without contamination from tissue juices. The collected blood sample must be promptly processed and sent to a laboratory that is experienced in testing for AHF. The type of hemophilia that affected Brent's cousin was type A, the result of a deficiency of AHF VIII in his blood. To determine if Brent had hemophilia type A, the laboratory must assay the factor VIII in his blood. Most hospital laboratories are not set up for AHF testing. A blood sample is usually sent to a reference laboratory for factor VIII assay when hemophilia is suspected. The most practical method for sampling a newborn's blood for testing is by catching the blood from the umbilical cord after it has been severed from the infant. The umbilical blood sample is free-flowing, and the source of blood is from the infant, not the mother.

Gwyn had informed the doctor and the nurse before her son was born that her nephew was affected with hemophilia. She instructed them that if her expected baby was a male, he should not be circumcised

---

5   One-third or one-fourth of males born with hemophilia are the first instances in their family.

6   Circumcision is completed on newborn male infants with a Gomko clamp, which clamps off the foreskin, rather than the amputation utilized in older males.

because there was a chance that her son might have hemophilia even if there were no signs of bleeding at his birth. She also informed both the doctor and the nurse that if her infant was a male, a blood sample must be collected from the umbilical cord after it was severed from the baby for testing for hemophilia. Neither the doctor nor the nurse honored her request. No sample was collected from the umbilical cord of her newborn son. After her son was born, Gwyn did not know if he was affected with hemophilia or if he was free of the bleeding disorder that affected his older cousin.

The explanation for not following the mother's request, for collecting a sample of umbilical cord blood at birth to be tested for hemophilia, remains unanswered. It is unlikely that the doctor and the nurse intentionally ignored the mother's request. That would be unethical. More likely, the explanation had a logistical basis. For example, when a test for hemophilia is to be performed on a blood sample, a special test tube—a prothrombin tube—is necessary. The collected blood sample must be kept cold by placing it on ice and promptly processed for analysis. Conditions may not have been arranged prior to delivery since babies are not born at scheduled times.

"Isn't he cute?" exclaimed Pierrette, a visitor friend of the mother, who came to the hospital to rejoice over the birth of the new baby. "Doesn't he look just like a little Buddha?" The newly born little boy had a red round face and a serious countenance—if newborns can be serious. He was named Brent McCann Perry. Brent died at age seventeen in 1993, the result of an infectious disease.

Brent was fortunate to have been born when modern medicine facilitated treatment of his uncommon medical disorder, which predictably should have allowed him to live many years. Advances in medicine in Brent's era were remarkable; however, the gains were polluted with havoc. How did this happen? Was this a mystery? Was this the way life was meant to be for some persons? The doctors who treat hemophilia were aware that pooling plasma from hundreds, sometimes thousands, of donors was risky. One contaminated donor would contaminate the entire large lot made from the pooled plasma. Yet they accepted medicine made from the pooled lot, reasoning that it was a trade-off, with the benefits outweighing the risks. Was it the impact of the doctor's treatment that caused Brent's death? Is the doctor guilty?

Discovery of Hemophilia in Spokane

On the second day of his life, Gwyn carefully carried her newly born son, swaddled in a blue baby blanket cozily tucked into an infant carrier basket, from the hospital where he first opened his eyes and made his first cry, to the little house on West 32nd Street. His father, Lee, and his two sisters—Paula, age six, and Colette, age four—were anxious to help take care of him.

The family did not know if Brent had hemophilia or if he did not. The opportunity to test for hemophilia with a sample of cord blood had been missed. Because of the difficulty of obtaining a free-flowing blood sample to test for hemophilia from his tiny veins, the doctor recommended waiting to see if signs of unusual bleeding appeared. If he was a few months older, the doctor reasoned, obtaining a blood sample for a test would be easier. Six months later, on the morning of April 2, 1976, Gwyn lifted her infant son from his crib. He was wide-awake. She kissed the top of his fuzzy head and then laid him down on the changing table. "Oh, you are a good baby," she said to him as she unsnapped his flannel pajamas and pulled them off over his head.

"Oh my God!" Gwyn shrieked when she discovered extensive purple blotches discoloring her baby's chest along the lower ribs, extending from the front to the sides of his chest. She rolled him over and noted that the marks were also on his back. She inspected them closely and thought they resembled bruises. He was not crying as if in pain. "Come here quickly!" Gwyn screamed at her husband. "Look at your son. He's all black and blue!" Terrified, the parents wrapped their infant in a blanket and rushed to the doctor's office in Spokane. On that April day, two days before Brent was six months of age, they recounted to the doctor that the day before their infant son had been pushing with his small stockinged feet while sitting in a jump-up swing that was suspended in the kitchen doorway, laughing while bouncing up and down.

After undressing and examining the infant, the doctor quietly declared that the purple discoloration of Brent's little ribs in his chest did not resemble the nature of bleeding he expected to see if the baby had hemophilia. He told Gwyn that other possible causes may have produced the bruises. For example, he said, leukemia, a cancer of the blood, often first appears as bruises of the skin in infants. He also mentioned "battered child syndrome"[7]; however, the doctor did not infer that Gwyn or her husband had beaten their infant son. This unfortunate condition was newly recognized in pediatric circles and was on the tip of most pediatricians' tongues.

The doctor successfully obtained a sample of blood from Brent's little arm vein, which was processed and sent to a special laboratory to be tested for factor VIII, the clotting factor deficient in hemophilia type A. While the needle was still in place in the vein, after the blood sample had been withdrawn, the doctor infused Brent with concentrate, even though hemophilia had not been diagnosed. The unusual bleeding into his chest was suspicious enough to warrant the infusion, knowing that hemophilia was present in the infant's male cousin.

Several days later, when the doctor received the report of the results of the blood test, he immediately called Gwyn to his office to notify her of the test results. He said he was surprised and dismayed when he discovered that he must report to Gwyn that her son had severe hemophilia, the same disorder that affected his eight-year-old cousin. The factor VIII in Brent's blood was less than 1 percent of the normal

---

7   During the 1960s and 1970s, in the medical offices of pediatricians, an awareness of babies who had been injured by a parent was prominent: battered child syndrome. Often a baby was mistakenly suspected of being the victim of battered child syndrome before the correct diagnosis of hemophilia was established.

amount, which established the diagnosis of severe hemophilia type A. Brent was given his first infusion of concentrate in 1976, in Spokane, to arrest bleeding in his chest.

From that moment on, for the rest of his life, although a normal child, Brent's life would be different from those of other little boys. Gwyn was pleased that she did not know that her son was affected with hemophilia until he was six months of age. Some people refer to a person who has hemophilia as a hemophiliac, a word Gwyn detested. She did not want her child labeled. Her infant son was not a hemophiliac—he was Brent. The six months of not knowing he had hemophilia gave her a chance to bond with him. Not fearing for him, she had cared for him as a normal baby boy during those happy six months.[8] Nature seems to feel that way too. Even infants who are born with severe hemophilia often do not bleed after birth. Sometimes no signs of bleeding appear for several months. In some instances, infant males born with hemophilia do not reveal signs of abnormal bleeding until they begin to crawl and walk, as late as one year of age.

---

8   From discussion with Gwyn McCann August 31, 2007

Signs and Symptoms of Hemophilia

The signs and symptoms of hemophilia are the result of a deficiency of the blood to clot normally (Genetics Home Reference 2009). A person's blood repeatedly circulates over and over again, confined to the inside of the blood vessels. The route of the circulating blood is a constant, endless, very long trip, night and day, year after year. And yet the blood does not leak from the tubes that allow it passage. If blood escapes from the tubes, that is called a hemorrhage. A common sign of a localized hemorrhage is a bruise, such as a black eye from a damaged blood vessel. After an injury or a ruptured blood vessel, blood escapes from the tubes into the tissues, where it decomposes and becomes discolored. Hemophilia families refer to hemorrhages as bleeds.

Why don't bleeds occur more often in people who do not have bleeding disorders? If a person were to grasp a sharp knife and slash across the back of his hand, he usually would not bleed to death. His body is protected by three processes to prevent blood from leaking outside the blood vessels, a process referred to as hemostasis. After a blood vessel is severed or broken, the first thing that happens in hemostasis is the release of adrenalin by the tissue surrounding the blood vessel. Adrenalin produces an immediate contraction, vasoconstriction, shrinkage of the blood vessel. The second thing that occurs within a few seconds is the formation of a seal at the site of injury by platelets, which plug the rent in the blood vessel wall. Platelets circulate in the blood and are attracted to an injured blood vessel wall by the exposure of the tissues in the blood vessel wall. Third, and more slowly, fibrin is laid down into the platelet plug. Fibrin acts as cement to hold the platelet plug in place while healing occurs. However, if significant amounts of fibrin were constantly present in circulating blood, blood clots would form, and a stroke or heart attack would result from excessive clotting. To prevent unwanted clot formation, fibrin must be activated from its precursor condition before it can be laid down.

One of the precursors of fibrin formation is antihemophilia factor, or AHF. AHF is necessary to form an effective blood clot at the site of a blood vessel injury. A person who has hemophilia has a deficiency or a defective AHF. His platelet plug does not cement in place; it does not retract. It is soft and mushy rather than firm. After the platelet plug forms at the site of a damaged blood vessel in a person who has hemophilia, oozing slowly begins around the soft plug and continues at the injured site.

Hemostasis—the control of blood flow

1. Release of adrenalin at site of injury
2. Formation of a platelet plug
3. Deposition of fibrin in platelet plug

Persons who have hemophilia experience episodic, recurrent oozing of blood into their tissues. In cases of severe hemophilia, the bleeds may occur spontaneously, without noticeable preceding injury (Genetics Home Reference 2009). As a result of bleeding, serious complications occur, with damage to muscles, joints, internal organs, and even the brain.

The genes that control production of the clotting factors—AHF F8 and F9—are located on the X chromosome. The mutant hemophilia gene X^h is recessive to the normal gene X^H. For a female to have hemophilia, both of her X chromosomes would need to carry the mutant gene.

Males have only one X chromosome, received from their mother, which is paired with a Y chromosome received from their father. Males who have the normal clotting factor gene are X^HY. Males who inherit a mutant clotting factor gene from their mother are X^hY. There is no hemophilia gene on the Y chromosome. As a result, when present, the recessive mutant hemophilia gene is expressed in males, resulting in hemophilia. Females who have a mutant hemophilia gene, X^hX^H, are hemophilia carriers without signs of hemophilia.[9] They can transmit their mutant hemophilia gene to their daughters, who will also be carriers of hemophilia, or the daughters may receive the normal gene from their mothers and be noncarriers, X^HX^H. For men who have hemophilia, X^hY, none of their sons will have hemophilia since they receive only their father's Y chromosome. However, all daughters born to men who have hemophilia will be carriers of hemophilia, X^hX^H, since they receive their father's X^h chromosome.

Brent was born with a defect of AHF factor VIII. Treatment consisted of replacement of AHF with intravenous infusions of factor VIII concentrate, beginning in 1976, to return the clotting activity to near normal so the injured blood vessel could heal properly.

---

9   Hemophilia does rarely occur in females, such as in Turner syndrome (see below: "A Girl with Hemophilia"), from lyonization or if a hemophilia carrier female marries a man with hemophilia.

Hemophilia in the McCann Family

Table 1. McCann family individuals

0001	Brent Perry	b. 1975 d. 1993	male, hemophilia
0002	Colette	b. 1971	female noncarrier, tested 1980s at OHSU
0003	Paula	b. 1969	female noncarrier, tested 1989–1991 at OHSU
0004	Rich		male, hemophilia
0005	Ann		female, noncarrier
0006	Margaret		female, hemophilia carrier, has an infant son, 0100, affected with hemophilia
0007	Henry		male, unaffected
0008	Bill Carson	b. 1966 d. 1991	male, hemophilia. First child in the family to have hemophilia discovered when he bled after circumcision.
0009	Ted		unaffected male.
0010	Jeff Carlson Jr.	b.1960 d. 1961	male, the firstborn child, died at nine months, congenital hydrocephalus—possible intracranial hemorrhage
0011	Blanche		female, hemophilia carrier
0012	Jacob		male, unaffected
0013	Harold		unaffected male, spouse of 0006
0100	Wendell	b. 2007	male, hemophilia
1000	Gwyn McCann	b. 1946	female, hemophilia carrier, born in Detroit, MI, one son, 0001, with hemophilia
1001	Darrel		unaffected male, first husband of 1000

1002	Lee Perry		unaffected male, spouse of 1000, father of 0001
1004	Lea McCann	b. 1952	female, hemophilia carrier, mother of son, 0004, who has hemophilia
1005	Joseph		unaffected male, husband of 1004
1006	Larissa McCann	b. 1949	female, hemophilia carrier, grandmother of 0100
1007	Cary		unaffected male, husband of 1006
1008	Louise McCann	b. 1942	female, hemophilia carrier, had a son, 0008, with hemophilia
1009	Jeff		unaffected male, husband of 1008
2000	Prudence Zorn McCann	b. 1916	b. Detroit, MI, female hemophilia carrier, mother of four hemophilia carrier daughters. No ancestors, relatives or siblings with hemophilia
2001	Eric McCann	b. 1911 d. 2008	unaffected male, born in St. Marys, Ontario
2002	Emily Zorn		female noncarrier
2003	Hannah Zorn		female noncarrier
2004	Alice Zorn		female noncarrier
2005	Hollister Zorn		unaffected male
3000	Vance Zorn	b. 1885 d. 1968	unaffected male
3001	Pentecote Cance Zorn	b. 1887 d. 1977	female, maternal great-grandmother of 0001, born in Detroit, MI

Although Gwyn did not know that her newborn son had hemophilia when she brought him home from the hospital after his birth when he was two days of age, she was less shocked with the discovery of his bleeding disorder than the doctor was for she was aware that her sister, Louise, three years older, had a son affected with hemophilia.

During the years following the discovery of hemophilia in the McCann Family, tests have been offered and completed on different blood samples collected from members of the family to establish and confirm the diagnosis of hemophilia after signs of bleeding occurred, and to identify females who might be at risk of transmitting the hemophilia mutant gene to their male and female offspring. The method of the testing has evolved over several years, initially from being useful but not completely accurate, to more accurate tests following the development of molecular testing procedures. Combining the information from the results of tests and information from the actual observations in the McCann family, improved knowledge of the inheritance of the hemophilia gene in the family has evolved. Parents in the family were informed that if they had a son with hemophilia, the child could receive medicine that would prevent bleeding, allowing him to achieve a near-normal life expectancy. They were assured that tests could identify females who might transmit the hemophilia gene to their children. Neither of these measures, intended to avoid the problems suffered by hemophilia families in past generations, were accurate in the McCann family.

After the unexpected discovery that Brent's cousin, Bill,[10] had hemophilia, revealed after he was circumcised and bled, a sample of Bill's mother's[11] blood was tested. She was identified as a female carrier of hemophilia. Subsequently, her three sisters, her mother, and her grandmother were tested after blood samples were collected in California, where the family lived at that time, and sent to Johns Hopkins University. The reports from the tests stated that the three

10   Table 1, individual 0008
11   Table 1, individual 1008

sisters,[12] their mother, and their grandmother were not carriers of hemophilia. The McCann family assumed that Bill's hemophilia was caused by a new mutation rather than inherited. After the discovery that Brent was affected with hemophilia like his cousin, the McCann family, including all four of the sisters, was retested. The blood samples were again sent to Johns Hopkins, in 1975, to be tested with improved methods that were regarded as more reliable than the methods available in the 1960s. With the development of improved methods for testing, family studies reveal that when no family history of hemophilia is present and a male is born for the first instance of hemophilia in the family, the mother is usually a carrier of hemophilia. Using the newer methods of testing, the mother of the four sisters—Prudence Zorn McCann, 2000, table 1—Gwyn's mother, was identified as a carrier of hemophilia. The three sisters of Prudence and their six daughters and her brother were tested and they were normal. Pentecote, 3001, table 1, was also tested, and she was normal; she did not carry the hemophilia trait. Apparently, Prudence had a new mutation, the first instance of the appearance of the abnormal hemophilia gene in the family. She probably was conceived with a mutation on the X chromosome that she received from her father's sperm. During the months and years that have followed, the four sisters have produced four male descendants who have had hemophilia.[13]

Theoretically, tests are useful for identifying women who are carriers of hemophilia, which allows them to decide if they wish to have children, if they are willing to accept the risk of begetting a male affected with hemophilia, or if they want to avoid having biological offspring who may have the bleeding disorder. In reality, most women who are from families that include an affected male independently decide upon their reproduction regardless of genetic testing. As exemplified in the McCann family, the older tests for detecting hemophilia carriers were

12 Table 1, individuals (sisters) 1000, 1004, 1006; (mother) 2000; (maternal grandmother) 3001

13 Table 1, individuals 0001, 0100, 0004, 0008

not accurate. Newer tests that utilize molecular testing are believed to be more accurate.[14]

Although Gwyn and her sisters were informed that they were not carriers of hemophilia after the initial tests were completed, but subsequently all four of the sisters produced descendants with hemophilia, they were not disturbed to a high degree with the information from carrier testing, even though it was erroneous. They believed that they, not the doctors, not the laboratories, were the ones who had the children. All the doctors and laboratories were doing the best they could, with intentions of being helpful. Producing offspring, regardless of the outcome, was the parents' responsibility. They attempted to use the best information available at that time.

---

14 With older tests, individual 0006 was informed that she was not a carrier of hemophilia. After she married, she was retested with new molecular tests and discovered to be a carrier of hemophilia. She and her husband are the parents of individual 0100, a little boy who is affected with hemophilia.

New Carrier Tests for Hemophilia

Table 2. McCann family

Number	Name	Sex	L/D		Hemophilia	
0001	Brent Perry	M	D	hY	hemophilia	male ∎
0002	Colette	F	L	XX	noncarrier	female O
0003	Paula	F	L	XX	noncarrier	female O
0004	Rich	M	L	hY	hemophilia	male ∎
0005	Ann	F	L	XX	noncarrier	female O
0006	Margaret	F	L	hX	carrier	female ⊙
0007	Henry	M	L	XY	unaffected	male □
0008	Bill Carson	M	D	hY	hemophilia	male ∎
0009	Ted	M	L	XY	unaffected	male □
0010	Jeff Carlson Jr.	M	D	XY**	?	male ?
0011	Blanche	F	L	hX	carrier	female ⊙
0012	Jacob	M	L	XY	unaffected	male □
0013	Harold	M	L	XY	unaffected	male □
0100	Wendell	M	L	hY	hemophilia	male ∎
1000	Gwyn McCann	F	L	hX*	carrier	female ⊙
1001	Darrel	M	L	XY	unaffected	male □
1002	Lee Perry	M	D	XY	unaffected	male □
1004	Lea McCann	F	L	hX*	carrier	female ⊙
1005	Joseph	M	L	XY	unaffected	male □
1006	Larissa McCann	F	L	hX*	carrier	female ⊙
1007	Cary	M	L	XY	unaffected	male □
1008	Louise McCann	F	L	hX***	carrier	female ⊙
1009	Jeff	M	L	XY	unaffected	male □
2000	Prudence Zorn McCann	F	L	hX*	carrier	female ⊙
2001	Eric McCann	M	D	XY	unaffected	male □
2002	Emily Zorn	F	L	XX****	noncarrier	female O
2003	Hannah Zorn	F	L	XX****	noncarrier	female O
2004	Alice Zorn	F	D	XX****	noncarrier	female O

Number	Name	Sex	L/D		Hemophilia	
2005	Hollister Zorn	M	D	XY	unaffected	male □
3000	Vance Zorn	M	D	XY	unaffected	male □
3001	Pentecote Cance Zorn	F	D	XX	noncarrier	female O

* After test reported as noncarrier in 1960s, had hemophilia descendents.

** Born with hydrocephalus, died at nine months

*** Tested following the birth of her hemophilia son, 0008, reported as a carrier

**** Six female offspring of 2004, 2003, and 2002 tested in 1980s; noncarriers XX noncarrier female; XY unaffected male; hX carrier female; hY hemophilia male L living; D deceased

After Brent was diagnosed as having hemophilia, the second instance of hemophilia in the family, inheritance rather than a new mutation explained the appearance of the disorder. The entire family was retested by collecting blood samples, which were again sent to Johns Hopkins Medical Center in Baltimore. The second testing was completed in1976, when improved methods that had been developed were regarded as more accurate to identify females who carry the hemophilia gene, compared to the previous tests of the 1960s. Of the four sisters in the family, three have had sons affected with hemophilia, and one has had a grandson with hemophilia. All four sisters are carriers of the hemophilia trait caused by the mutant hemophilia gene they inherited from their mother rather than a normal hemophilia gene. The mother of the four sisters, Gwyn's mother (Individual 2000, figure 1), Brent's maternal grandmother, was confirmed to be a hemophilia carrier by the newer test method. She had a normal, unaffected brother and three sisters.

The first tests to identify female carriers of hemophilia consisted of measuring activity of factor VIII. A female with less than 50 per cent factor VIII activity was assumed to be a carrier of hemophilia. The second generation of carrier testing consisted of measuring the amount of factor VIII protein immunologically, which was compared with the factor VIII activity. The basis of this test assumed that factor VIII was being produced, but it was inactive. Neither of these approaches is completely accurate because of lyonization.

Lyonization refers to the inactivation of one of the female X chromosomes (Vogel and Motulsky 1986, 75). Females possess two X chromosomes, whereas males have only one X chromosome, which is paired with a Y chromosome. Yet females do not produce twice as much product as males from a gene located on the X chromosome. An $X^H X^H$ female does not produce twice as much factor VIII when compared with a $X^H Y$ male. In females, one of the X chromosomes is lyonized, (turned off). In a female carrier of hemophilia, $X^H X^h$, if the mutant gene (h) is turned off, the expressing gene (H) on the active X chromosome would produce as much factor VIII as a normal male.

Most recently, tests for identification of female hemophilia carriers include molecular analysis, which directly characterizes the hemophilia factor VIII gene (F8) rather than the product of the gene. The most common mutation of F8 is the intron 22 inversion, detectable with Southern blot analysis (Oldenburg and El-Maarri 2006).

According to the new test results, none of the grandmother's three sisters were hemophilia carriers. The suggestion that the maternal grandmother had a new mutation, the first instance of the mutant hemophilia gene's appearance in the family, appeared to be correct. The explanation that the grandmother was conceived when a normal egg from her mother was fertilized by a sperm bearing the mutant gene received from her father also explains the origin of the hemophilia trait in the family. When a male is born with hemophilia, genetic tests can be completed to characterize the mutant gene that causes his hemophilia (Oldenberg and El-Maarri 2006). Not all persons with hemophilia have the same genetic mutation, even though the signs of the disorder may be the same. Different molecular changes in the hemophilia gene can result in the same characteristics and symptom of hemophilia. With the molecular information from the test results completed on an affected male within a family, female carriers of the mutant gene can be identified using prenatal tests completed during their pregnancies. There are medical reasons for knowing before birth if an expected child will have hemophilia. If a mother is to give birth to an infant affected with hemophilia, if the birth is difficult and complicated, it is advisable to deliver the baby via Caesarian to avoid the increased the risk of intracranial hemorrhage.

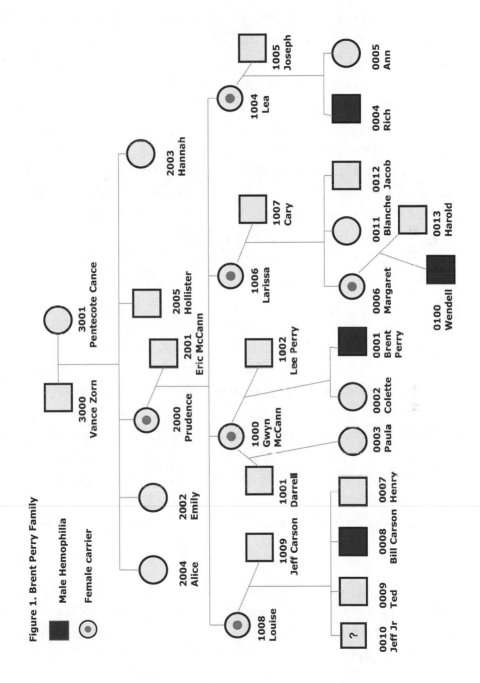

Figure 1. Brent Perry Family

Move from Spokane to Portland, Oregon

When hemophilia was discovered in Brent, his parents realized he would require many doctor visits and medication to treat recurrent bleeds. He didn't bleed all the time, not continuously; instead, the bleeds were episodic. He bled when he bumped into something. His parents discovered that for each episode, Brent needed to go to the doctor and get a shot of medicine into his tiny veins to help his blood clot normally and stop the bleeding. His mother was caring for three children at home at the time. She had moved from California to Spokane with her first husband, divorced him after they had one child, and then married Brent's father and had two more children including Brent. She was busy at home taking care of Brent and his two sisters.

Brent's father didn't keep a job very long. He was frequently seeking a get-rich-quick scheme, abandoning a steady job if it didn't interest him, but he was a good father and gave Brent a lot of attention. There was always a shortage of household money. Gwyn needed a practical way to care for the members of her family, especially Brent. She began calling different places within the Western states to identify a place where Brent could receive good hemophilia treatment. She knew that Brent's cousin, Bill, had to have shots, infusions of medicine, when he had bleeding, not just once but sometimes as often as once or even twice each week. His mother, Brent's Aunt Louise, took him to a hemophilia clinic in Atlanta, Georgia, where the medicine he needed was available. Most doctors and clinics and pharmacies did not keep a supply of the medicine, which was expensive. Most doctors hadn't seen a case of hemophilia.

Gwyn talked on the telephone with hemophilia treatment centers in Seattle, San Francisco, and Los Angeles, seeking information that would lead to a treatment plan for her son. She was searching for community support for the practical management of hemophilia care. Her husband was out of work, she had two daughters to care for, her son would need expensive medicine—not just once but forever—and she had a household to maintain. She disliked the concept of moving her family to a large city such as Los Angeles or San Francisco. Brent's parents discovered that a Portland, Oregon, hemophilia clinic could provide medicine and medical care for boys who had hemophilia, without worrying about the cost. The clinic provided comprehensive care, including a staff that addressed all aspects of hemophilia: dental, psychological, orthopedic, physical therapy, and financial—as well as infusion treatments for bleeds. Hemophilia care in Oregon was included in their crippled children's program.

In the autumn of 1976, when Brent was eleven months of age, the Perry family packed up all their belongings and household goods. With their two daughters and Brent in the car, Gwyn and Lee drove 350 miles to Portland, Oregon, from Spokane. That was before U.S. 395 from Ritzville to Pasco was a four-lane highway, before most cars had air-conditioning.

"Wave good-bye to that tree," Gwyn said to her daughters. "You will not see another tree in Washington until we reach Oregon, across the Columbia River." She was referring to the dry eastern Washington climate, a contrast with the rainy Portland weather. Thirty miles south of Spokane marks the last tree and the beginning of the Palouse, a treeless region of gentle hilly wheat fields. "Just look over there," Gwyn exclaimed, pointing eastward as Lee drove the car south toward Ritzville. "You can see the tip of Steptoe Butte." She was referring to an isolated pointed promontory rising skyward to guard the Palouse.

As they passed through the Tri-Cities of Pasco, Kennewick, and Richland, Gwyn told her daughters, "Many of the houses in these three towns are the homes of scientists and engineers who work at Hanford, where the atomic bomb was made." She reassured Paula, saying, "Don't worry, the days of making atomic bombs have passed. No one is going to nuke us now."

The family continued south toward Oregon. "That is Horse Heaven Hills, once the home of wild stallions, maybe even Black Beauty,"

Gwyn remarked as she pointed to the endless long, low mountains stretching westward along the Washington side of the Columbia River that separate Oregon to the south and Washington to the north. Brent's sister Colette was too young to understand everything her mother pointed to, but Paula thought the sites were interesting.

The days seemed brighter after the family moved. Lee had promised his wife he would get a regular job in Portland. When they were settled into their new home, the parents and Brent visited the hemophilia treatment center up on the hill in Portland (Plate 1). Gwyn was impressed with the compassion shown by Sue Underwood, the nurse at the clinic. Sue was a large, friendly woman with an accent revealing her Tennessee heritage, which made Brent's mother feel at ease. Without the rushing around often noted during a scheduled clinic appointment, Sue and Brent's parents visited and talked about caring for him whenever he needed treatment. Gwyn also met Isabella, the person in charge of finding a way to pay for Brent's treatments. She revealed to his parents the necessary steps to become eligible for the financial help to pay for the medical care Brent would need, including the concentrate for infusions, the clinic visits, hospital care if needed, and even dental care. Sue introduced Brent's parents to Dr. Anton Taillefer, director of the hemophilia clinic, emphasizing with her Tennessee accent the pronunciation of his French name: \tī-fer\. Gwyn was encouraged when Dr. Taillefer examined Brent and concluded that he was in perfect condition, saying that they were going to keep him that way. He was not fragile.

A management plan was developed so his parents knew what to do when Brent had a bleed. The plan for the treatment of hemophilia followed an evaluation by experienced specialists, including doctors, nurses, a dentist, social worker, physical therapist, psychologist, and a financial planner. A written document was generated that listed the medical and social issues, followed by recommendations for treatment during the interval until the next evaluation. By examining the details of the management plan, the parents knew precisely what course to follow whenever a bleed occurred. They received information about the signs and symptoms of different kinds of bleeds, such as elbows, knees, and ankles. Other families in the clinic were instructed in the method of infusion of concentrate at home.

Infusions for a Toddler with Hemophilia

The hemophilia treatment center was not the place where Brent received all his care as a small child. For the usual medical treatments for colds, baby shots, and earaches, his parents took him to Dr. Jim Hunter, a Portland pediatrician. Dr. Hunter was a doctor recommended by the treatment center, for he would accept hemophilia children in his practice. He was different. Many doctors would not want a child with hemophilia in their office. Most baby doctors' waiting rooms are filled with well babies or children who need baby shots—but not the kind of shots Brent needed. The doctors don't want a kid coming into their waiting room, unscheduled, in agony from a painful bleed, not able to sit still and wait his turn to be seen. Most baby doctors' waiting rooms are baby mills, not treatment rooms, not places for truly sick or suffering children.

After Brent began walking, falling to the floor was eventful. Stand up, fall down. A child without hemophilia can fall down a hundred times each day with no consequences while learning to walk. Sometimes after Brent fell or bumped into something, a large purple bruise appeared. Whenever a bleed occurred, Brent was taken to the treatment center for a shot, an infusion of concentrate into one of his veins to replace the clotting factor, AHF, the stuff missing in his blood. Without AHF in his blood, a bump or slight injury caused bruising or swelling, signs of hemophilia.

Brent did not like shots, which was revealed by his yelling and crying as soon as he was held down. He fussed and fretted. He would turn his head away from the nurse as if he wanted to be rescued from torture by his mother or father. Tears welled up in his eyes and spilled down over his cheeks. He turned pink from crying, and his nose ran. The nurse and the doctor—and maybe another strong-armed man, sometimes Arnold Deaton, the physical therapist—would grab his arm tightly and hold it out straight while a tight rubber tourniquet was stretched around it above his elbow, which made his little blue vein pop up while he was sitting in his dad's lap. The nurse swabbed the skin at the site of the needle puncture with cotton soaked in alcohol, and then the doctor stuck a thin needle into the vein. The needle was connected by plastic tubing to a plastic syringe that contained a small amount of a clear liquid that the doctor and nurse said would stop his bleeding. The fluid, less than an ounce, was slowly shoved into his vein, after the tourniquet was released, without much sensation. Sometimes Brent detected a funny metallic taste in his mouth while the concentrate was running into his vein.

After the shot, the needle was pulled out of the vein, and a cotton ball, a "bunny tail," was firmly pressed in place, with the pressure of his dad's thumb applied over the hole in his skin to prevent leakage of blood. After a couple of minutes, the cotton was removed and a Band-Aid, often bearing a cartoon of Bugs Bunny, was applied. Although most individuals who are subject to a needle stick for a blood sample, or who receive an intravenous injection or infusion, are familiar with the procedure, Brent's situation was different. He would receive intravenous infusions all his life, which meant that if his parents were to assume giving his infusions in the future, they must become familiar with details of the procedure.

Only a few days after Brent's first checkup at the hemophilia treatment center, while he was still wobbly on his legs as he learned to walk, he stumbled in the living room, fell forward, and whacked his forehead on the low coffee table in front of the blue sofa.[15] A knot

---

15 In toddlers with hemophilia, forehead bleeds are common when they are learning to walk.

on his forehead soon swelled up. His father grabbed ice cubes from the freezer and wrapped them in a washcloth that he gently pressed against Brent's forehead. Brent's parents quickly wrapped him in a blanket. The family piled into the car and rushed to the treatment center. Dr. Taillefer and Sue gave Brent a shot of concentrate into his small arm vein.

The next day, the knot, sticking straight out, was still there. The swelling continued. Brent was returned to the clinic and given another shot. His veins were not prominent. Access was difficult. Dr. Taillefer had to poke him twice before the tiny needle was inserted into his arm vein. Brent yelled and cried, which made his mother feel horrible, while his father remained calm and helped hold his son's arm for the infusion. Dr. Taillefer used a tiny twenty-five-gauge needle, which was designed to start an IV in a small vein on top of a baby's head, a scalp vein needle. It had two small green "ears" for a grip and was often called a "butterfly" because of its resemblance to those winged critters. The shot wasn't really painful, but since he wasn't old enough to talk, Brent let his opinion be known by pitching a fit, thinking that maybe those doctors and nurses would stop and never do that to him again.

After repeating the shot on the third day, the doctor and the nurse talked with Gwyn and Lee, and they agreed that the walnut-sized knot wasn't disappearing with the shots. However, the shots probably kept the knot from spreading across Brent's small forehead. They decided to discontinue giving Brent shots and wait and see what happened. He could have worn a small helmet to protect his forehead from another bump. Instead, Gwyn was told her son could wear a baseball cap with a stiff bill, which would insulate him from another blow to the forehead if he fell forward again. However, Brent's dad didn't wear a baseball cap, so why would they expect Brent to wear one? The nurse recommended a soft, thick headband, which Brent tolerated. The knot in the middle of his forehead became delineated and firm; it continued sticking straight out. Colette and Paula said their little brother looked like a unicorn. That hornlike knot lasted three months before it softened and disappeared.

The Frenum Bleed

Two months after Brent's first birthday, his mother noticed that his spit was pink. The bib covering the front of his fuzzy little blue pullover jersey was bloody where he had drooled. Gwyn was alarmed when she realized her son was bleeding from his mouth. His breath smelled bad. When she changed his diaper, his poop was black. She remembered the information she had received at the hemophilia treatment center.[16] Blood loss after circumcision, a nose bleed, or a mouth bleed is serious, a threat to life for infants who have a small blood volume because the blood is lost to the outside of their bodies. If not stopped, blood loss over a few days will lead to anemia, followed by heart failure and then death. Some of the deaths in hemophilia families in the old days were in infants who bled from their mouths. Older children who have hemophilia seldom bleed from the mouth. Gwyn wrapped Brent in a blanket, fastened him into an infant seat buckled into the rear seat of the car, and drove to the hemophilia treatment center up on the hill. When they arrived at the clinic, the front of his shirt was bloody. He was a mess. He was whisked directly to the second-floor treatment room.

A nice feature of the clinic was that his mother wasn't required to stop at the front desk for a financial interview, which was usually required in most medical offices. When you go to the doctor's office, they don't typically ask you what's wrong … where do you hurt? They say, "Do you have your insurance card with you?" Not at the hemophilia clinic. Gwyn telephoned the clinic before they arrived; they went right past the front desk. The doctor and nurse were in the treatment room immediately after their arrival, not one minute of waiting. They had already mixed the medicine in preparation for a shot. Dr. Taillefer called to Dr. Purcel Manson, a dentist whose suite was a few steps along the hallway. Together the two doctors looked into Brent's bloody mouth. He

---

16 When a baby has a nosebleed or bleeds in the mouth after biting his tongue or lip, he swallows the blood, which produces bad breath and black stools.

was on his back, lying in his mother's lap, feet toward her, legs spread apart, his head extended downward, away from her.

"Aha! There it is. There's the bleeder," the doctors exclaimed after blotting the inside of Brent's mouth with a cotton ball. The doctors were excited. You would think they'd stumbled upon a buried treasure. A bright lamp lit the inside of his mouth. They noted a tiny drop of bright red blood oozing from the labial frenum. The frenum is that thin little web inside the upper lip, extending to the gum centered behind the upper two front middle teeth.

"Your son has a frenum bleed," the doctors said to Gwyn.

"You did the right thing by bringing him in to the clinic," Dr. Taillefer said. "Frenum bleeds are common in toddlers who have hemophilia. They fall forward and strike their mouths on something, which makes a tiny tear in the frenum. Bleeding in the frenum cannot be treated with cautery or sutures, for they will produce more bleeding. Cautery will stop the bleeding, but in a day or two, the cautery site will break down and more bleeding will occur. The frenum is wet and in motion, and a Band-Aid won't stick or stay in place. Pressure cannot be applied by squeezing that little slippery place between your thumb and forefinger. The best way to treat a bleeding frenum is with an infusion of concentrate, a shot."

Frenum bleeds usually require only one infusion. Infused concentrate quickly restores the clotting activity of the blood, within minutes. Concentrate does not heal the wound. Doctors and nurses do not heal the tiny tear in the frenum. An infant quickly repairs his own body. Medicine, doctors, and nurses only help create the conditions for the body to heal itself.

Reviewing histories of hemophilia families frequently reveals the death of an infant in a family, such as a grandmother's brother or an uncle who was a child many years ago. Mouth bleeds, such as a torn frenum, may have led to death from blood loss in the years before concentrate was available for treatment. Prior to 1960, 90 percent of the males affected by hemophilia in the United States were less than eighteen years of age. Where were the older hemophilia males? They were dead. Their life expectancy was short. Most of the hemophilia males did not live to old age before 1960.

In addition to mouth bleeds, a recognized cause of death in hemophilia males who lived in the last two centuries was bleeding into their heads—intracranial hemorrhage. One instance often cited was Leopold, the first person to have hemophilia in Queen Victoria's family, her fourth son, her eighth child, born in 1853 (Appendix II). Leopold died March 28, 1884, at thirty-one years of age, one day after a head bleed. At the order of his doctor, he had gone to Cannes in February because of joint pain.[17]

The doctors and nurses held Brent down so that he couldn't move, while he screamed, with bloody spit coming from his mouth, as the nurse jabbed him in the arm.

After the needle entered Brent's vein, the red color of blood could be seen rising in the thin transparent plastic tubing connected to the syringe containing the medicine. The rubber buff-colored tourniquet was snapped from his arm. The nurse infused the medicine into his vein within sixty seconds. The needle was removed, a cotton ball was applied with thumb pressure by his mother over the tiny needle site, and he sat up. Brent ceased crying, and within a minute, his spit was clear. He began to smile. His mother recognized that at his age, he did not associate needles and restraints with anything beneficial for his body. It was as if he thought that holding him down and giving him a shot was nothing but punishment. Perhaps he thought he had done something wrong to deserve such unpleasant treatment. Brent began to associate the shots with his bleeds. However, he wasn't old enough

---

17   Some historians maintain that Leopold died after too much claret and morphine following a knee bleed. He slipped and fell in the yacht club in Villa Nevada, in Cannes. He died the next morning, some say from a burst blood vessel in his head. Perhaps both circumstances caused his death.

to understand that the cessation of bleeding was attributable to the shot. Brent's reaction was typical of most young children who require multiple intravenous infusions.

Gwyn learned to acknowledge Brent's anxiety, understanding that he became nervous whenever he needed a shot. Both Gwyn and Lee learned that they must be strong and remain calm whenever he had a bleed, and not become hysterical while he endured the restraint and the shot. They needed to comfort him and reassure him without reinforcing his anxiety.

Brent discovered that going for a car ride to the clinic meant restraint and a shot, which he objected to by crying and withdrawing. The bleeds were unpredictable. But Brent also learned, with the understanding and compassion from his parents, that the infusions were part of his life. For most people, such incidents are frightening and unpleasant. But for Brent they were normal. He didn't suffer much from the tiny needle stick. He protested more against the restraint, being held down against his will, than the needle stick. He especially didn't like it when he was wrapped up in a full-length blue restraint, with one arm sticking out, flattened onto a stiff board and fastened down tightly with Velcro straps. It was better when the doctors and nurses let him sit on his dad's or his mom's lap for his shot. He hated it when the doctor or nurse missed the vein on the first stick and tried a second time. He detested it when they fished around with a needle in his arm … or when some big person jabbed his or her elbow into his belly while trying to hold him still for the shot.

Brent's reaction was typical of most young children who require intravenous infusions. After several infusions, they relax and come to regard needle sticks as part of their normal life.

Acquiring Knowledge and Experience about Hemophilia

Brent's parents eagerly absorbed information about hemophilia. They discovered the signs that indicated an early beginning of a bleed. They knew Brent wouldn't tell them if he had a bleed before it became very painful. Often it was too late for stopping the bleed early and avoiding pain. At the end of the day, his parents checked him over, inspected his body, before putting him into nightclothes at bedtime. They kept him in double diapers to prevent butt bleeds, which might happen if he fell backward and suddenly sat down hard on a toy wooden block lying on the floor. The low coffee table with hard, angled corners was stored in the garage, to be retrieved when he was older. An effort was made to avoid trips to the clinic in the middle of the night. Youngsters who have hemophilia do not develop a bleed at night when they are quiet in bed. A bleed that begins in the daytime may not be noticed until nighttime. Sometimes it was necessary to telephone the doctor on call at night. If the doctor and Brent's parents concluded that a midnight infusion was necessary, he was strapped into a car seat for the short trip to the pediatric area of the hospital for an infusion of concentrate. The medicine was already prepared for his infusion when he arrived. A prearranged plan had been developed so that his family knew what to do to avoid a painful bleed. Brent was not allowed to go barefoot. He wore padded clothing. The most important feature of the plan to avoid pain was infusion whenever there was restricted motion in an ankle, elbow, or knee, before signs of swelling appeared. The nurses at the hospital accepted Brent's parents' requests for an infusion without delaying for more pronounced signs of a bleed, such as swelling or redness.

After Brent was up and about, old enough to walk and explore the house, the locations of the bleeds changed from his mouth and skin to his arms and legs. An early sign of a joint bleed was lack of movement, a stiff ankle or elbow. If he wouldn't walk or move his arm, that would be an early indication of a bleed into an elbow or ankle joint. The intent of his parents was to detect early signs, before the bleed had progressed, and stop bleeding with an infusion. If they waited until swelling and discoloration were noticeable, that was too late for early treatment. Pain and stiffness overcame him if the bleeding wasn't stopped early. And how those bleeds into his ankle or knee hurt! The pain was terrible and lasted so long—not just a few minutes but hours … or days.

The secret to successfully treating bleeds of hemophilia is early infusions. A practical way for giving infusions at the earliest sign of a bleed, the doctor and nurse told Brent's parents, would be for them to learn how to give their son infusions at home. The strategy for the best treatment of bleeds in hemophilia includes immediate access to concentrate, allowing an infusion to be given at the earliest sign of a bleed. Delay of infusion of concentrate occurs if the child must be bundled up and driven from home to the clinic or the doctor's office and then wait his turn to be seen by the doctor. Most doctors do not have concentrate in their offices. They request the medicine from the pharmacy. Most pharmacies do not keep concentrate in their supply of drugs and medicines; it must be ordered from a supplier.

If an infusion was necessary in the middle of the night, that meant a trip to the emergency room, the ER. During the night, the ER is a busy place. Brent's sisters couldn't be left home alone, so they came along for those midnight ER adventures. They brought their little cases of dolls and coloring books and teddy bears. Their small, colorful bags contained games and books to read. Paula even brought her little record player to listen to Judy Garland singing "Over the Rainbow."

ER experiences were extraordinary for Brent's family. He was an infant who did not appear gravely ill. The policy of the ER included attending to the most ill patients first. The family had to wait their turn before care was provided for Brent, before he was infused for a bleed. While in the waiting area of the ER, they were alarmed when they heard the sound of a struggling child suffering from croup on a hot summer night. They witnessed the admission of a child bleeding from the mouth from a dog bite. Their attention was drawn to the entrance of the ER, where a man with a gunshot wound was wheeled in from an ambulance, accompanied by four Portland policemen. An old woman was wheeled by on a gurney draped with a white sheet after she'd succumbed to a fatal heart attack. There was never a quiet moment in the ER. Brent's parents worried about

Brent while they waited for him to be seen. They also worried about their other children. However, Colette and Paula never complained when they were hustled from their snug, warm beds at night, nor did they question why a trip to the ER was necessary. They thought going to the clinic in the daytime and to the ER at night was not unusual; it was normal … normal for their family. Sometimes trips to the clinic meant they would miss school. Every once in a while, the hemophilia treatment center wanted Brent to come there for an all-day checkup. They called it an annual comprehensive evaluation. That day was a real pain in the butt! Brent's parents had only one car. For them to be with him while trying to deliver his sisters to school didn't work well. His sisters missed school when his mother hauled him to the clinic for the all-day checkup.

The details of assuring an available supply of concentrate for infusions for treating bleeds in hemophilia must be worked out in advance, before Brent was brought to the clinic for treatment, to avoid pain and suffering. The secret to early treatment is identifying a dependable, readily accessible supply of concentrate. In September of 1980, when Brent was five years of age, Sue Underwood, the clinic nurse, asked Brent's father if he would like to learn how to give the shots to his son. She said she and the doctor had talked it over and decided that the best way for Brent to get medicine early, before the bleed was too painful, would be for his parents to keep the magic medicine at home. The nurse said they could keep concentrate in their home and bring it with them whenever they brought him in for a shot, an infusion. That way, there would be no delay while waiting for the medicine to be brought from the pharmacy to the ER in the middle of the night. Or, if his family was traveling, they could take the medicine with them to assure that Brent could receive an infusion in any ER along their route. But even better than just having the medicine at home to take with them to the ER, they could learn how to give the shots for his infusions at home.

Brent's mother trembled and said she couldn't give her son a shot. "I don't think I could poke a needle into my son's arm," she quietly confessed. But his father spoke right up and said he could. But even if his mother couldn't bear to give her young son a shot, she could help Lee with all the other necessary steps, such as mixing the medicine and holding Brent on her lap with her arms around him while her husband stuck Brent with the needle and infused the medicine. One person can't give an infusion to a small child by himself. It takes teamwork. Brent's parents, with his sisters, were a good team.

Lee and Gwyn learned home infusion treatment from the nurse. They attended the clinic for six separate instruction lessons. Sue gave them instructions for mixing the water and medicine, pulling it from the vacuum bottle and pushing the mixed medicine out of the syringe. After a session or two, they practiced pushing the medicine through the tubing and butterfly needle stuck into a ripe orange. They weren't really shooting medicine into oranges; they were practicing with saline (salt water).

"Okay, let's get Dr. Taillefer," Sue announced. "They're ready." When Sue believed Brent's parents were ready to give a shot into the vein of a real live person instead of an orange, she grabbed either Myrna, the other nurse, or Dr. Taillefer. This time, she grabbed Dr. Taillefer.

"You are the guinea pig for us today?" Gwyn laughed as she watched Dr. Taillefer roll up the sleeve of his shirt and sit in the treatment room chair for a poke into his arm. The doctor was sitting in the same chair Brent's parents had sat in many times while holding him on their lap. Lee snapped a tourniquet around the doctor's bare arm, swiped alcohol across the skin, and grasped the butterfly needle by the two green ears.

"Okay, here I go," Lee nervously remarked. After pausing for a brief moment, as he tuned pale and then pink, he poked the tiny needle into the middle of the doctor's bulging arm vein.

"Don't be nervous, Lee," the doctor reassured him. "I'm used to this. The poke is harder on you than it is on me."

"Wow," Brent remarked with a grin, "Dad's giving the doctor a shot."

"Congratulations," Dr. Taillefer enthusiastically proclaimed to Brent's father. "That was perfect. You did a fine job. It didn't hurt at all. I didn't feel the needle stick." Lee withdrew some blood from Dr. Taillefer's prominent arm vein while Gwyn clamped the tubing. Lee changed syringes and shoved some saline into the doctor's vein after Gwyn released the tourniquet. After Lee pulled the needle out of Dr. Taillefer's arm vein, applied thumb pressure with a cotton ball to the puncture sight, and finally applied a Band-Aid, the doctor said to Brent's parents and Sue, "You are ready. You did a good job. But before you infuse Brent at home, for the first couple of infusions, we'll have you infuse him here with Sue. When you are ready, you can do it at home."

Not only did Brent's parents learn how to give shots for infusions, they were also taught the required sterile technique for preventing an infection at the place in his arm where they would stick him with the needle. The medicine was stored in two small bottles. On the inside bottom of one bottle was some dried almost-white powder. The other bottle was filled with water, which was sucked out through a needle into a syringe and then inserted through the small rubber stopper of the medicine bottle. After removing the aluminum covering and wiping the stopper with alcohol, the water and medicine were mixed, which reconstituted the concentrate for an infusion.

"Bubbles are bad," Sue said. "After inserting the water into the bottle containing the powdered medicine, don't shake the bottle," she warned Lee and Gwyn. "Just role the bottle gently in the palm of your hand until the white stuff is dissolved. Avoid bubbles. Alternate the veins. Don't give a shot into the same vein one day after another shot. After poking a vein with a needle, the vein needs to rest for a few days. It is best not to use the same vein day after day; the vein needs to recover. Those veins must be kept in good shape. They're very important. They are Brent's lifeline." But whenever Lee tried to give Brent a shot in another vein other than his favorite arm vein, he often missed. If he missed more than two or three times, the family would go to the hospital pediatric area or the hemophilia treatment center.

They learned how to store the medicine, not to leave it in a sunny window where it might become overheated and loose potency. After Brent received a shot of medicine in his arm vein, his parents were required to learn how to dispose of the needles they had used. They must be certain that the garbage man would not accidentally be stuck with a sharp needle that had been in someone else's veins. After the infusion, needles and syringes were dumped into an empty blue Maxwell House coffee can. Brent's parents were told that the medicine contained hepatitis virus. "It is very important that no one else is accidentally stuck with one of the used sharp needles," they were reminded. Needles were bent before they were put into the can, to prevent reuse just in case a druggie found them. The lidded coffee can full of needles and plastic syringes was labeled HAZARDOUS WASTE and disposed of in a special area.

Accountability and Eligibility

Accountability was important. To allow Brent's parents to keep medicine costing thousands of dollars at home, they must keep records. A bottle of concentrate containing one thousand units of factor VIII activity, costing ten cents for each unit, cost one hundred dollars. If they kept twenty bottles at home, the value of the inventory amounted to two thousand dollars, a large amount of money in the 1970s.[18] The hemophilia treatment center purchased the concentrate from the pharmaceutical manufacturer and dispensed it directly to Brent's parents without going through a pharmacy. Therefore, the cost was kept low, at wholesale price.

The hemophilia clinic provided medical care for more patients than just Brent. Little patients, small children, required less medicine than adults. On average, the amount of AHF in one infusion was ten units for each pound of body weight. The amount of AHF in each infusion depended on the severity and location of the bleed. After receiving a blow to the head, twenty units per pound of body weight was infused, compared to ten units per pound for a finger bleed. If a child was struck on the head by the seat of a swing on the school playground, he would be immediately infused with twenty units per pound of his body weight. Usually 10 AHF units per pound of body weight was the general guideline for the amount of AHF units for an infusion to treat most bleeds. A twenty-five-pound infant required 250 units. A twelve-year-old boy weighing one hundred pounds would be infused with 1,000

---

18   In 1977, $2,000 was equivalent to $8,720 in 2008
     (RE: http://www.measuringworth.com/indicator.html).

units. Parents of a child infused at home were required to learn many details about the indications for treatment.

The most desirable feature of home infusions was the promptness of an infusion at the earliest sign of a bleed, before pain, swelling, immobility and disability set in. The expense of treatment was reduced by eliminating costs of visits to the ER and doctor. Knowledge of appropriate indications for infusions and proper handling of concentrate and supplies was necessary for families infusing AHF at home.

Brent's parents did not have medical insurance. Medical insurance was offered by some employers to their employees, but Brent's father was not employed most of the time. Sometimes a family who has a medical problem that requires recurrent treatment can find a doctor who will take care of them regardless of their ability to pay for the care. There are doctors who are interested in the boy or man who has hemophilia because they recognize that he needs a regular doctor who gets to know him.

In 1977, if the person was less than twenty-one years of age, the Crippled Children's Division (CCD) paid the doctor for providing his hemophilia care, if the parents were enrolled for benefits. The payment the doctor received from CCD for providing his care was less than the amount of his usual fee, but some doctors accepted the lesser payment. For families who had no medical insurance, the cost of the medicine was paid by the hemophilia treatment center, which received support from Title V of the Social Security Amendment for Children with Disabilities, referred to as CCD funds. Each state within the United States receives CCD funds. Allocation of the funds differs between the states. Oregon decided to include the cost of hemophilia care under their Title V allocation. That is the reason Brent's parents moved from Washington to Oregon—to improve their access to hemophilia care and to identify a plan to meet the cost of his lifelong requirement of concentrate. In 1977, the State of Washington did not include the cost of hemophilia as a condition covered by their CCD program.

With many patients receiving home infusion, a large inventory of costly concentrate was distributed to their homes. Accountability to the funding source was necessary to assure responsible use of the funds so that funding would continue in the future. When a person turned twenty-one, he became eligible for the Hemophilia Assistance Program (HAP). For men who had no medical insurance, HAP paid for the concentrates. Funds for HAP were derived from the Hemophilia Foundation of Oregon and from a ten percent markup on the sale of concentrate.

All patients were billed for the cost of the concentrate. If a patient had medical insurance, the insurance company paid for the medicine. If the patient's family had no insurance, CCD funds paid for the medicine. Regardless of the funding source, for a family to be provided with a supply of expensive concentrate to be kept at home to manage the recurrent bleeding episodes, one of the criteria that must be met beforehand was accountability. Brent's parents were reliable and filled out a form each time he had an infusion to treat a bleed. The completed forms, the bleed sheets, were returned to the clinic at the time of his annual checkup for review by the doctors and nurses.

By age three, Brent sat in his mother's lap in the kitchen while his father gave him a shot. Gwyn kept the medicine in the refrigerator. However, the bottle of water for mixing was kept at room temperature. This helped the medicine mix faster, and it didn't need to be shaken so vigorously to go into solution, thereby making it ready for use sooner than if the added water was cold. Brent didn't want to delay once his parents decided he needed a shot. The intention was get it over with as soon as possible. Gwyn pulled the medicine bottle from the refrigerator and mixed the room temperature water with the medicine by swirling the bottle in the palm of her hand, without vigorous shaking to avoid bubbles. When the medicine was dissolved, she handed the bottle of concentrate to her husband, who withdrew the contents into a syringe for injection.

Lee was pretty good at hitting his son's vein, but sometimes he missed on the first poke. That made him nervous, but not Brent. Brent knew his father was doing his best—he was human. The shots were harder on his parents than they were on him. Nearly always, when he missed on the first attempt, Lee was successful hitting the vein the second time. Brent had a favorite vein inside the bend of his right arm. But Lee remembered that Sue had instructed them to give the shots in different veins rather than always infusing in the same vein.

Dr. Taillefer, Dr. Watson, and Sue were all good at hitting the vein. At times, Brent's mother told him, they had to give a baby, or another boy just like him, who had poor veins, a shot to stop the bleeding. If the child had no visible arm veins, they gave shots in the top of the foot. And sometimes, Gwyn said, they even give a shot into one of the baby's veins on top of his head, into a scalp vein. Some parents never wanted to give their sons shots. Brent's parents were better at giving shots than some of the other parents were, so they began giving him infusions at home at an earlier age than most parents did for their boys. Usually, boys are four or five years of age before their parents give them the medicine at home. Although the doctor or nurse may have been better at hitting veins than Brent's father, Brent preferred his father. The doctor didn't see Brent as often as his father did, and Lee knew his son's veins better than anyone else. He knew just where to stick the needle to draw blood each time.

Usually Brent had an infusion at home once or twice each week, sometimes three times in one week. Occasionally two or three weeks passed without an infusion. If he had a shot at the first sign of a bleed, usually only one infusion was necessary. But if Brent had a bad bleed into his ankle, he often needed a follow-up infusion the next day.

One of the other parents began talking with Brent's parents when they attended the clinic. He suggested to Lee that since Brent required an infusion once or twice each week and the shot had a lasting effect for three days, why not give him a shot before he bleeds, and then he would never have a bleed? Why not infuse him regularly every three days? The interested parents proclaimed that when hemophilia is discovered in a child, if he is started on infusions while still a small baby and receives medicine on schedule throughout his childhood, he will grow up without any damage to his joints or risks of serious internal bleeding. They reminded Brent's parents that diabetics receive insulin regularly before they become ill; they don't wait to have low blood sugar before they get insulin. Why not treat hemophilia preventatively?

Brent's father confessed to the other father that he didn't know if he could successfully hit Brent's veins that often.

The other parent replied by saying that Brent could have a porta vein if venipunctures were difficult.

The man explained that a porta vein is a small, round, flat device, about the size of a quarter that is placed by a surgeon beneath the skin of the chest. It is connected to a vein with a small plastic tube that is inserted into the vein and remains there continuously. At the time of an infusion, the skin over the porta vein is cleaned with alcohol. An infusion needle is inserted, and concentrate is injected. Some of the other treatment centers across the country use them frequently and start small babies on prophylaxis,[19] the man enthusiastically informed Brent's parents. He explained that the intention was to avoid complications caused by hemophilia, allowing a child to grow to adulthood, by keeping the clotting protein in his blood from falling to zero, at a level that would prevent him from bleeding.

Lee told the man he had heard about those porta vein devices—and that sometimes they become infected and cause a serious threat of blood poisoning. Brent's mother proclaimed they didn't want to be confronted with another medical problem.

The man agreed that unfortunately, infection is a risk with porta veins. But he offered that the risk of infection is less than the benefits from prophylaxis, saying that everything in life is a trade-off. He said he just wanted to be sure Brent's parents had heard of them.

The clinic in Portland seldom used porta vein devices. They didn't recommend prophylaxis as often as other treatment centers did. The Oregon hemophilia treatment center favored demand treatment, an infusion of concentrate after a bleed. Brent's parents were grateful that AHF replacement medication was available for their son as concentrate, regardless of the method of application.

---

19 By preventing head bleeds, prophylaxis reduces deaths in hemophilia children under the age of five years.

New Treatment for Hemophilia

Before 1964, there was no AHF replacement treatment for stopping bleeds in hemophilia. Boys who were affected suffered and became deformed from recurrent joint bleeds. Their life expectancy was short. Often they became crippled and couldn't attend school. In 1964, Dr. Judith Pool, a doctor-scientist at Stanford University discovered cryoprecipitate (cryo), which was effective in treating bleeds in hemophilia. Her remarkable discovery heralded a new treatment of hemophilia. It was the first major treatment advance to open a new doorway to a normal life for persons affected by hemophilia. With infusions of cryo, it was possible to achieve a life without suffering, deformity, and premature death. Cryo was made from the plasma obtained from Red Cross volunteer blood donors.

Dr. Watson related to Brent's parents that Roger Norman, a young Oregon boy who had hemophilia, was stricken with a bleed inside his head, into his brain. He became unconscious and lapsed into a coma. Before 1964, the outcome of such an event was death. The recently discovered cryo was administered to Roger at Emanuel Hospital in Portland before and during brain surgery. Roger survived. Cryo was a miracle. Logistical problems with cryo were its storage and its availability. It required a special freezer that most people did not possess in their homes, and the Red Cross couldn't make enough cryo to treat all the persons with hemophilia. Hyland Laboratories, a pharmaceutical manufacturer, began making a lyophilized concentrate from the blood obtained from paid donors. Using a process that was advanced a step further than producing cryo, the AHF was concentrated into a powder contained in a small glass vial that could be reactivated by adding water. The freeze-dried product did not require a special refrigerator or freezer for storage. This meant that concentrate could be stored at home, making the medicine available immediately. However Hyland's concentrate wasn't always available.

In 1971, Parke-Davis,[20] another pharmaceutical company, introduced Humafac. Humafac was also made from the plasma of paid blood donors. The volume of the reconstituted concentrate was only seven milliliters, less than two teaspoons, which was a desirable volume for small patients, allowing the infusion to be quickly completed. Parke-Davis was best known to many persons as a source of vanilla. Many of the older remedies for treatment of various illnesses were extracts of natural substances, including vanilla beans. When the Parke-Davis representative came to the Oregon Hemophilia Treatment Center, he brought with him several pint-size bottles of pure vanilla extract. He said he filled the dark brown glass vanilla bottles from a barrel of vanilla located in his garage. But more importantly than vanilla, he assured the clinic that Parke-Davis could provide a dependable, uninterrupted supply of Humafac. That promise was important. The treatment center wanted to avoid starting a patient on home infusion and then discovering that concentrate was not available for continued treatment

When Parke-Davis introduced Humafac in 1971, the treatment center began providing families instructions for procedures to infuse their sons at home. They recognized that the best way of treating bleeds in hemophilia included immediate access to concentrate for clotting factor replacement infusions, without delay, at the earliest sign of a bleed. The benefits of home infusion of concentrate had been demonstrated by hemophilia clinics in California and New York. Delays in treatment occurred if the child must be taken to the doctor's office or an emergency room for an infusion. Treatment was entrusted to the parents, with

---

20 Parke-Davis was acquired by Warner-Lambert in 1970, which was sold to Pfizer in 2000 (RE: http://en.www.wikipedia.org/wiki/Parke-Davis).

backup from the treatment center. A doctor was always on call to provide advice to the parents whenever they had questions concerning the infusions. Communication with the hemophilia treatment center and a dependable, uninterrupted supply of concentrate in the home, which the parents knew how and when to infuse, improved the lives of persons with hemophilia. Compared to how things were at the beginning of the last century, in addition to concentrate for infusion, other factors contributed to improved care in the 1950s and 1960s: telephones, modern housing, and improved roadways. Dependable sources of concentrate and improved living conditions in communities dramatically elevated the outlook for children born with hemophilia. They no longer had extended absences from school. They didn't lie in bed day after day, suffering in agony. Boys with hemophilia who received concentrate would no longer become crippled by adulthood. They looked forward to becoming adults rather than dying as children.

Roland Arnette, a student from Reed College who was studying in Dr. Taillefer's laboratory reviewed the family trees of the families that had an affected relative in previous generations. He collected the year of birth and the year of death for persons who had hemophilia in the late 1800s and 1900s. Life expectancy was sixteen or eighteen years before the 1950s. By 1980, after concentrates became available, life expectancy for hemophilia was more than fifty years of age and was approaching near normal (Stafford et al. 1980).

Life expectancy in hemophilia

- Prior to the 1960s, most persons born with hemophilia didn't live to adulthood.

- After concentrates became available in the 1970s for treating bleeds, life expectancy in hemophilia exceeded fifty years of age.

Commercial production by pharmaceutical manufacturers of a dependable supply of concentrate depended upon the procurement of plasma derived from paid blood donors. In contrast, American Red Cross production of cryoprecipitate was not derived from paid donors, whose life situations encourage them to sell their blood for survival. Instead, each unit of cryo was produced from one Red Cross volunteer who regularly donated his blood. The unpaid Red Cross donors were healthy, and their lifestyles excluded known risk factors such as hepatitis or intravenous drug usage. Cryo was not produced from the pooled plasma of hundreds of donors. Each unit of cryo was produced separately. Commercial sources of plasma were collected from hundreds of persons who sold their blood, including homeless persons who needed the money and may not be healthy. The hundreds of units of plasma collected by the pharmaceutical manufacturers from the blood of paid donors were mixed together, pooled into one lot, and processed as one large batch.

Brent's parents wondered why the Red Cross did not produce concentrates from plasma collected from healthy, screened volunteers. Wouldn't concentrate be safer if it were made from the plasma derived from their selected donors?[21]

They were informed that plasma from regular established volunteer Red Cross blood donors would be safer than plasma from paid donors. The Red Cross had been asked that if they are responsible for the nation's blood supply, why didn't they make all the cryo and concentrate for infusions required for treatment of persons with hemophilia. Dr. Stephen Hunt, director of the Portland Red Cross blood bank responded saying that the Red Cross didn't have the equipment or the manpower to make all the concentrate needed to treat all the persons who have hemophilia.

---

21 Hyland Pharmaceutical eventually produced commercial concentrate using plasma from Red Cross volunteers. This concentrate was marketed displaying the Red Cross label and sold by the Red Cross.

Nature of Bleeds

As Brent grew older and his body became bigger, he required an infusion each week, sometimes twice a week. Once in a while, he could go two or three weeks without a bleed requiring an infusion. The nature of Brent's bleeds changed and settled into his joints. When he was three and a half years old, his ankle was very painful. He couldn't walk or move his foot. From the top of his foot up into his leg, there was swelling. His ankle was stiff. It hurt so badly, he cried all night long. Kids with hemophilia can't have aspirin to relieve the pain. Aspirin zaps the platelets and increases bleeding after an injury. That was Brent's first joint bleed. He had to have a shot.

Gwyn and Lee brought their suffering young son up to the hemophilia treatment center, where the physical therapist, Arnold Deaton, made a splint for his painful ankle. Arnold was a soft-spoken friendly cowboy from Greybull, which is in northern Wyoming. He had long hair like Buffalo Bill and wore cowboy boots. Brent's parents were instructed to spread a towel over Brent's foot and ankle and cover the towel with crushed ice to take away the pain. Not just a few cubes taken from the freezer and wrapped in a washcloth. Instead, Lee was instructed to cover the ankle with twenty pounds of crushed ice wrapped in a large towel to cool the ankle. He could buy bags of crushed ice, he was told, at a truck stop. Brent had another shot the next day.

Each time Brent received a shot with an infusion of concentrate, Gwyn pulled a spiral-bound notebook, which had a green cover, down from the top of the refrigerator where it rested. She wrote the date, location of the bleed, and how much concentrate Brent received. She kept that record book for more than seven years. She also filled out the bleed sheets, which were returned to the clinic, where a supply of concentrate was dispensed. The bleed sheets resembled a multiple choice examination. Gwyn marked on the paper with a number two lead pencil, blackening in one of the boxes to indicate the location of Brent's bleed: right ankle, left elbow, mouth, finger…. She selected and marked one of the locations among forty choices. Whenever the family received a new supply of concentrate, they were required to turn in the bleed sheets at the clinic. The records were a method of accountability, a testament for the use of medicine they had infused. The doctors and nurses at the clinic studied the bleed sheets and noted where Brent had been bleeding. They said the bleeding places should be random, not in just one part of his body. They told Lee and Gwyn that before a baby begins to walk, there are usually few bleeds in hemophilia. Once an infant begins walking, he begins falling, and bleeds occur. At that time, being upright, the joints that bear weight are the places where bleeds most often appear. The knees and ankles are the most frequent places of bleeding, but the elbows bleed too.

Brent's father asked the doctors why the hips aren't the most common place for a bleed if the location of the bleed is determined by weight bearing.

The doctors acknowledged that Lee was correct about weight bearing, but they explained that the type of joint also affects the bleed. The hip is a ball-and-socket joint. The knee is a gliding joint and more vulnerable to injury that results in bleeding. The knee can get twisted, or it may slide around. Shoulders do not bleed as often as knees, elbows and ankles. The temporomandibular joint (TMJ), the jaw joint, seldom bleeds, despite enormous forces exerted on the joint. There is no weight bearing on the TMJ. The joints of the spinal column, which are weight bearing, seldom bleed in hemophilia.

From the frequency of shots for infusions of concentrate given for different places in Brent's body, the doctors and nurses at the clinic noted, by reviewing the bleed sheets that a pattern was developing.

His bleeds were not randomly distributed among his joints. The most common place he was bleeding was his ankles. Brent's knees and elbows seldom bled. His hips were okay. His ankles, both of them, became his target joints.

Gwyn asked the doctors and nurses why her son developed ankle problems instead of knee or elbow problems from recurrent bleeds. She was told that every person is different. Although all humans are similar in many ways, physiological responses to injuries are different. Perhaps Brent had joint laxity in his ankles, they said. He may have been born that way, which caused his ankles to tilt a small amount. His ankle joints were not level, and as a result, they didn't bear weight centrally as they should have. Lee thought that sounded like a good explanation when he remembered that Brent did not have ankle bleeds until he began walking. The doctors, nurses, and the physical therapist said Brent must always wear high-topped shoes, not shoes that are low cut. He should never go barefoot. They also recommended that Brent wear supports for his ankles. The supports they suggested resembled the thick blue stockings made from the kind of material wind surfers wear in their wet suits. The ankle supports for Brent were better looking than some of the braces he noticed on other kids who came to the clinic. Some of the older boys and men were wearing knee braces. Some of the men in the clinic had difficulty getting up from their chairs. They walked stiff-legged. Some were on crutches. Some couldn't bend their elbows.

Blood inside a joint is not only painful, it's also harmful. When the joint space is filled with blood, it cannot escape, and the blood decomposes. White cells (leukocytes) in blood contain proteolytic enzymes,[22] which digest tissues inside the joint. The lining of the joint, the synovium, reacts as if it were angry, resulting in thickening and inflammation, a synovitis. The white blood cells in the decomposing

---

22 Proteolytic enzymes, also known as proteases, lyse or digest proteins. Leukocytes, the white blood cells, contain the proteases elastase and cathepsin G.

blood release enzymes that destroy the cartilage covering the ends of the bones in the joint. The cartilage breaks down over time, leaving a narrow joint space with bone on bone, without a cushion of cartilage between the bones. Bone on bone is very painful. The result of a bleed into a joint is stiffening and decreased motion from the thickened synovium, leading to a painful degenerative osteoarthritis from loss of cartilage. The progression of degenerative joint changes depends upon the age of the child when the bleed occurs. Only one bleed into an infant's joint can result in irreversible damage. Recurrent bleeds into a joint before a child is mature often lead to progressive loss of joint function. The joint becomes stiff, movement is lost, the muscles waste away, and the person becomes disabled.

Compared with a young child, a bleed into a joint of an older person, such as a forty-year-old man, is less devastating than a joint bleed in a child. The grown man will have pain but not as much destruction from a joint bleed.

Clinic Visit at the Hemophilia Treatment Center

A man who appeared to be about fifty years old was sitting in the clinic waiting room on a day when Brent arrived for his annual comprehensive checkup. He was dressed neatly, wearing a dark blue blazer with an Optimist pin stuck in the left lapel. He said hello to Brent's parents, introducing himself as Tom Dameron. He related that he had hemophilia, but he could not infuse himself at home because his elbows were too stiff, which prevented him from reaching his arm veins with his hands. He was at the clinic to see the bone doctor, the orthopedist. He had difficulty rising from his seat because his knees were stiff and wouldn't bend. He walked aided with an adjustable aluminum crutch with a black rubber tip. He told Lee he was going to talk to the doctors about an operation to take out one of his knees and replace it with an artificial joint made of metal and plastic. Surgery was possible in persons who had hemophilia, since concentrate infusions restored their blood clotting to normal, allowing them to withstand surgery. Some of the older men were getting knee joint replacements.

The talk in the clinic waiting area that day was about Jack Peterson, a man who came to the hemophilia treatment center from Alaska. He was a forty-five-year-old man, a bookkeeper who worked for the state of Alaska in Juneau. He could no longer walk more than a few steps. He wanted new knees so he could go for hikes again. The Oregon doctors replaced both of his knees in one operation. That was a big operation, more than six hours, with four orthopedic surgeons operating at one time. The doctors reasoned that it would be less expensive, require less concentrate, and involve only one recovery period if they replaced both knees during one operation rather than two separate operations.

Visits to the clinic were different on different days. The first Wednesday of each month was "Bone Doctor Day" (Orthopedic Day). Some clinic days, only young kids were seen. During other days, the clinic was filled with persons of all ages who had hemophilia, including many disabled adults. After Brent completed his checkup with the hemophilia doctors and the dentist, he was whisked into the bone doctors' examination room. On Orthopedic Day, the bone doctor was present. In fact, two bone doctors, Dr. Daren North and Dr. Chris Anderson, were checking the arms and legs of everybody. Some bone doctor days, Dr. Charles Parrish and an orthopedic resident doctor were also in the clinic, making it four bone doctors at once. Fastened onto the wall of the small room was a row of flat green metal boxes, just below the height of the doctors' faces. Those interesting boxes were lit with fluorescent lights that illuminated Brent's black-and-white X-ray films.

"That's Brent's ankle joint," the doctors told Gwyn. They pointed to another box and said, "Look right here. There are his elbows and his knees. All of his joints look normal." The bone doctors conferred with Arnold Deaton, the physical therapist, who measured how much Brent could move his joints, a test he called "range of motion." They peered over the numbers from the test results, X-rays were viewed, and the doctors gently pumped Brent's arms and legs back and forth.

They looked for such signs of damage as quadriceps atrophy, or decrease in the space normally present in the knee joint. They moved the joints to detect crepitation[23] and to test for muscle strength. Brent's joints were not destroyed like those of older men.

Brent's parents referred to that clinic visit as the day of "two old Toms," Tom Dameron and Tom Guerara. Tom Guerara was a short, round Italian who dressed dapperly in pin-striped trousers, a dark blue blazer over a button-up light yellow dress shirt, and a red cravat. He had a trimmed gray moustache, neatly combed wavy gray hair, a round belly, and a New Jersey accent. His talk seemed rather proper, almost formal. He didn't like kids. He'd never had any of his own, although he had a pretty wife; they elected to adopt a child. Tom had been a tool and die maker in New Jersey before he and his wife moved to Oregon. He could no longer stand before machines because his knees were nearly frozen, caused by bleeds in his youth, before concentrate was available. His wife said he became cranky after he retired from the machine shop. They decided to move to Oregon to be near their adopted daughter.

Another man in the clinic that day was Bill Harrison, from Idaho, who came with his wife, Esther, to the clinic to see the bone doctors. Bill was seventy-five years old. He had survived many bleeds from hemophilia in the days before concentrate was available. As a young boy living on an Idaho farm in the flat southwestern part of the state, in the 1930s, without indoor plumbing, electricity, and running water, but plenty of rattlesnakes, little care was available for treating hemophilia. Bill recalled the early years of his life, when he had a bleed as a child. After days of suffering, he was loaded into the rear seat of the car, an old square four-door Chandler with running boards and a big spare tire mounted on the rear. His dad drove over the dusty, bumpy, unpaved gravel road into town to the doctor's office. The doctor stuck a needle into his dad's arm

---

23 A grinding sensation during movement, when joint surfaces are rough.

vein and one into Bill's arm vein. He connected the needles with a tube, which allowed the father's blood to run into his son's vein. However, the small boy began shaking violently and became so ill from the direct blood from his father that the doctor had to stop the transfusions. Bill survived, grew up, and married Esther, a nurse, who learned to infuse her husband when concentrate became available for home infusion. Bill, who had difficulty walking, a result of destroyed ankle and knee joints, had developed a prosperous insurance company business. Bill and Esther also had an adopted daughter. They decided not to have any biological children because they were afraid that if they had a daughter, she might bring a grandson with hemophilia into the world.[24]

Gwyn and Lee were impressed to learn that not all men who had hemophilia in the old days died young; some survived to adulthood. All three of those older men had the same medical disorder that Brent had: hemophilia. They were born and raised in the days before any concentrate was available. Their bodies revealed many telltale signs of lack of treatment for repeated bleeds during their youth, ending up with crippling in their later years.

For their checkups, the doctors directed the older men to undress and wear white dressing gowns that opened and tied with a string in the back. "Do you have any idea how difficult it is for me to undress and then redress? Do you know how hard it is for me to reach down and untie my shoes?" Tom Guerara complained, scolding the younger doctors, whom he regarded as insensitive to his needs.

"I can't unknot or retie my necktie," Tom Dameron added, frowning. "My elbows won't bend. Can't we skip the undressing and the gown? Is looking at my knees and elbows for the benefit of the doctor or for me? For me, I don't need to undress. I already know my joints are shot."

"I wear cowboy boots, shitkickers," Bill Harrison cheerfully added with a smile. I can't reach down to my shoes, and I couldn't untie them

---

24 None of the children born of men who have hemophilia will be affected. Males do not transmit the hemophilia gene to their sons. All their daughters will be carriers of hemophilia.

even if I could reach that far down. With cowboy boots, my dear wife, Esther, can pull them off."

The experiences of these older men revealed some of the effects of hemophilia in persons raised before concentrates became available—a remarkable contrast compared with youth of Brent's era. Descriptions of older men with hemophilia reveal what Brent could have anticipated if he had been born before concentrates were in use.

On the way home from the clinic, when they were in the car, Lee talked with Gwyn about the older men they'd seen at the clinic. "I'm thankful my son was born during the days when AHF concentrates are available," he said. "He won't grow up to become crippled like those unfortunate fellows. They are nice men. Think of all the suffering and pain they have been through. Can you imagine what their lives were like without any treatment? I feel sorry for them. "Wow!" Lee exclaimed, shaking his head. "Four bone doctors and none of them get paid for checking Brent in the clinic. They do it because the joint and muscle problems caused by hemophilia are interesting to them."

"And they do it to gain experience in replacing knee joints," Gwyn said. She went on repeating to her husband what the bone doctors had told her. "The doctors told me big changes are occurring in joint replacement. One of the reasons is that new types of metal and plastics are available that can be placed in a person's body without a reaction … without rejection. Another reason results from the Japanese taking over the watch making industry. Inexpensive Japanese battery-powered watches have replaced more expensive Swiss-made wind-up watches."

Brent was getting old enough to understand his parents' conversation. "Are you kidding, Mom?" Brent said. "What do watches and knee joints have in common?"

"Nothing. They have nothing in common," Gwyn replied, looking at her son. "What happened was that the Swiss lost their watch making business to the Japanese, but they had many skilled technicians who had know-how. The Swiss decided to change from making watches to joint replacements, creating a new industry for their skilled, experienced, innovative craftsmen. A Swiss company named Zimmer became the provider for nearly all the joint replacements, Dr. North told me."

"Golly, Ma, I learn something new from you every day."

"Yeah, you bet," Gwyn said, smiling, knowing she was a source of information that her son and husband found interesting.

Gwyn recounted that when an orthopedist replaced a knee joint, the Zimmer man, dressed in surgical scrubs and wearing a mask, shoe covers, and a surgical head cover, entered the operating room, bringing all the components for the new replacement knee. The doctors didn't know which size of knee replacement parts a person needed until they were in the middle of surgery, with the knee joint open before them. The Zimmer man prepared a table with all the sizes laid out at the time of surgery. The doctor would say, "Give me an upper number three or a lower number six." The part was handed to him to fasten into the open knee space where the joint used to be.

It was similar to a Lego set. The orthopedist chiseled and ground notches in the bone. The selected joint parts were snap-locked into the bone notches. The new knee joint popped into place, just like snapping two pieces of Lego together.

Since the Zimmer man brought all the knee replacement parts to surgery, the hospital didn't need to purchase lots of instruments, tools, components, and supplies that they would never use. They even brought a machine to line up the legs. The feet must point correctly. One foot could not point sideways with the other foot pointed straight ahead. One leg couldn't be shorter than the other after surgery.

A Spinal Cord Bleed

At the hemophilia treatment center, other people, in addition to doctors and nurses, were helpful to Gwyn. When she had a question or a problem, she depended on a number of people for help.

Hanna, the social worker, checked to make sure Brent's family had everything they needed at home to manage hemophilia. When he was old enough to go to school, Hanna met with Brent's schoolteachers to answer questions about hemophilia. Arnold Deaton, the cowboy physical therapist, gave Brent pep talks about saving his ankles. Isabella assured his parents that the cost of his hemophilia care was included in his treatment plan. Don Porter, the dentist, examined Brent's teeth and made sure he brushed them without bleeding from his gums. He reminded Brent to floss after brushing his teeth.

One of the benefits of the hemophilia treatment center was the information and advice parents received from one another. Brent's parents met Andrew and Mary Singer one day while sitting in the clinic waiting area before his checkup. Like Brent's parents, who had moved from Spokane to Portland, they had recently moved from Prineville, in the sagebrush country of central Oregon, to a new home in Eugene, in the Willamette Valley. Andrew was a fair-complexioned man with blond curly hair, a round belly, and a big smile. He drove a big red and white Kenworth True Value Hardware truck, delivering supplies such as sprinkling cans, bicycles, nails, stepladders, barbecue grills, and lots of other stuff, supplying True Value Hardware stores in Oregon, California, and Washington. His passion was trucks. He owned two other trucks and hired drivers to operate them while he drove the company-owned Coast to Coast Truck. The Singers had two sons with hemophilia. Their youngest son, Wendell, was Brent's age. When he walked, his right foot dragged as if it didn't work properly.

Wendell's mother confided to Gwyn that Wendell had bled into his spinal cord when he was a year and a half old. She told Gwyn that he had been jumping up and down on the bed in their home in Prineville, and he fell backward over the foot of the bed, landing flat on his back on the floor. Four days later, he couldn't get up out of bed. He was unable to walk. He had a stiff neck and a fever of 106 degrees. Dr. Thompson, his country doctor, thought he might have meningitis. The doctor tried to perform a spinal tap, a lumbar puncture, by inserting a long needle into the center of the little boy's back, into the spinal canal, to withdraw spinal fluid to analyze for meningitis. The doctor was frustrated when he couldn't obtain any spinal fluid. Not only was the desperate attempt unsuccessful, but soon afterward, a huge purple circle appeared on the boy's back around the place where the spinal needle had been inserted into his backbone. His mother recalled that it looked as if someone had painted a large purple target on her son's back. The doctor knew the little boy needed an infusion of concentrate, but he couldn't find a vein where he could insert the needle. The doctor desperately made an incision in the skin on the inside of the forearm of the child to free up a small vein, a cutdown for the IV needle, without success.

The doctor telephoned the hemophilia treatment center and requested help. Myrna took the call and shouted at Natasha to find Dr. Taillefer right away. She instructed her to tell him that Dr. Thompson was calling from Prineville. He had an emergency. After coming to the telephone and talking with the doctor in Prineville, Dr. Taillefer quickly telephoned the National Guard at the Portland airport and related that there was a sick little boy out in the desert, and he needed help right away. The commander of the National Guard said to come right out to the air base, where a helicopter and its crew would fly the doctor to Prineville.

The helicopter pilot and his crew flew at a low altitude east of Portland, up the Columbia River and through the gorge, below the snow-covered peaks of the Cascade Mountains, just above the power lines to the long, high bridge that spans the river at Biggs. The pilot, after talking with his radioman through their headphones, changed to a southerly course, flying at a low level and following the Deschutes River to Lake Billy Chinook, where the Crooked River joins the Deschutes. The helicopter followed the Crooked River to Prineville at the base of the Ochoco Mountains. The pilot made a couple of low passes over the town and concluded that he could avoid the power lines. The side cargo door was open, and the crew was on the lookout for electric wires or trees, guiding the pilot through their intercoms in their helmets, while a swirling cloud of dust was blowing away from the downdraft of the overhead whirling blades. He safely set the helicopter down in the high school parking lot. Andrew Singer, the little boy's father, was among the many people who rushed to the high school when they saw the military helicopter—painted green, brown, and black camouflage colors—touch down on the asphalt near the school building.

After the rotors stopped, Dr. Taillefer slid in beside Andy—into the cab of his blue Chevy pickup truck—for the swift ride to the home of the little boy, where his mother and the country doctor, Dr. Thompson, were waiting with other family members. Dr. Taillefer's movements were a little guarded, for he was walking on a badly sprained left ankle. One day earlier, he had fallen out of the pear tree in the orchard behind his home. His stiff ankle was black and blue, swollen, and painful. His shoe was tight, which prevented tying the shoelace. He had an Ace wrap around the swollen ankle. The doctor recognized that he had a bleed into his ankle, just like men have from hemophilia. It was painful to walk on it. He knew a little bit what it would be like to have hemophilia. But he also recognized he could not sit still just because of a sprained ankle. When a doctor is needed, he has to go.

After arriving at the Singers' home, the Portland doctor and Dr. Thompson quickly examined the little boy, who was motionless, lying straight on the bed, in the back bedroom of the small one-level house. The two doctors conferred with each other, and then they told the parents of the very sick little boy that their son was in grave danger. His belly was distended, going up and down when he breathed, rather than his chest expanding, a sign of paradoxical respirations. His knee jerks were absent, hyporeflexia, a sign of impending neurological deficit. He was nearly comatose. Working together, the two doctors opened their medical bags and brought out a scalpel, alcohol swabs, and Novocain. They quickly revised the cutdown, successfully inserted a small needle into the arm vein, and infused concentrate. After the infusion, the IV tubing into the vein was kept open with a saline drip.

"We must move Wendell to the university hospital immediately," Dr. Taillefer solemnly told his distressed mother and father. "He is in danger. He has a bleed into his back that is putting pressure on his spinal cord. We must stop the bleed as quickly as possible, and we can't succeed here. The National Guard helicopter will quickly fly him back to Portland."

Carefully, Wendell was lifted and carried to the seat of a van, where he was stretched out while he was delivered to the helicopter waiting at the high school. "I'm sorry, Mrs. Singer, but we cannot let you ride with us in the helicopter back to Portland. Dr. Taillefer will be at his side constantly, and he will give your little boy the best care possible. As soon as we take off from the schoolyard, why don't you and your husband leave in your car for Portland? Give us your telephone number in case we need to call your home," the understanding helicopter pilot said to the worried parents.

After the little boy was secured inside the helicopter, the doctor conferred with the crew, fastened himself into a seat next to the child, and fitted his gray head into a helmet. The big rotors began to move as the pilot started the engine after the crew checked to be certain the crowd of people was a safe distance away from the aircraft. Inside the helicopter, the noise and vibration prevented talking except through headsets built into the helmets. The IV that had been started in the little boy's veins was kept open with a slow drip. The drops in the IV drip chamber of the tubing from the suspended bottle of saline were counted. The drip rate was adjusted so that the tubing would not need changing for the duration of the flight from Prineville to Portland. Listening to the heart rate was impossible, but the small child's pulse could be felt in his tiny wrist and the rate of his breathing counted.

As the helicopter returned toward Portland, low, dark, ominous clouds appeared, signaling bad weather. The crew was advised by the air base to return north rather than cross the Cascade Mountains, a shorter route but with worse weather. The pilot flew just above the Columbia River, where the visibility was best, to avoid the bad weather over the

Cascades, carefully rising above the large orange balls identifying an electrical transmission power line crossing the river. The motionless child's breathing did not change; the IV drip continued uninterrupted during the flight. Although the doctor was nervous in his concern for the child, he was reassured by the security provided by the National Guard airmen, who were extending themselves to help the gravely ill little boy. Being in their hands within the interior of the helicopter was comforting, a sensation of protection. As dusk was settling, the lights reflecting from the Willamette River in the city of Portland welcomed the helicopter home. The pilot made a circle around the university hospital and then gently set the craft down on the helicopter pad near the CDRC Building, the location of hemophilia treatment center. An ambulance was waiting beside the pad.

"Thanks to you and all of your crew and to the U.S. Air Force National Guard for all of your splendid service," Dr. Taillefer said to the crew after the blades had stopped swinging overhead, allowing conversation again without shouting. "You just saved a little boy's life."

"You're very welcome," the pilot replied with a smile. "We hope the little boy will have a good life ahead. We are keeping his parents in our thoughts. It is a great pleasure and a privilege to help someone in need. We are glad we could help." No paperwork was required; the air force did not prepare a bill for their service.

As he rode in the ambulance the short distance to the hospital entrance, bringing the sick little boy for care, Dr. Taillefer saw the helicopter swoop up and away into the darkening sky as it returned to the Portland Air Base, near the Columbia River. *I've always known I could count on the military when I need help*, he thought, remembering the last time he had an experience with a helicopter—when he was a rifleman with the infantry in Korea. *The military always brings me a feeling of security, as if I have come home.*

Wendell was quickly moved into the surgical suite of the hospital, where the neurosurgeon and his resident assistants were waiting for his arrival that evening. The head of hematology, Dr. Waxman, and his resident assistant, Dr. Thomas Collins, infused additional concentrate into the IV tubing. Dr. Taillefer changed clothes, donning a green surgical scrub suit, surgical hat and mask, and shoe covers. He scrubbed his hands and arms with a disinfectant solution and cleaned his fingernails with a sharpened wooden stick, standard procedures, before entering the surgical operating room. The anesthesiologist prepared an additional vein at a second cutdown site in the other arm for intravenous administration of medicine and necessary drugs used during surgery. By then, Wendell was paralyzed in all four extremities; he was quadriplegic. The neurosurgeon inserted a needle into the little boy's spine, a lumbar puncture, where dye was injected. X-rays after the dye was injected, a myelogram, revealed a block in the spinal canal in the upper back and neck. The neurosurgeon and his residents, all wearing green scrub suits, masks, gloves, and gowns, draped green surgical barrier sheets over the little boy. He had been placed prone on his abdomen on the operating table, his backside upward. In the cool, subdued operating room, below a centrally placed large maneuverable operating room light, his head was turned to his left side. The anesthesiologist carefully induced sleep while controlling the child's breathing with a respirator connected to a mask placed over the child's face. Usually for general surgical anesthesia, an endotracheal tube is inserted into the throat. Inserting a tube into the trachea of a person who has hemophilia has a risk of producing a bleed in a crucial area of the body. Therefore, a face mask was used for administering the gases for anesthesia rather than inserting a tube into the child's windpipe.

After the skin of the back was prepared with a scrubbing solution for sterilization, the surgeons made a midline incision over the upper spine and back of the neck. The infusion of concentrate apparently was effective in restoring the clotting of the blood. There was no excessive bleeding. The surgeons removed the bones of the spine covering the spinal cord, a laminectomy. Within the spinal bones, the spinal cord was uncovered and visualized. A lump the size of a walnut was discovered; it was a hemorrhage, and it was compressing the cervical spinal cord. When the spinal cord was decompressed by removing the bones over the spinal canal, it immediately began to pulsate, caused by the heart beating.

"Hurray!" all the doctors cheered. The spinal cord was alive. It had not been crushed and destroyed by the pressure of the hemorrhage. Their skills and efforts had paid off; the chance for recovery was good!

The parents arrived at the hospital after their long drive from Prineville. They were delighted with the doctors' optimistic report. The chance that their son would walk again, rather than become a paraplegically crippled child, was favorable. After three hours in the surgical recovery suit, Wendell was moved into the pediatric intensive care unit (PICU), where he was carefully monitored by experienced nurses who watched over him constantly.

In the morning, in the PICU, the nurses noted that their eighteen-month-old patient was oozing bright red blood from his arm around the cutdown site, despite a continuous infusion of concentrate. He had received enough concentrate to increase his factor VIII level to 100 percent of normal. However, when Dr. Waxman measured the factor VIII from a blood sample, the amount of factor VIII activity was less than 1 percent of normal. He followed that measurement by mixing one milliliter of the boy's plasma with plasma from another person. After mixing the two plasmas together, Dr. Waxman calculated that one milliliter of Wendell's plasma inactivated the factor VIII activity in fourteen hundred milliliters of normal plasma. The little boy had an inhibitor—a strong inhibitor to factor VIII. When another person's factor VIII was infused into him, his body reacted and destroyed the factor VIII with an amnestic antibody response. The doctors wondered why this eighteen-month-old child had a strong inhibitor to factor VIII. He wasn't born with an inhibitor. Inhibitors to factor VIII develop in about one out of fifteen boys who have been infused to treat their hemophilia. They questioned whether the child had been infused with concentrate prior to his present spinal cord bleed.

"Remember," Dr. Taillefer reminded the other doctors, "this is not the first time this little boy has been infused with factor VIII concentrate. No. And it isn't the first time he has been brought to this hospital for surgery."

Dr. Taillefer related that the child was discovered to have hemophilia when he was five weeks of age. At that time, he began vomiting, forceful vomiting—referred to as projectile vomiting—after a feeding. When he burped after he was nursed, the milk in his stomach shot clear across the room, resembling the trajectory from a water cannon. His country doctor, the same doctor who takes care of him in Prineville, Dr. Thompson, sent him to this same hospital because he thought he might need surgery. He arrived at the hospital on July 11, 1973, a year and a half before the present hospital admission. When he was examined, a knot was felt in his belly, the so-called olive sign. An opaque liquid dye was injected through a small tube that had been inserted through his mouth and down into his stomach. The X-ray revealed that only a thin stream of the opaque liquid emptied from the stomach into the intestine; a finding known as the string sign. He had a muscular obstruction at the emptying part of his stomach, pyloric stenosis. His brother, George, had already been diagnosed with hemophilia. Before this little brother was taken to surgery to open the emptying portion of his stomach, he was tested for hemophilia and discovered to be just like his brother: he had hemophilia. He was infused with concentrate before, during, and after surgery, performed one and a half years previously, to relieve the obstruction to the emptying of his stomach, a pyloromyotomy. Apparently, he was also immunized by the infused AHF, and he formed antibodies to factor VIII.

As soon as Dr. Waxman confirmed the undesirable presence of an inhibitor to factor VIII in Wendell's blood, the concentrate necessary to prevent him from bleeding was changed from Koate to Konyne.[25]

---

25 Koate and Konyne were AHF concentrates manufactured by Cutter Biological. Koate was infused for treating factor VIII deficiency. Konyne was for treatment of factor IX deficiency. However, Konyne contained enough prothrombin complex that it restored clotting activity in factor VIII deficient persons and was used to manage inhibitors.

Within a few minutes after Konyne was infused, the bleeding oozing around the cutdown site in Wendell's small arm ceased. During the next days after surgery, Wendell began to move his arms and legs, and he responded to his mother and father, who were at his bedside in the PICU. On the fifth day after surgery, the amount of Konyne infusion was decreased. He began bleeding internally, into his stomach. He had developed a stress ulcer. Konyne, the concentrate, was increased, and the bleeding ceased. Wendell recovered from the surgery on his spine while receiving infusions of Konyne for two weeks. His parents brought him home to his family in Prineville.

"Now," Mary Singer said to Brent's mother, "he is a normal little boy. He does have a long scar from the surgery on his back and up the back of his neck. And he drags his foot when he walks, but we hope his walking will improve and his limp will go away with time."

"You must have been through a lot of worry," Gwyn said. "You have two sons with hemophilia. Is there anyone else among your relatives who have hemophilia?"

"No, our two boys are the only persons in our family who have hemophilia. We worry about George, Wendell's brother," she said as George rose from the chair where he had been reading a magazine.

Gwyn noticed that when George, age eight, walked, he also limped like his younger brother, as if one leg was shorter than the other. She turned to Mary and looked at her quizzically.

"Well, you see, George had a bad bleed into his hip that destroyed the hip bone where it fits into the hip socket. He also has an inhibitor to factor VIII and takes Konyne for bleeds like Wendell does. Although George limps, he doesn't complain. He wants to grow up and someday drive a big truck like his daddy drives. He loves trucks, and he worships his daddy," Mary related to Gwyn with a woman-to-woman smile. "Our sons do not sit back sheltering themselves from hemophilia. For them, every day has meaning, and they are eager to discover whatever lies ahead in their future. Kids are strong if they are given a chance."

Gwyn continued looking into the face of Mary Singer, as if she were searching for more information, as the two women, both mothers of boys with hemophilia, sat next to one another in the chairs of the waiting room of the clinic.

"I see you have noticed my eye," Mary Singer said softly to Brent's mother.

Gwyn had noticed that Mary, a pretty brunette woman with fine facial features and a soft voice, had a left eye that did not track correctly when she looked directly at her.

"A few months ago, I had a brain tumor," Mary Singer related to Gwyn. "The neurosurgeons discovered a tumor on my optic nerve, and they had to remove my left eye. Now I have a fake eye; my left eye is a glass eye. I can't see out of it. It doesn't follow well with my good eye, my right eye. But it looks okay when I look straight ahead."

"Oh my God!" Gwyn exclaimed when she and Brent were back in the car on their way home from the clinic. "And I thought we had a difficult time in our family because of hemophilia. I was wrong. Think of other people. There is the Singer family, two sons with hemophilia. Both have inhibitors; one has destruction of his hip; the other had a spinal cord bleed; and the mother has a brain tumor. Sometimes I think God puts several cases of suffering within one family so that most families are spared of grief. He groups bad things so that most families only know good things. That's God's way," she proclaimed.[26]

Before treatment for bleeding in hemophilia became available, before cryoprecipitate or concentrates, a bleed into the central nervous system, the spinal cord, or the brain of a person with hemophilia was

---

26 Later, Gwyn recalled that she realized that God—or nature or some other invisible force that she didn't understand—does mysterious things in other ways. For although the Singer family was confronted with many challenging hardships, the two Singer brothers, who have hemophilia, did not succumb to AIDS or hepatitis. Gwyn's son, Brent, became HIV infected from the concentrate and died of AIDS. The Singer brothers, like Brent, were infused many times and have remained well. "Why is that?" Gwyn puzzled.

fatal, as it was for Leopold, the son of Queen Victoria, who was born with hemophilia. With the new medicines available for infusions to replace the deficient clotting proteins of the blood in hemophilia, central nervous system bleeds could be successfully treated, as they were in Roger Norman in 1964, and a few years later in Wendell Singer from Prineville. Bleeds into the head or spinal cord were no longer universally fatal as they had been until the 1970s.

When Brent was five years of age, while making a visit to the hemophilia treatment center, Gwyn noticed a young man sitting in a chair in the waiting room. The man was tall and thin, with long brown hair that curled over his shoulders. He visited with Gwyn. He spoke softly, which prevented Brent from hearing all his words. He informed Gwyn that he was twenty-one years old and lived north of Portland in the small town of Vader, located in the forest of southwestern Washington. On his right leg, he was wearing a brace fastened with Velcro straps. His leg was thin; the muscles were atrophied. The brace included a flat, shiny metal strip on the inside and outside of his leg, with a rear hinge in the middle, at the level of his knee joint. He removed the brace before going into the examination room. When he walked without the brace, he lurched up and down. The left leg, his good leg, was two inches shorter than his right leg. He said his name was Brad and shyly confided to Gwyn that when he had knee bleeds as a young boy, the blood in the knee joint stimulated the femur, the thigh bone, to grow faster than his normal leg.[27] As a man, his legs were not of equal length. He was wearing a two-inch lift fastened to the bottom of his left shoe to lessen his limping. The long-leg knee brace kept his knee from buckling and dislocating, he said. He told Gwyn that he expected to be reprimanded by the doctor and physical therapist. He had not followed their instructions to complete quadriceps knee exercises to prevent his muscles from shrinking while wearing the brace. He said

---

27 Blood is not normally present within the joint space. When a bleed occurs into the knee joint of a growing child, the growth center at the end of the bone, the epiphysis, is stimulated, resulting in overgrowth.

the clinic staff directed him to do leg lifts ten repetitions ten times each day. But he admitted that the quadriceps exercises were not enjoyable; they were terribly boring. Instead of doing exercises when he had pain in his knee, he said he had been giving himself a shot of concentrate for an infusion.

The Hemophilia Treatment Center

The Oregon Hemophilia Treatment Center was where Brent's parents gathered their supply of concentrate and the other supplies necessary for infusions, such as disposable needles and plastic syringes, Band-Aids and alcohol wipes. When Brent attended the clinic at the center for his annual checkup, several people met with his parents. One person who talked with them was Isabella. Her assignment in the clinic was to identify a method to pay for the concentrate and supplies that Brent required for treating hemophilia. Isabella was a social worker and an administrative assistant. She was an advocate for persons like Brent who had hemophilia, assuring them that they would receive whatever medical supplies they needed. The clinic received funds from the Oregon CCD hemophilia budget to pay for the medicine. The cost for the X-rays, laboratory tests, and checkups by the doctor and dentist were paid by CCD. The doctors and dentists, including the orthopedic doctors and the blood specialist, were not paid for their services to the clinic. They were there, bringing their experience, because they were interested in the problems of hemophilia and getting to know persons like Brent. Most doctors create a little niche for themselves, a special interest that helps them discover the meaning of life, a medical interest that serves as their professional passion.

Brent's mother was impressed by the hemophilia treatment center and wondered how the center came about, how everything was paid for. Would payment for her son's medical care, necessary if he was to avoid pain and threatening bleeds, continue in the future? She asked questions and got to know people when they attended the clinic at the center. When she saw them repeatedly, she became friends with the nurse, the social worker, the financial counselor, and others. She was eager to discover the origin of the center.

There was a pediatrician, a doctor who cared a lot about children, who gave up his practice in Medford, Oregon, moved to Portland in the 1960s, and became the director of Oregon's Crippled Children's Division. In Oregon, CCD was not just an agency, it was an entity, located within a building on the campus of the medical school. Included within CCD were thirty separate clinics for children with special needs. The faculty who staffed the clinic held academic appointments in departments of the medical school, which has been renamed OHSU.[28] CCD was renamed CDRC. The pediatrician and one of the hematologists at the medical school were concerned that boys with hemophilia became disabled from recurrent bleeds. The destiny for boys who suffered pain and disability, who became crippled in adulthood, was not acceptable. Something needed to be done about it. The doctor, Dr. Dick Sleeter, and the hematologist, Dr. Rutherford Skyles, working together, started a hemophilia clinic in 1966. The goal was to prevent crippling. Dr. Dick Sleeter appointed a pediatrician, Dr. Betty Skilling, as director of the new clinic. After two years, Dr. Skilling went away on sabbatical leave. Shortly after her departure, in April of 1968, Dr. Dick Sleeter called Dr. Taillefer to his office.

Dr. Anton Taillefer had arrived in Oregon a year and a half earlier, after completing a research fellowship at the University of Glasgow, Scotland, in 1966. He moved to Portland, a destination he had not previously visited, without knowing any acquaintances, by sailing from John Brown's Shipyard on the Firth of Clyde, aboard the Empress of England, crossing the Atlantic with his wife and family to Montreal. Across Canada, on Canadian National Railway, he brought his wife and four young daughters to Vancouver, British Columbia. From there, the

---

28 OHSU: Oregon Health Sciences University; CDRC: Child Development and Rehabilitation Center

family boarded the train to Portland, where they began their life. Their first night in Portland, they lodged in a single room at the Hoyt Hotel, a hotel that no longer exists. From the train station, they walked to the nearby hotel, to their second-floor room, directly above the dance floor on a noisy Saturday night. A few days later, they found an apartment in Tigard.

In 1968, Dr. Dick Sleeter called Anton Taillefer to his office and asked him how he and his family were doing since they'd moved to Oregon. He asked if they were happily settled into a house in Portland after their voyage from Scotland.

Dr. Taillefer admitted that they were struggling. He and his wife and four young daughters were living in an apartment along Fanno Creek in Tigard. His wife was pregnant with their fifth child, and the crowded two-bedroom apartment was too small for their family, especially when their family kept growing in size.

With insight and understanding of the responsibilities of a large family, Dr. Dick Sleeter replied that he too was Catholic. He was seated comfortably behind his large wooden desk, leaning backward in a swivel chair, puffing on his dark brown burl pipe, feet propped up on the desk. Dr. Sleeter commented that Dr. Taillefer's annual salary as an assistant professor was sixteen thousand dollars, not a lot of money for a family of seven. He said he would refer him to Mrs. Burdick at Portland Teachers Credit Union for some financial help. Dr. Sleeter always referred his staff to Mrs. Burdick for financial assistance. Nearly everyone on the staff at CCD had a loan with PTCU at one time or another. Dr. Sleeter asked Dr. Taillefer if he had a student loan to pay off.

He did. Although he had received the GI Bill for help toward medical school tuition, he had accumulated an eight-hundred-dollar loan debt that must be repaid. He was not from a doctor's family nor any other privileged family with financial means. He had grown up on a farm in Iowa before studying medicine and going abroad.

While inspecting Dr. Taillefer's resume, Dr. Sleeter noted that he'd served as a rifleman in Korea. He asked him if he'd saved money while he was in the army. He commented that while Dr. Taillefer was serving in a combat zone, there wouldn't have been any place to spend his pay unless he gambled it away playing poker.

Dr. Taillefer didn't play poker while in the infantry in Korea. Every payday, the first sergeant cleaned out the money bet by the rifle company's poker players. The sergeant had a big bankroll. He was a rich man. Dr. Taillefer was not. His pay was sent home to be saved, but he didn't quite save enough to pay for medical school, although he had the benefits of the GI Bill after he was discharged from the army.

Dr. Dick Sleeter smilingly confided that he was fifty-five years old before his student loan was paid off. He then reminded Dr. Taillefer that he had been appointed to start a genetics program with Dr. Gaylord Case in Oregon. Dr. Sleeter confessed that he did not know what medical geneticists actually do. Medical genetics was a new specialty in pediatrics. When he'd attended medical school at the University of Iowa, there were no course subjects that discussed genetics. Genetics, as part of medicine, had come about only recently. He asked Dr. Taillefer if he would like to provide care to patients with a genetic disease. Most genetic diseases have no treatment—no cure. Dr. Taillefer was puzzled and asked what medical disorder Dr. Sleeter was referring to.

"Hemophilia," Dr. Sleeter replied.

Dr. Taillefer reminded his director that he was not a blood specialist. He was a pediatrician. He assumed a hematologist would be more appropriate to serve in a clinic that cared for people with a bleeding disorder.

Dr. Sleeter replied, while smoke curled upward from his pipe, that he wanted someone who was interested in the total child, not just his blood, to direct the clinic. Boys with hemophilia have orthopedic problems as well as psychological and dental problems. They suffer, they miss school, and they get hepatitis. They have a short life expectancy; often they die before they are old enough to marry. He said he was aware that Dr. Taillefer was a generalist, interested in children, even though he had completed specialized training in genetics. He knew that Dr. Taillefer had cared for some hemophilia patients with Dr. Harold James when he served as the chief resident at The Children's Hospital in Washington, D.C.[29] He had excellent training and medical experiences at the University of Minnesota, the San Diego County Hospital, Children's Hospital in Washington, D.C, Stanford Medical Center, and the University of Glasgow. He was also in the general practice of family medicine a short time in Robbinsdale, Minnesota, in 1965. Dr. Sleeter was satisfied that the thirty-eight-year-old Dr. Taillefer was well qualified and had a respectable background to direct a clinic that cared for extended needs of children. Besides, the directorship of the hemophilia clinic would only be for six months, until Betty returned from sabbatical leave. After she returned, Dr. Sleeter informed Dr. Taillefer, he could resume his genetics activities in medicine, whatever that might be.[30]

Dr. Betty Skilling decided to get married. She did not return to the clinic from Sabbatical leave. Dr. Taillefer became the permanent director of the clinic.[31] Although his directorship was by default, he was pleased to become a clinic director and accepted his assignment with professional honor. He was not trained as a hematologist; however, three hematologists served on the staff in the clinic. One of them, Dr. Rutherford Skyles, who had staffed the clinic from its beginning, was in charge of the laboratory that performed the blood tests related to hemophilia. Shortly after Dr. Taillefer accepted directorship of the hemophilia clinic, Dr. Skyles unexpectedly backed away from medicine before customary retirement age. He hung up his stethoscope and took up the violin. Elmer Waxman, one of Dr. Skyles's students, had recently completed studying hematology with Dr. Sam Rappaport

---

29 Renamed Children's National Medical Center
30 Dr. Dick Sleeter was particularly cordial to Dr. Taillefer. Both doctors were born and raised on Iowa farms.
31 Later, in 1976, the clinic was designated a hemophilia treatment center.

at the University of Southern California (USC). He returned to his native Portland to become the director of hematology at the medical school, replacing Dr. Skyles. He accepted a staff position in the clinic. Dr. Marshall Patterson, a hematologist in private practice in Portland, formerly director of the Portland Red Cross blood bank, served as another of the hematologists on the staff of the clinic. When Dr. James Watson completed his fellowship in hematology at the University of Indiana, he also joined the hemophilia clinic staff. Later, upon the appointment of Dr. Ned Strong to the staff, four hematologists served in the clinic at the hemophilia treatment center.

When Dr. Taillefer became director of the Oregon Hemophilia Clinic, the only available medicine for treatment of bleeding in hemophilia was cryoprecipitate (cryo), derived from plasma, for hemophilia type A patients who were deficient in factor VIII, and whole plasma for treating men and boys who were deficient in factor IX, type B hemophilia. Cryo was a great advance in treating bleeds. However, its utilization was cumbersome. Treatment of a bleed in a one-hundred-pound boy required ten bags of frozen cryo, which had to be ordered from the Red Cross blood bank, thawed, pooled into one plastic bag, and suspended from an IV stand while it slowly dripped into the person's vein. Since the cryo was not purified, many persons developed allergic reactions to the components in the plasma. Cryo was not convenient for infusions at home. Further purification of the components in plasma that contain the AHF clotting factor, resulted in the successful production of lyophilized concentrate. The new concentrate was stable in a small vacuum bottle. AHF clotting activity was easily reconstituted by adding a small volume of water or saline, with little risk of an allergic reaction. The new concentrate was produced by Hyland Pharmaceutical. However, its supply was limited, which prevented its dependable utilization for home infusions. The scene changed in 1971 with the introduction of Humafac by Parke-Davis. That new medicine was available as a dependable source of concentrate for infusions at home.

By nature, most persons want to avoid going to the doctor. When a person is afflicted with a chronic disorder that will affect him day after day and be present from birth until death, attending the clinic time after time is drudgery. When a person is suddenly stricken with appendicitis, the doctor removes the appendix at surgery, the person recovers, there are no residuals, and the illness is over, gone. Not so with hemophilia. It will always be there. Before concentrates became available, there was little relief from the suffering and pain of hemophilia by going to the doctor or to the clinic. Since the introduction of concentrates for treating bleeds, persons affected with hemophilia have come forward, enthusiastically attending the clinic when they discovered there was a way they could manage their own treatment for bleeding episodes. They no longer had to fear death from an intracranial hemorrhage. The many times of lying in bed agonizing with pain in their knees night after night were gone. They could safely undergo surgery without fear of bleeding to death. After replacing defective clotting factor, injections of Novocain could be given for dental work. At the dentist, patients were protected with an infusion of concentrate, avoiding pain and swollen and discolored faces and jaws from bleeding at the injection site. Sue, the nurse, instructed parents and grown-up men in the procedure for infusions at home. After their training sessions, they were provided with a supply of concentrate. When the concentrate was consumed at home, the supply was replaced in order to maintain a dependable source of clotting factor for infusions.

Cost of Hemophilia Care

I n 1972, Sue remarked to Dr. Taillefer that some of the families who were supplied with concentrate from the clinic had medical insurance.[32]

The concentrate dispensed to the families was expensive. If a patient received an infusion of one thousand units of AHF, costing ten cents for each unit, that amounted to $100, a sizable sum of money in the early 1970s.

The frequency of infusions at home to control recurrent bleeding episodes was once, twice, sometimes three times within one week. For a person infusing twice each week, the weekly cost at $200 added up to $10,400 each year. If the clinic supplied concentrate to fifty patients for home infusion, the annual cost equaled $520,000.[33] After reviewing the bleed sheets the families completed at home whenever an infusion was given, the frequency of infusions was noted to vary between individuals. Infants were infused infrequently, perhaps once each month. Teenagers were infused the most often, peaking at age thirteen, when they averaged ten to twelve infusions each month. Adults were infused less often. One hundred and fifty infusions in a person each year was common. After

---

32 Prior to the 1970s, during Dr. Taillefer's training, the cost of medical care at the clinic was paid by the state or county. Patients were not billed for services or supplies. Itemized costs, such as a Band-Aid, a cotton ball, or an aspirin, were not tabulated, in contrast with profit-making fee-for-service designs of hospital administrations beginning in the 1980s.

33 In 1972, the cost of $10,400 for an individual equaled $51,000 in 2008; $520,000 for inventory in 1972 was equivalent to $2,675,000 in 2008 (RE: Measuringworth 2009).

several years of home infusions, hemophilia patients began to break the one-thousand-infusion barrier when they were infused more than one thousand separate times. The number of persons joining the one-thousand rank slowly expanded and soon was no longer exceptional.

The hemophilia center was required to be fiscally responsible to the budget allocated from CCD. If a patient's family had medical insurance, a request for reimbursement could be sent to the insurance company, requesting payment for the cost of the medicine, Sue and Dr. Taillefer reasoned. At that time, in 1972, the medical business office at CCD did not send bills to patients requesting payment for services or supplies. Until then, the medical school hospital and clinics and CCD were part of the State of Oregon system and did not bill for services. Times changed with the introduction of medical reimbursement. Hospitals and clinics are no longer controlled only by doctors. Policies were dictated by persons of a different specialty, hospital administrators. With the increased role of hospital administrators and increased number of subscribers to medical insurance, attention has become directed toward billing for services and collection of fees from medical insurance. The hemophilia clinic fell into step with the fiscal changes, which have changed the delivery of medical care, and began billing for services if a patient was a subscriber of a medical insurance plan. Medical insurance evolved, while tied to employment rather than universal insurance for everyone. Many areas of financial concerns appeared to confront the hemophilia clinic. Most prominent was the evolvement of categories of patients: those who were insured and those who had no medical insurance, children and adults. Children who were residents of Oregon were eligible for hemophilia treatment through CCD funds. The clinic was confronted with the dilemma of identifying a method to pay for the cost of hemophilia treatment for those individuals over the age of twenty-one who had no medical insurance, or for persons who were not Oregon residents.

During the first year that the hemophilia clinic mailed statements to insurance companies, requesting reimbursement for medical services for dispensed concentrate, $250,000 was collected, equivalent to $1,286,000 in 2008 (RE: Measuringworth 2009).[34] The hemophilia clinic was the first clinic in CCD to usher in the era of billing insurance companies. Eventually, billing insurance for medical care reimbursement became a major activity of the delivery of medical services for every clinic. As time has passed, the cost of a clinic visit has become dictated by the amount insurance will reimburse rather than the fee set by the provider, an indication that medical care has become a commodity rather than uniquely a method for relief from suffering. Unfortunately, the reimbursed funds received from the first attempts at billing insurance companies in 1972 did not directly benefit the clinic. There were no provisions for reimbursement in the clinic's budget. There was no account for depositing the payment received from insurance. The money collected from insurance companies was directed to the medical school's general fund, for roof repairs or improvement of sidewalks rather than for direct patient care. Sue and Dr. Taillefer were confident the hemophilia program could benefit in the next year's budget if they demonstrated to the administration fiscal responsibility with this first attempt at reimbursement.

All the people on staff at the treatment center were shocked and saddened when they returned to the clinic Tuesday morning, August 22, 1972, and discovered that Dr. Dick Sleeter wasn't upstairs sitting in his high-backed swivel chair at his desk, puffing on his pipe. While walking with his wife along the Metollius River at Camp Sherman in central Oregon, where he loved to fly-fish for rainbow trout, he suddenly fell to the ground. His pipe was no longer smoking. He was dead. The doctor that children and faculty loved so much died of a sudden heart attack, a reminder that life for everyone is transient, not permanent, not

---

34 In 1972, $250,000 in sale of concentrate was recorded as received from medical insurance for sale of concentrate at the Oregon Hemophilia Clinic. In 2008, the cost of concentrate dispensed from the Hemophilia Center amounted to $20,000,000.

to be wasted but to be cherished. His assistant, Dr. Byron Morrison, was appointed by the dean of the medical school to replace him as director of CCD.

Dr. Taillefer was notified in June, 1976, that the office of Maternal Child and Health (MCH), part of NIH, intended to provide funds for hemophilia. Such an announcement was a surprise. The government traditionally had a policy of not funding categorical illnesses. Hilton Wassil from MCH traveled from Bethesda, Maryland, to Portland, arriving at CCD on Monday, June 7, 1976. He explained that MCH was intending to fund hemophilia treatment centers but not to pay for hemophilia care. The goal was to develop comprehensive treatment plans to assure that hemophilia care was available to all the children residing within each of the ten health regions of the United States. Hemophilia clinics were invited to apply for a grant from MCH by September 1, 1976, just three months away. Those clinics awarded grants would be designated regional hemophilia treatment centers. The grant from MCH would provide funds for such personnel as secretaries, financial counselors, and administrative assistants; computer services; office supplies; and travel expenses. The grant would not pay the salaries of doctors, dentists, or nurses, or the cost of concentrates for infusions.

Only one grant would be awarded within each of the ten health regions of the United States. To apply for the grant, the applicant was required to have the unanimous support of the other existing medical treatment facilities in his region. Compared to the less-recognized program in Portland, Seattle, Washington, just 175 miles north, had a more nationally recognized hemophilia clinic at the Puget Sound Blood Center. However, discussion with the director of the Seattle hemophilia clinic, Dr. Lawrence Body, revealed that the Seattle clinic was a private organization and did not intend to apply for the federal grant. Agreement between Seattle and Portland gave the go-ahead to apply for the Region X Comprehensive Hemophilia Treatment Center grant, which would serve the Pacific Northwest region of the United States. Region X includes Alaska, Idaho, Washington, and Oregon. By prearranged discussion and agreement, no other facility—no other hospital or clinic in Portland, Seattle, Spokane, Anchorage, or Boise—applied for the hemophilia grant in Region X. There was no competition for the funds within the region. Instead, agencies in those communities were asked for letters indicating their support for the proposed hemophilia treatment center. They agreed and endorsed Portland's proposal and willingly provided letters of support for the designated regional center. Letters of support for the Oregon CCD grant application were received from the Red Cross blood bank as well as the CCD programs in Washington, Alaska, and Idaho.

Dr. Taillefer assembled a group of fourteen staff, who retreated Friday, August 13, 1976, to a rented house on the Pacific Coast in Oregon to write the application for the MCH grant titled Region X Comprehensive Hemophilia Center Program. The goal of the grant proposal was to identify all the children and men with hemophilia living within the region—and to assure Maternal and Child Health that they were receiving optimal care. Providing medical care for every person with hemophilia in the region was not the goal. Rather, the intent was to identify access to proper care for every person affected with hemophilia. Present with their thoughts and suggestions for the application were the physical therapist, hematologist, orthopedic surgeon, nurses, social worker, geneticist, dentist, psychologist, secretary, administrative assistant, assistant director of CCD, and computer data manager (plate 2). The group finished the grant writing during a three-day weekend. During the retreat, ideas were discussed; the suggestions were condensed, organized, and set onto the required grant application forms.

After returning from the beach, all the personnel assisted in the tasks of grant preparation. Documents, letters of support, logistics, budgets, goals, and methods—the multiple components—generated a two-inch-thick proposal that required copying and stapling many pages of papers together. Twenty-one copies of the grant were required to be shipped to MCH to allow outside reviews by designated health-care experts. The application was shipped as a hand-carried parcel by United Airlines to Bethesda, where it was delivered overnight and placed on the desk of the granting agency on the Wednesday September 1 deadline.

One month later, on Friday, October 1, 1976, a telephone call was received from Bethesda, Maryland, announcing that Oregon's hemophilia grant application was approved. Dr. Taillefer, the project director, was informed that instructions would be received for revisions suggested by the reviewers and required by MCH. The award, which was intended to be funded for five years, required comprehensive annual progress reports and annual resubmission of budgets.

Instructions for revisions required by MCH for the Region X Hemophilia Grant in 1976:

1. Attend biannual meetings of the hemophilia centers' directors.
2. Submit quarterly progress reports.
3. Revise the budget to comply with the amount of the award.
4. Meet twice each year with Seattle's Puget Sound Blood Center director.
5. Appoint members from the community to a hemophilia advisory board (nonmedical).
6. Assist in the creation of a hemophilia medical advisory board.
7. Develop a system for uniform data collection.
8. Devise a method for evaluating outcomes of the project.
9. Conduct annual outreach hemophilia clinics in Alaska, Idaho, and rural areas of Oregon.

The announcement that the Portland, Oregon, CCD clinic was designated the federally funded hemophilia treatment center for Region X was followed by a flurry of activity. One of the first assignments was to negotiate between the funding source, MCH, and the business office of the medical school, an agreement to bypass the indirect costs for administration of the grant. The medical school traditionally received 40 percent of the funds of an awarded federal grant as indirect costs. Those funds were used to pay for the administration of the grant, support for the library, maintenance of medical records, billing and insurance, and payment for housing and utilities. Successfully, the director of CCD, Dr. Morrison, negotiated with the dean of the medical school to allow full funding to be awarded to the hemophilia treatment center, with no indirect costs subtracted from the total amount funded. The funds were entirely directed toward improvement of hemophilia care. The major expenditure of the treatment center was the purchase of concentrates for dispensation to patients. Funds from the grant were not designated to pay for the cost of concentrate. The cost of the concentrates for treatment was provided by allocation of funds from CCD. The concept included receipt of start-up-funds from CCD to purchase an inventory of concentrates for treatment of bleeding episodes in persons affected with hemophilia in Region X. The concentrate was distributed directly from the treatment center, not from the hospital pharmacy. Persons who lived close to the center were supplied with concentrate when they attended the clinic. For those persons who lived a distance from the center, who were evaluated in the outreach clinics in rural regions of Oregon, Idaho, and Alaska, concentrate was shipped to them as express mail. CCD developed a billing system that facilitated reimbursement from medical insurance companies. Receipts from reimbursement, which included a 10 percent markup as a handling expense, were utilized to purchase additional concentrate, which successfully allowed the creation of an inventory used to supply hemophilia persons throughout the region.

A dependable source of concentrates was a central feature of the treatment center. Pharmacies, hospitals, and doctor's offices did not maintain a supply of concentrate. The cost of the inventory was too expensive for them to stock on their shelves. If they ordered a supply for a patient who moved away and who did not appear at the pharmacy to claim the concentrate, the pharmacy would be confronted with a large expenditure, a loss. The hemophilia treatment center enjoyed the confidence of the administration of CCD as well as the university hospital. The Hemophilia Medical Advisory Board, a group separate from CCD, composed of members appointed by the Oregon Hemophilia Foundation and the University of Oregon Medical School Administration, reviewed the policies of the treatment center and the purchase of concentrates. Added to the wholesale cost of the purchase price of concentrates, a 10 percent handling fee was approved by the Medical Advisory Board. Funds generated by the handling fee provided a method for the purchase of concentrate in instances where there was no identified method of payment for a person with hemophilia. The treatment center purchased concentrate directly from the pharmaceutical manufacturer, avoiding distribution and handling costs by an intermediate distributor. Guidelines and regulations mandated by the State of Oregon were followed, which required submitting the purchase of concentrate to pharmaceutical suppliers for bids. Bids submitted by suppliers of concentrate were carefully considered before acceptance.

The purchase price was only one consideration when accepting bids from pharmaceutical suppliers. Hemophilia patients were displeased if the brand of concentrate they were infusing was frequently changed. The medicine they were utilizing was directly infused into their bloodstream through their veins, which is psychologically different from swallowing a pill in the treatment of most medical disorders. Hemophilia patients were reluctant to change from one brand of concentrate to a different brand just because the treatment center was coaxed into purchasing a different brand because of a price reduction. From a medical point of view, no difference was detected between the different brands of concentrate that affected the health of the persons receiving the medicine. The only difference noted was patient preferences.

As access to medical information for consumers changed through increased media activity, such as advertising and direct consumer contact by the pharmaceutical manufacturers, conflicts of interests became increasingly frequent. Prior to 1960, advertising a pharmaceutical product or a doctor's services was considered unethical. In contrast, publicity of pharmaceutical products through advertising became commonplace in the 1970s. By the 1980s, advertisement for drugs and services saturated television, newspapers, and magazines. Because of the cost of concentrate, a great amount was at stake for the pharmaceutical companies. Competition was intense. Although the pharmaceutical companies who manufactured concentrate provided a great product that benefited persons affected with hemophilia, sometimes their tactics— such as when they contacted patients or provided financial incentives to prescribing physicians—were reprehensible. The intense competition between the drug companies who produced the concentrate, with an emphasis on marketing rather than safety, may have contributed to the contamination of their products with hepatitis and HIV.

Dr. Taillefer was aware of pharmaceutical competition whenever the calendar indicated it was time to receive annual bids for supplying concentrates. On one occasion, when presenting their bid for supplying the inventory of concentrate to the center, two sales representatives from Alpha Therapeutics appeared with a wooden crate. Within the crate were lemons the size of cantaloupes and avocados nearly the size of pineapples. "I raised these lemons and avocados on my own ranch in sunny Southern California. Take them. They are for your family. We thought you would like them. We brought them for you." The sales representative of the drug company announced with a wide, friendly smile.

The attractive fruit was accepted from the drug company and donated to the cafeteria.

Accepting Hemophilia
as Part of Normal Living

Brent's first year of school was at Mt. Tabor Elementary School in southeast Portland. The school was named for Mt. Tabor, a forested small mountain only a few blocks from the school entrance. He learned that the rocky hill was an active volcano until only six hundred years ago. Portland is a city with old volcanoes that are no longer spewing steam into the sky, within its borders. Brent was only four years and eleven months of age the first time he walked through the schoolhouse door in September 1980, one month before his fifth birthday in October. Oh, yes, he remembered that day! He was excited but scared. He didn't know anyone, none of the other kids. He was rather short compared to some of the other kids. The girls were as tall as the boys.

"I wish I had kept him home another year so he would have started school when he was a year older," Gwyn said.

Brent went through kindergarten and first grade at Mount Tabor. He was not absent from school because of a bleed. Brent liked school. He ate lunch in the cafeteria, which was fun. Sometimes he brought his lunch when his mother had no money to give to him to buy a meal ticket. His father didn't always have a job, so there were some things the family had to do without. But his father was a good guy. He liked to take Brent places like the G.I. Joe's store to look at all the outdoor and camping stuff, such as kayaks, tents, hiking boots, and knives. His sisters were nice to Brent. Lee and Gwyn enjoyed taking their kids to the beach. Lee said that if they went to the beach, Brent must wear his high-topped shoes to prevent an ankle bleed. Brent knew what his father meant, but heck; it's no fun to run on the beach in shoes. He pleaded with his father to allow him to run in the sand at Cannon Beach near Haystack Rock. Brent and his two sisters could run forever on the wide sandy beach when the tide was out. They would scare the seagulls that landed on the seashore and watch them sail up into the blue sky over the ocean waves. They searched to discover who could find the prettiest piece of driftwood. They searched for sand dollars and agates. They could even fly a kite in the ocean breeze.

Lee said to his son, "Okay. But if you get an ankle bleed after you take your shoes off, it's going to hurt. It will be painful."

"Yeah, I know. I want to try running in the sand anyway."

After they played at the beach, Brent and his sisters piled back into the car. They were hungry. "Let's go for pizza," his sister Paula cried out. Pizza was a great idea. But when they stopped the car, Brent couldn't get out. He couldn't walk. Lee had to carry his son into the pizza parlor. All the time they were sitting in the booth waiting for pizza, Brent was in pain. He was squirming around, twitchy, trying not to cry. Brent knew he should not have run without shoes in the sand. But it was worth it. After climbing back into the car, his ankle hurt all the way home. It was tight, stiff, and swollen.

Finally, when they arrived home, Lee covered his son's painful ankle with a towel and gently piled crushed ice over it. He gave Brent a shot in the arm for an infusion of concentrate. Pierrette, Brent's mother's friend from Spokane, was visiting with the family that day and had gone with them to the beach. She had known Brent since the day he was born. "Look at me," Brent said to Pierrette. "See. Watch me get a shot. I'm not afraid." The medicine was mixed and ready for Lee to give Brent a shot. But he missed the vein. Missing made Lee nervous, but not Brent. He didn't cry. He didn't fuss. He sat up straight and held his arm out for his father to try again. He smiled and said, "Dad will hit it on the next poke." And he did. The ice numbed his ankle, and he went to sleep. When he awakened, the pain was less but still present. His ankle hurt less the next day.

Hemophilia was no longer a mystery. Brent didn't question why he had bleeds. They were normal for him, part of his life. That's just the way it was. He realized he had to accept the cards he was dealt. He knew what it was like to have a bleed … and that the pain would be over after a shot. He knew that if he had pain and swelling, it wouldn't last forever. His parents had received hemophilia lessons at the hemophilia treatment center, and they knew what to expect. Brent wasn't frightened. He had been attending school regularly, not missing classes because of unpredictable bleeds. Brent and his family were in control of their lives. After the ankle bleed at the beach, if he wanted to play hard, his father gave him an infusion, before they left home, to prevent his ankles from swelling and becoming painful.

Moving

Move from Portland

Brent's third year of school, the second grade, began in Pasadena after his family moved from Portland to California in 1983, when he was eight years old. His father unexpectedly announced that there was a new job opening in Los Angeles. His proclamation wasn't a sensational surprise. Lee often changed jobs. He was a restless man, always hoping for a better life for his family, but not quite knowing how to make that happen. For the trip by car to California, they packed a supply of concentrate and all the other stuff necessary for an infusion so that Lee could give Brent a shot during the journey if he had a bleed.

After they arrived in California and were settled in their new Pasadena home, Gwyn telephoned the treatment center. She wanted to enroll Brent in the California hemophilia treatment program at UCLA in Westwood Village. But they had no medical insurance. His care was transferred to the Los Angeles County Hospital in downtown Los Angeles.

The hospital wanted more blood tests from Brent. Whenever a person changes doctors, they always want new tests. Why can't the doctors believe what they are told? Gwyn told them her son had hemophilia. They said they needed test results for their records. "We acknowledge that your son has hemophilia," they said to Gwyn. "We just want to confirm the diagnosis."

LA Times Talks about a New Illness: Gwyn Gets Scared

In the autumn of 1983, Gwyn read a newspaper article in the *Los Angeles Times* about a strange new illness affecting homosexual men. The article also mentioned that several persons with hemophilia were exhibiting signs of the new illness. The article worried Gwyn. When they returned to the Los Angeles hemophilia treatment center at the county hospital for a checkup, Gwyn asked a nurse if she was worried. The nurse brushed off Gwyn's comments and concerns. Gwyn remarked to her husband, after she returned home from the clinic, that the people in the treatment center were not very nice to her. They treated her as if she was a troublemaker. The nurses were not understanding about her worries. They thought she was one of those overprotective mothers.[35]

"The hemophilia clinic at the Los Angeles County Hospital is a terrible place. I wish I never had to go back there," Gwyn remarked to her husband.

The job that Lee thought was waiting for him in Los Angeles didn't develop. He was always searching for a job. His ideal vision included making a lot of money without working hard. He wasn't lazy; he was just unconventional, not a man who could resign himself to the regular workplace. He didn't locate a job that he could accept. Finally, after Brent began his second year of living in California, his parents decided that California, the Golden State, wasn't so golden after all. The family missed their friends. They were lonesome. California wasn't their kind of place. The air was terrible, and they seldom saw the sunshine. It was blotted out of the sky by gray smog. They were homesick for Oregon and wanted to move back to Portland.

In the autumn of 1984, Lee quickly took charge, rented a U-Haul truck, and announced that they were leaving California and moving back to Oregon. The children were excited and happy to help pack and load their stuff into that big truck. Everything they owned—all their clothing, furnishings, pots and pans, beds, and shoes—was piled into the truck, including Brent's box of small toy race cars he had collected. For the last time in their California home, Lee gave Brent an infusion in the kitchen. Except for the white refrigerator and electric cooking stove, which were left for the next tenants, the kitchen was empty, cleared of furniture, dishes, and pots and pans, which were packed into the truck. A clean green bath towel was spread on the stove top for Brent's armrest during the infusion. They infused 946 AHF units of Koate HT into his arm vein, a prophylactic infusion that would prevent a bleed and avoid stopping for an infusion during the long car trip to Oregon.

Return to Oregon

The Perry family set out from their California home, heading northward, back to Oregon—Lee driving the U-Haul truck, Gwyn following behind his truck in their old Pontiac with Brent and his two sisters and lots of stuff. Following Lee's truck was not easy for Gwyn. Gray smog cut the visibility to the length of a football field. Paula, riding up front in the passenger seat beside her mother, kept her eye on the truck up ahead by noting the U-Haul logo on the back of the truck. Ascending the section of I-5 known as "the Grapevine" was difficult because of the huge slow-moving trucks that clogged the right and middle lanes, blocking the visibility of the U-Haul truck. They finally emerged from the dense Los Angeles smog and hectic traffic and headed up I-5 toward Portland, one thousand miles north. They kept moving, traveling for two days, stopping only for gas or to use the bathrooms in a gas station or at the rest stop. They ate corn dogs and soup in the convenience stores at the gas stations. Gwyn told Brent he couldn't dip his corn dog in mustard. She feared a mess of yellow mustard in the car. Lee didn't have enough money for motels at night, or for eating in restaurants along the way. They didn't have a bath. They didn't brush their teeth. It wasn't always easy for Gwyn to keep the truck ahead in sight on the busy I-5 Interstate. She couldn't see the truck after dark, so they stopped for the night at a rest area. They slept in the car the best way they could. It seemed like a long time to Brent, as if they would never get there. As a child, he didn't question the practicality or the feasibility of the adventurous move from California back to Oregon. If the return was planned by his parents, it must be okay.

Brent was jammed into the rear seat with one of his sisters. His two sisters took turns sitting up front beside their mother in the passenger seat. Brent had a sketch pad, a box of sixty-four crayons—new, no broken ones—and three of his favorite small toy cars he'd grabbed out of the shipping box in the truck. His sisters brought several books and two of their favorite board games. A gallon jug of water, paper cups, and a plastic lidded Tupperware container with carrot and celery sticks and thin slices of salami were on the floor behind the front seat. Before they arrived in Portland, Brent yearned for some real food.

An annoying problem plagued them: the car had no air-conditioning. Therefore, the windows were rolled down for ventilation. When the windows were down, Brent couldn't hear what his mother said from the front seat, nor could he hear his sister sitting next to him in the backseat when she tried to read to him from their books. They had to yell at one another to hear above the sound of the wind roaring in through the open windows. When Brent tried to make a drawing with his crayons on the paper pad, the sheets were blown everywhere. Somewhere along the interstate, a bunch of motorcycles came from behind and pulled up along the left side of the car. The windows were rolled down. The riders looked at Gwyn, grinned, and shouted at her, but the noise of the wind prevented Brent from hearing what the riders were shouting. Those heavyset guys wore blue and red bandanas on their heads, no helmets. Most of the riders had beards and moustaches. They wore sleeveless blue denim jackets with pictures of pirates on their backs, enclosed by the words HELLS ANGELS. Gwyn didn't wave at them or smile. She kept looking straight at the road ahead of them. Finally, after nearly ten miles, the motorcycles, about twenty of them, passed ahead with a loud roar. Some of the riders waved as they rode ahead; one blew a kiss at Gwyn.

Crossing the northern border of California, over Siskiyou Pass to Ashland in Oregon, brought hope that the Perrys might arrive in Portland soon. They were getting closer to home. The air was sparkling clear, no more smog, giving the sensation that it was safe to take a deep breath again. When the family finally arrived at the house of Gwyn's friends in Portland, they were completely exhausted, dirty, hungry, and had no place to stay. They couldn't move into a home; they didn't have a home. Their friends could see that they were exhausted. When they offered an overnight in their comfortable house, their spirits were elevated, as if a heavy burden had been lifted from them.

At last, after a warm shower and brushing his teeth, Brent was pleased to crawl into a bed with clean sheets, a soft pillow under his head. He went to bed happy.

The next morning, after a good night's sleep, Lee wanted to change into fresh clothes that were stuffed into one of the boxes in the truck. He opened the front door of his friend's house to see that the new day had begun with a beautiful morning. He started to descend the stone steps that led to the driveway and to the street where the truck had been parked at the curbside the night before. He had to blink his eyes. Then he blinked them again. He couldn't believe it. The truck was gone, nowhere to be seen. Lee frantically raced around the neighborhood, looking in every direction. The big orange and white U-Haul truck was not in sight. Desperately, Lee rushed back up the steps, into the house, into the bedroom and woke up his wife. He painfully informed her that the truck was missing.

"Oh, my God!" Gwyn shrieked. "Didn't you lock the doors of the truck last night after you parked it on the street?" She was trembling and crying.

Brent's father somberly confessed, while gazing downward at the floor, that he didn't recall locking the truck before he went into the house to go to bed. He was tired last night. Gwyn rose from the bed and frantically threw her friend's dark blue terry cloth housecoat over her shoulders. She rushed to the telephone and called the police. Within a few moments, a police car arrived, and two tall policemen walked up the steps and into the house. They were uniformed and wearing thick black leather belts. From his belt, one policeman wore a holster over his right hip, where the shiny butt of a big pistol was visible. The other police officer, who was taller and left-handed, wore his holster over his left hip. The left-handed policeman began writing on a pad of paper as Lee and Gwyn told them what happened. The right-handed policeman asked questions. They wrote down the description of the truck and its contents on their pads. After gathering information, they opened the front door of the house, descended the steps, and returned to their black-and-white Ford Crown Victoria police car, with PORTLAND POLICE painted on the doors. They filed a police report on their radio, listing the stolen U-Haul truck and the contents. The policemen walked back up the steps to the house and softly told Gwyn that they would return as soon as they discovered any information about the truck. Slowly they drove away from the front of the house, down the gently sloping neighborhood street, while surveying the neighborhood.

"Those were nice guys," Brent said. "I've never been up close to a policeman before. They have big guns."

"It's a good thing we have policemen," Gwyn replied. "I'm glad they were here to help us."

A short time later, the same two policemen drove back up the street, parked their police car in front, and returned to the house. "Lady," the right-handed policeman softly said to Brent's mother, "we found the missing truck."

"Oh, thank God!" Gwyn exclaimed with a big smile. "Thank you. Thank you so much."

"But, ma'am," the policeman continued, while his left-handed partner stood in the doorway, "the truck is empty. The truck was abandoned. Empty ... all the contents removed."

The Perrys were dazed and shocked by what the policemen told them. Suddenly, they realized that they had no place to live. No employment. No possessions. Everything they had owned was gone, even the family photographs and the baby books. Nothing was left. Not one item. That was a very bleak day. How could life change so quickly? The day before, they were gloriously happy upon their return to Oregon. This day was such a contrast, one they had not anticipated.

Through the kindness and benevolence of friends and relatives, after a few days of grieving and struggling, the Perrys found a home in Oswego, a pretty suburb on the south side of Portland, near the Willamette River. Brent liked the modern wooden house set beneath towering cedars with tall, straight trunks as thick as the width of their dining room table. There were other trees, alders, dogwood, Douglas firs, and vine maple. A little creek gently tumbled down a shallow ravine below the back of the house. Dark green sword-leaf ferns grew along the bank, their erect fronds appearing to wave a welcome to Brent. At the far end of the living room, a cheerful fireplace further enlightened the homey, welcome feeling. And Lee located a job. Temporarily. They started over. Brent's parents welcomed dishes, furniture, and clothing from their friends and family. They purchased new clothes. Brent selected a cool pair of tan short pants and a long-tailed white shirt, which he wore without tucking in.

Part II

The Appearance of a New Disease

Something Is Wrong with the Concentrate

Myrna's Call

The Perrys settled into their new home. Brent and his sisters enrolled in school. Brent was nine years old in September 1984 when he began attending the third grade at White Pine Elementary School in Oswego. He liked the new school. However, he had recurrent bleeds, time after time, a reminder of hemophilia. The school and his house had changed, but Brent had not—hemophilia was not in abeyance. The location of his bleeds on his body were not random. Most bleeds were in his target joints, his ankles. Although he was only nine, he could give himself a shot. Gwyn and Lee had patiently worked with him, teaching him how to mix the medicine, pull it from the bottle with a twenty cc syringe, and infuse it into his vein. Brent's parents helped him when he gave himself a shot.

On Tuesday, September 25, 1984, Gwyn received a telephone call from Myrna Campbell, the nurse from the treatment center. Gwyn had telephoned Myrna to let her know they were back in town. Myrna solemnly informed Brent's mother that the lot of concentrate that Brent had been using for infusions had been recalled by the drug company that had made it. The word "recall" was soon to be dreaded by Brent, his family, and everyone else who had hemophilia. A man who had hemophilia and had been infused with the medicine from the same lot that Brent used had become ill. The man with hemophilia had become affected with the new mysterious disease that no one knew much about, the disease that had been discovered in homosexual men who went to the bathhouses of New York and San Francisco. The pharmaceutical manufacturer of the medicine recalled the entire lot, demanding that all the unused concentrate be returned to the manufacturer.[36]

Alaska Outreach

In 1986, the Oregon Hemophilia Treatment Center personnel organized and conducted a hemophilia clinic in Alaska. An effort was made to identify all Alaskans who had hemophilia. They met with twenty Alaskans who had hemophilia, examining them and reviewing their medical histories.

> Designation as a federally funded Region X Hemophilia Center included a responsibility to identify persons who had hemophilia and produce an individual written plan for each person, describing his medical condition and the care he was receiving in his community of residence within Region X. Region X included Alaska, Idaho, Oregon, and Washington.

The state's resident population was known to include more than three hundred thousand white persons and sixty thousand Alaska natives, which included Aleuts, Indians, and Eskimos. Half of the natives were males, totaling thirty thousand persons. Considering the expected frequency of hemophilia, one of ten thousand male persons, there could be three

---

36 Whenever a virus was suspected in concentrate, or a person became ill who was infusing concentrate, the pharmaceutical manufacturer attempted to recall the entire lot of hundreds or thousands of unused bottles of concentrate.

Alaska native persons who had hemophilia.[37] Prior to this date, there were no reports of Eskimos who were affected with hemophilia, although the medical diagnosis had been identified in American Indians.

Dr. Hunter Ramsley, the director of Alaska's Maternal and Child Health Services, had contacted all the physicians in the entire state, announcing the arrival of the group from Oregon, who would be visiting different towns. Dr. Ramsley informed the Alaska medical doctors that the Oregon outreach team wanted to meet anyone who had hemophilia and provide an evaluation without any financial cost. Alaska is a large state with few towns and not many roads. That meant traveling to remote areas would be difficult and time consuming. Dr. Aaron Kingston, a hematologist whose office was located in Anchorage, alerted his patients that he was aware that hemophilia specialists from Oregon wanted to see them.

For individuals with hemophilia, arrangements were made for scheduling evaluations in their doctor's offices, in a hotel, or sometimes in the homes of the patients. One man who had hemophilia was evaluated in a tavern where he was employed as the floor sweeper. Two men were examined after their fishing vessel tied up at the wharf at Homer. Another man with hemophilia was examined on Kodiak Island after the bush airplane he was piloting landed at the Kodiak Airport. On their journey to Fairbanks, the doctor and nurse passed the Malamute Saloon in Ester, seven miles south of Fairbanks, where, seventy-seven years earlier, Robert Service had composed several poems in the Cripple Creek Gold Camp, later named the Ester Gold Camp, including "The Cremation of Sam McGee" in 1907.

Two teenage boys who had hemophilia were located and evaluated in their homes in Fairbanks. During subsequent hemophilia expeditions to Alaska, two Eskimo children, brothers, in the remote village of Chevak, near the Bering Sea, were discovered who had hemophilia (Plate 8).

---

37 Hemophilia is reported with the same frequency in all races and populations. The frequency varies with age groups and levels of medical care, but the incidence, which is the rate at birth, does not vary.

First Sign of a New Disease: Stories about the Arrival of AIDS

Dark Hours: Recalls of Concentrate

During 1984 and 1985, recalls of concentrate were frequent. Nearly all the manufactured lots of concentrates that had been purchased from suppliers were recalled. Whenever signs of the new disease appeared in a child or man who had been infused with concentrate to treat his hemophilia, the entire lot of the concentrate he was using was recalled by the manufacturer. Everyone who received concentrate from that lot was contacted and advised to return the un-infused concentrate to the clinic. But the recalls were too late to avoid harm by preventing infusion of a suspected but unidentified infectious substance. The concentrate had already been infused into many persons by the time of the recalls. Logistically, maintaining a supply of concentrate throughout the region, for more than a hundred persons infusing at home, checking all the lot numbers, returning the unused concentrate and exchanging it for different lot numbers, which hopefully were safer, was a giant mess, almost an impossibility. The number of bottles of concentrate recalled and exchanged wasn't tabulated, but it was estimated to total ten to twenty thousand bottles. Not that many bottles of concentrates were returned; many had already been infused by the date of the recalls.[38]

The hemophilia treatment center personnel were demoralized in 1985. Gwyn felt horrible. She was devastated; worried that Brent would become ill and develop signs of the new disease. Brent's father was

---

38   Estimate from the Oregon Hemophilia Treatment Center

in bad shape psychologically. What could the Perrys do? Brent had bleeds, but he wasn't ill. Would he become ill? Was there a way to tell if he would become ill? Should he discontinue infusing concentrate to prevent a mysterious sickness that was creeping into persons like him who had been infused with the medicine?

The hemophilia community was terribly confused. The families that included a boy or man who had hemophilia formed a community (Resnik 1999). Not all the families actively submitted themselves into the community. Some persons with hemophilia maintained a low profile. Most of the families were anxious to discover resources for their concerns. National, international, and state organizations— including the World Federation of Hemophilia (WFH), the National Hemophilia Foundation (NHF), and in Portland, Oregon, the Hemophilia Foundation of Oregon (HFO)—promoted the welfare of their members.

The families and organizations from the hemophilia community comprised a strong, effective, active group for several reasons. Hemophilia is a lifelong disorder affecting infants, children, and adults. It is not a disorder that affects mainly elderly people, such as the dementia of Alzheimer's. By completing research in hemophilia, the understanding of other genetic disorders has been greatly enhanced. Knowledge gained from hemophilia research stimulates concepts applicable to other medical conditions. Hemophilia affects every type, class, and race of people; it is not limited to any one group or geographical distribution, although the two sexes, male and female, are not equally affected. Hemophilia is almost exclusively limited to males. The most adhesive force that binds the families and organizations together is the treatment, the concentrate. Hemophilia will never disappear, but its effects can be minimized with treatment, which is not common for many genetic disorders.

The hemophilia community was greatly concerned that the blood supply for the manufacture of concentrates had been contaminated with an unidentified infectious agent. This previously unknown and unwelcome infectious substance produced a new disease that was followed by death in those recipients of concentrate made from the blood collected from infected donors.

The families were faced with a difficult choice: was it worse to withhold infusions and suffer from bleeds … or choose to infuse and risk becoming ill with the mysterious disease? Beginning in 1985, the concentrate dispensed to persons affected with hemophilia was heat-treated, which destroyed the infectious substance, identified as HIV, and hepatitis viruses, removing the risk of viral pollution. In the process of producing concentrate from donor plasma, application of heat destroyed contaminating viruses. However, the Perrys and the other hemophilia families wondered if it was too late by the time the purification steps were invoked. They wondered if they had already been poisoned.

In 1986, when Brent was eleven years old, he became a sixth grader at Mead Middle School in Oswego. He attended school there during sixth, seventh, and eighth grades. Recurrent bleeds were treated with a shot, for an infusion of concentrate, without missing classes. Brent was pretty good at giving himself an infusion, but he continued to prefer that his father give him his shot. Most of his infusions were for ankle bleeds. Brent was well and unaware that he had already been infected with the virus that became known as HIV. He had neither signs nor symptoms of HIV infection.

Jason's Story

On Wednesday, February 19, 1986—a snowy, dark, cold winter night—Nurse Sue Underwood and Dr. Taillefer drove the car they had rented in Alaska to the home of Jason Cobb, a ten-year-old boy, an only child, who lived with his parents in their modern log home in the countryside near Eagle River, north of Anchorage. As the car slowly made its way up the driveway to the house, the occupants inside were alerted to the car's arrival by the crunchy sound of the tires on the packed snow. After being welcomed to the warm interior of the house, the doctor and nurse visited for a half hour with Jason's parents, mainly his father, to assess the child's setting and his parents' resources. After Jason became acquainted with the doctor and nurse, whom he had not previously met, and he was comfortable, he was given a checkup. The examination took place in the living room before a heater while attempting to respect Jason's modesty. The doctor inspected Jason's head and neck, and he looked into his ears and mouth with a light. He inspected the boy's gums and teeth. Dr. Taillefer noted the muscle strength and development of Jason's arms and legs. The elbows, wrists, hips, knees, and ankles were checked for range of joint motion. Straightness of his spine was noted. The abdomen was palpated, checking for an enlarged liver or spleen, and the doctor listened to his heart and breathing with his stethoscope (plate 3).

"What are those feathery creatures flying around in your house?" Dr. Taillefer asked Jason during the examination.

"Oh, Doctor, those are my birds, my pet birds," Jason eagerly replied. "See how they'll perch on my shoulder." A medium-sized blue and black feathered fowl with a yellow curved beak perched on his shoulder, one of several birds that had been flying about the house. "They have to get to know you before they will alight on you."

"Jason, you are amazing," Dr. Taillefer said. "You're really good with those pretty birds." Dr. Taillefer was thinking to himself that he didn't really want to get to know the birds; he didn't want them sitting on his shoulder.

Jason was born December 23, 1975, in New Jersey. In 1983, his father, Wayne Cobb, an entrepreneur salesperson, a handsome middle-aged man, was transferred to Alaska by the company that had employed him on the East Coast of the United States. He was to manage a new office supply store that was opening for the first time in Anchorage. Jason had been infused with concentrate many times to treat his hemophilia in Newark, New Jersey, before moving with his parents to Alaska. His father had been trained in home infusions, which facilitated the family's move to a rather remote area. Without his father's competence providing infusions for his son and a supply of concentrate, hemophilia would have prevented Jason from living in the countryside near Eagle River.

"The Oregon Hemophilia Treatment Center will ship concentrate to your home for Jason's necessary infusions. We have met with Dr. Ramsley, the state director of Children's Services for Alaska, and we have contacted Jason's doctor in Anchorage for approval. You already know how to infuse your son," Dr. Taillefer remarked, complimenting Jason's father. Jason's mother was quiet; she was pleasant but said very little and asked no questions.

"What did you discover when you checked Jason? What are your findings that we should know?" the boy's father asked the doctor.

"He is a nice boy," the doctor said. "His joints are in pretty good shape. However, he has limited extension of his right elbow and some atrophy of the quadriceps muscle in his left leg. Jason is below the average height of most ten-year-old boys. However, when he is twelve years-of-age, I predict that he will begin to shoot up, gain stature. As an adult, he will probably be of average height. There are two findings of concern. He says he has a sore mouth, and his gums are reddened. Brushing his teeth is painful. We will send you a pint bottle containing 0.12 percent chlorhexidine gluconate, a solution for rinsing his mouth. Jason should take a mouthful each morning and evening, swish the fluid around in his mouth for a full minute, and then spit it out. The mouthwash will help reduce inflammation of his gums, gingivitis, and help make his pain go away. But he should also be seen tomorrow by a dentist in Anchorage. Dentists are much better at solving mouth problems than medical doctors are. I am not good at diagnosing disorders of the gums or inside the mouth. He has changes I have never seen before in the lining of his mouth. Let's find out if the dentist recognizes what they are."

Dr. Taillefer continued talking to the parents, especially to the father, Wayne. "Your son also has a rash. He has places on his skin that look like eczema or even a bit like psoriasis. I don't know what caused the rash, but I wonder if it could be from all the birds flying around in your house. Maybe it's psittacosis."[39]

The next morning, Dr. Taillefer and the nurse accompanied Jason and his parents to the dentist's office in Anchorage. The dentist, after examining Jason's mouth, confessed that he did not know what caused the inflammation and sores on the inside of Jason's mouth. He obtained a small piece of the lining of Jason's mouth, the mucosa, from a biopsy, which was sent to the pathology laboratory for examination.

Dr. Taillefer was seeing the first case of AIDS he had ever seen, except he didn't recognize it. This would not be the last time he would be confronted with an AIDS victim. Since then, when he has seen other persons who developed AIDS, he has noticed similar skin problems, resembling psoriasis and eczema. And in the months and years ahead, he would see persons with excruciatingly painful mouths in hemophilia, in individuals who had been infused with concentrates and developed AIDS.[40] He also did not realize that this attractive, innocent ten-year-old boy would not live many more years.

Jason died January 6, 1987, at eleven years of age. An autopsy examination revealed that Jason's body, including his brain, was riddled with *Mycobacterium intracellulaire*, a pathogen often found in persons who die after HIV infection. Jason did not die from hemophilia. His death was caused by AIDS, the result of the medicine intended to prevent his death from hemophilia. The hemophilia treatment center was alarmed and confused after learning of Jason's death. They wondered what was confronting them. What were they supposed to know and do? Where could they turn for information and help? Was Jason's death a one-time

---

39 Psittacosis is an acute infectious viral disease affecting birds of the parrot family and is transmissible to humans.

40 Dry mouth develops in some AIDS patients when the salivary glands fail to make saliva. This painful condition may be partially relieved with artificial saliva.

tragedy, or would the clinic face more tragedies in the future? The clinic staff pleaded with one another, asking where they could get help.

A Second Case of AIDS: John's Story

Another young person who had hemophilia, who had been infused with concentrates, became gravely ill in 1986. John McAnulty, age sixteen, developed intractable diarrhea that did not respond to attempts at treatment utilizing customary medicines and measures. John's home was in a lovely white house in the forested West Hills of Portland, where he lived with his father, a Portland physician, his mother, and his younger brother. John was tall. He had a pleasant personality and a lively sense of humor. Over several months, he became emaciated. The emaciation seen in AIDS patients was later referred to as "slim disease."[41] He had been admitted to the University Hospital, where his medical care was managed by infectious disease specialists. However, doctors were not familiar with AIDS. The combination of antiviral medications, effective in subsequent years to prevent the progression of AIDS, had not been discovered. Finally, sadly, this youth tired of being in the hospital. He was exhausted, struggling to cling to life. He knew the end of his short life was near. He wanted to die, if he was meant to, at home, not in the hospital.

John died April 9, 1987, three months after Jason died, both of AIDS. Memorial services for John were the first that Dr. Taillefer attended for AIDS victims. In the months and years ahead, funerals were held for many more persons who had hemophilia and were overwhelmed by AIDS. John's mother was devastated. She was thankful she had a remaining son who was well, who had not endured the suffering that had plagued his brother. She felt some guilt in her son's difficult life. He would not have died of AIDS if he had not been infected from the concentrates used to treat hemophilia, which he'd inherited from

---

41 Slim disease was recognized in Uganda in the 1980s, characterized by diarrhea and weight loss associated with HTLV-III infection, subsequently called HIV infection (Serwadda, D. et al. 1985).

her. Although John's mother had previously been shy, at the memorial services for her deceased son, she appeared to be stronger than many of the other mourners who were grieving for the loss of John. John's parents were consoled by their son's responsible acceptance of his suffering. He was not tormented when confronted with death. They believed he discovered that the meaning of life is a personal inner thing that varies from person to person. At the age of sixteen, despite his awareness of a hopeless outcome, he displayed remarkable courage,

At the memorial services for John, Dr. Taillefer related to Susan McAnulty that he was sorry for her son's death. He said he was devastated knowing that he'd given her son medicine that had caused his death. Doctors who treated John, he said, meant well—they intended no harm—but they were wrong. The doctors intended to give John medicine to make his life better. Instead, their treatment took her son's life away. He painfully asked John's mother to forgive him and the other doctors.[42] Perhaps John's mother has felt a burden all during her son's life for giving him hemophilia. Her burden may be diluted with the guilt of the doctor who gave her son medicine that resulted in his death, as if guilt, if there is any, could be shared between the mother and the doctor.

Consideration of a mysterious disease contracted from concentrates manufactured from blood plasma was no longer a remote concept, the doctors and nurses at the treatment center fearfully realized amidst their bewilderment. The disease had arrived in their midst, confronting them. *What should we do? First Jason in Alaska and now John in Portland, their innocent young lives taken away prematurely, not from a medical disorder but from the treatment prescribed by the doctor who gave them contaminated medicine. Doctors are supposed to save lives, not to make people ill, not to take away lives.* These were the thoughts of the doctors and nurses in the clinic.

After experience with Jason and John, Dr. Taillefer and the other doctors and nurses in the treatment center recognized that their

---

42 From Dr. Taillefer's notes of April 1987

knowledge of the signs and symptoms of AIDS from HIV infection had been deficient. AIDS was a new disease. Their awareness of the signals of this new disease was a learning experience.

Early signs and symptoms of AIDS from HIV infection in children

- Failure to grow and gain weight
- Poor appetite
- Skin rashes resembling eczema
- Thrush and inflamed gums
- Weakness, loss of energy

Later signs of AIDS

- Diarrhea
- Slim disease
- Fatigue
- Depression
- Memory loss
- Dry mouth
- Pneumonia
- Depression

Bicycle with a Short Crank Arm: Roger's Story

Brent's mother dropped him off in front of the hemophilia treatment center and then pulled off to search for a parking spot. Parking a car was always a problem at the center. A special area was reserved for patients, but sometimes no parking places were vacant. Brent noticed a young guy shove his bicycle with fat, knobby tires into the bike rack in front of the center.

"That's a cool bike you've got there," Brent said. But the young man didn't answer. He began to walk away.

"Hey! Aren't you going to lock it up?"

The man looked back at Brent and said "Nah. I never lock it. Who would steal a junker bike like this one? Nobody, that's who."

Brent held out his hand and said, "I'm Brent."

The guy grinned and shook Brent's hand. "I'm Roger. Are you here for treatment too?"

"Yeah, for a checkup," Brent replied.

Gwyn heard the tail end of the conversation as she walked up after parking her car. "Hello. Would you like to walk with us into the clinic?" she asked Roger.

"Sure," Roger said to Gwyn as the three walked into the low brick and glass building, a modern building whose appearance some persons suggested resembled a mausoleum (plate 1). The hemophilia treatment center suite was located on the second level of the clinic building, accessible by an elevator. After leaving the elevator and turning right through a doorway, a small waiting area defined the location where Brent, his mother, and Roger met the nurse when they needed to pick up concentrate and infusion supplies.

The clinic was the supply depot for hemophilia concentrates. Down the hallway, through the swinging doors, the concentrates were stored in the cold room, a walk-in refrigerated room with a heavy, thick door that made a solid thud sound when it was slammed shut. The door had a safety latch, allowing a person to open the door from within if he or she was accidentally locked inside. Shelves within the cold room held boxes of concentrate sorted by brand and by the amount of AHF units. On one shelf were cartons of Cutter's Koate HP, and after 1985, Koate HT,[43] each containing twenty-four yellow boxes of glass vials of 250–400 AHF units. On a higher shelf, cartons contained boxes of 500 unit vials of concentrate, while the top shelves held cartons containing boxes of 1000 AHF unit vials. Across the center aisle within the cold room, an additional set of shelves, above

---

43   Koate HP, high-purity Koate, was replaced with Koate HT, heat-treated Koate, in 1985. Koate was produced by Cutter.

the black slate countertop, held cartons of Armour's Factor 8. The brown cardboard cartons contained blue boxes of glass vials of AHF in 250, 500, and 1000 unit sizes. The 250 unit sizes were for infants who needed an infusion. The 500 and 1000 unit sizes were for children and adults. Bigger kids needed more medicine according to their weight. Several other brands of concentrates were similarly placed in a designated area within the cold room. Koate was for infusions of type A hemophilia for persons deficient in factor VIII, the most common form of hemophilia. Konyne concentrate was for infusions into type B hemophilia persons, who are deficient in factor IX. In addition to AHF concentrates produced by Cutter and Armour, other pharmaceutical manufacturers of concentrates included Hyland, the American Red Cross, Parke-Davis, and Alpha Therapeutics.

Logistically, stocking all the brands in every size of concentrate produced by the pharmaceutical manufacturers was overwhelming. Nurses and doctors are trained and enjoy their medical specialties; they did not intend to become warehousemen. To be practical, inventory of only three brands of concentrate produced by Cutter, Armour, and the American Red Cross were maintained, rather than all the manufactured labels. Each of the manufacturers provided concentrates in different amounts of AHF units and with different expiration dates. Whenever concentrates were dispensed, a record must be entered, including the lot number and the expiration date. The inventories of concentrates in the cold room required monitoring. Concentrate dispensed and new supplies received were tabulated to assure a reliable supply without an overstock or a depletion.

The cold room was a repository for concentrates for the region. Maintaining a supply of concentrates was not necessary for community pharmacies. Having multiple depots of concentrates was not efficient or practical. By agreement, after discussion with the Red Cross and the Medical Advisory Board, the treatment center was selected to be the repository for concentrates to supply the community. Whenever a person with hemophilia was to undergo surgery, the hospital was supplied with concentrate dispensed from the hemophilia treatment center cold room. Large amounts of concentrates were necessary during the postoperative recovery period, such as following a knee replacement. All hemophilia persons within the region depended on the source of concentrates located at the hemophilia treatment center to treat their bleeding episodes. No one who needed concentrate was denied, regardless of ability to pay for the medicine dispensed.

In addition to the medicine, other supplies were provided, including alcohol wipes, Band-Aids, cotton balls, disposable syringes, butterflies for the infusion, and small bottles of sterile saline. Maintaining inventories of medicine and the necessary supplies for the infusions was a significant demand, requiring many hours of the treatment room nurses who maintained the concentrate distribution center.

Roger, twenty-six years of age, and Brent, age ten years, arrived at the clinic at the same time that day to pick up supplies of concentrate (plate 4). Brent's supplies were brought home in his mother's car. Roger's concentrates and all the other infusion supplies were carried home in the wire baskets that straddled the rear wheel of his old bicycle. Roger's mother had died of cancer when he was sixteen. Brent had a family: a mother and father and two sisters. Roger lived alone, a reminder that hemophilia spares no one. One of every ten thousand newborn males has hemophilia in all countries in the world, in all societies. No races are exempt from this disorder of bleeding, which has been recorded in history for many centuries. Brent and Roger were not the first instances of hemophilia in their family, and they wouldn't be the last. Others before and after them were affected with hemophilia.

Roger's mother, Elsie, had been a tavern operator (figure 2). Roger was raised in the tavern. He didn't know his father. His two older brothers, Jim and John Berry, had a different father. Both—like their mother's brother, Joe Krostag, who lived in Boise, Idaho—had hemophilia. Roger's mother's sister, Arvella Palmer, who lived in Tillamook, had a son, Wayne Palmer, Roger's cousin, who also had hemophilia.

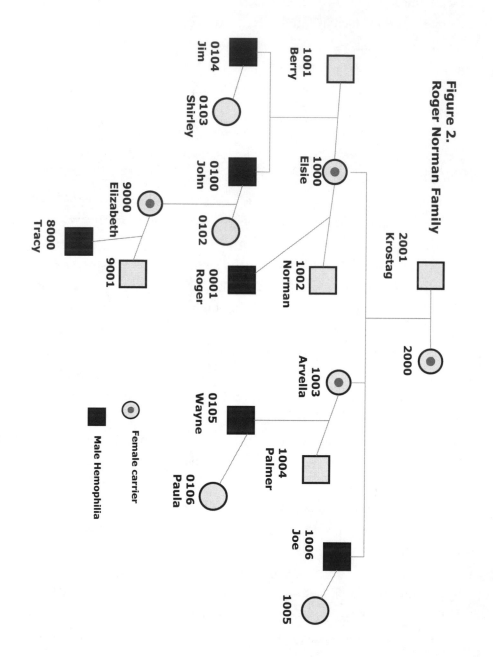

Figure 2.
Roger Norman Family

Roger and his brothers were born in their family's rural country home on the Pacific Coast, near Tillamook, Oregon. Roger was born September 3, 1959. He was not circumcised after birth because previous males in the family had been born with hemophilia.

Circumcision was not widely utilized before World War II. After the war, medical insurance became common, as it was tied to employment. Rather than pay higher wages, employers offered medical insurance to attract employees. The cost of the insurance was deductible from the employers' taxes. Medical insurance paid for circumcision, which became a bread-and-butter item for obstetricians. After the obstetrician attended the mother during childbirth, he returned to her bedside for a checkup. On the second day after birth, he routinely circumcised newborn males for the handsome fee paid by insurance, an easy way to make forty bucks. Although a baby's care is assigned to a pediatrician after discharge from the hospital, a ritual was established, dictating that obstetricians, rather than pediatricians, perform circumcisions.

Prior to widespread medical insurance in the United States, few males were circumcised. Others maintain that the rise of circumcision after World War II resulted from the experience of soldiers in battlefield conditions where poor hygiene prevailed, leading to increased infections. More recently, advocates of circumcision have cited increased urinary tract infections in uncircumcised males. That was not the case in the hemophilia clinic. Most males who are born into families with hemophilia are not circumcised. An increase in urinary tract infections was not observed in uncircumcised males attending the Oregon Hemophilia Treatment Center. The American Academy of Pediatrics has not issued a clear recommendation for or against circumcision.

Roger had bruises as an infant, but no infusion therapy to treat bleeds was available in the early 1960s. Blood transfusions and plasma were available but not helpful for treating hemophilia type A, the result of a deficiency of factor VIII. Plasma did help in hemophilia type B, the result of a deficiency of factor IX. Roger and his brothers had to wait it out whenever they had a bleed. Ice was used to relieve pain, and splints were applied to keep the joint motionless when there was a bleed into a knee joint. They had no analgesics, not even aspirin, which increases bleeding. When they were old enough to walk, these youngsters used crutches and rested an arm or a leg whenever they had a bleed. Roger and his brothers lay awake at night, sometimes for many successive nights, enduring agony and intense pain when they suffered from a muscle or a joint bleed. Sometimes the pressure after a bleed into an arm or leg intensified so greatly that compression shut off the circulation and the bleeding ceased, but the pain continued. Fortunately, Roger had not been subject to a fasciotomy, which was performed in some other persons after a bleed.[44]

In 1965, when Roger was a young child, only five years of age, he became unconscious, lapsing into a coma. No one knew what caused the coma. He had not been ill, and meningitis was not suspected. He was brought in an ambulance along the winding Wilson River Highway, Oregon Highway Number 6, through the coastal mountains, past Jordan Creek and Lee's Camp, from Tillamook to Emanuel Hospital in Portland. Roger had a bleed into his head, an intracranial hemorrhage. Shortly before that time, in 1964, cryoprecipitate became available for treating bleeds in hemophilia.

Roger underwent neurosurgery after he was infused with cryoprecipitate to restore his blood-clotting activity during surgery. The skull of the child was opened after the infusion. A bleed into the brain tissue was discovered. The neurosurgeon aspirated the blood clot that had formed after Roger was infused with cryo. Unfortunately, removal of some of the softened brain tissue by aspiration was necessary in order to remove the blood clot from the damaged brain. Roger survived, one of the first persons with hemophilia in the United States to have brain surgery and survive, while receiving cryoprecipitate. He was infused

---

44 A fasciotomy is made by surgically slitting the fascia of an arm or leg to release pressure, resulting in an appearance similar to a burst hot dog that has been overcooked.

daily with cryo through the postoperative period in the hospital, which promoted his blood to clot normally during the time his brain and skull healed. Following his discharge from the hospital, he returned to his home in Tillamook to convalesce with his mother and brothers. However, less than a year later, in 1966, when he was six years of age, a second head bleed occurred. He was again hospitalized and underwent a second craniotomy while receiving cryoprecipitate for removal of an intracranial blood clot. He was infused with cryo and recovered while hospitalized. He was discharged and returned home. When he developed a third and then a fourth intracranial hemorrhage, he did not receive surgery. Instead, he was hospitalized, infused with cryo, and administered intravenous medication to reduce swelling of his brain.

During the first five years of his life, Roger received only supportive treatment for his recurrent hemorrhages, no medicine to stop bleeding. From age five to fourteen, 1965–1973, he was infused with cryoprecipitate during surgery or for life-threatening bleeds. While in second grade, he moved from Tillamook into the city, Portland's West Hills, with his mother. At the treatment center, Roger was the first person with hemophilia to be instructed in procedures for infusing himself and keeping concentrate, Humafac, at home for infusions. In 1973, when he was fourteen, despite brain damage from intracranial bleeds during his childhood, he learned the methods of home infusion. The residual from damage to Roger's brain included a learning disorder, epileptic seizures, and visual impairment with tunnel vision. He had no peripheral vision, he could only see straight forward. Roger did not complete school. He was classified as being disabled. However, Roger would not accept an image of himself as being disabled.

When Roger's mother, Elsie, died from cancer, Roger became a homeowner at the age of sixteen. He lived by himself in southwest Portland, in the single-story three-bedroom house left to him by his mother. It was a rust-colored house, with shingled siding, set up on a grassy knoll with access via a steep asphalt-paved driveway.

The wood trim around the doors and windows was painted green. With the reddish siding and the green trim, a Christmas effect was suggested. He maintained the small house, including cutting the large lawn, cleaning the leaves from gutters, removing the moss from the roof. He completed all the indoor chores necessary to maintain a tidy home, such as vacuuming the rugs, cleaning the windows, and washing the dishes. He cooked for himself, although his diet was not healthy. For breakfast, Roger said, he often prepared packaged Eggo waffles in the toaster. After the waffles were toasted, Roger smeared them with butter and submerged them in maple syrup. He gleefully referred to the toasted waffles as cardboard waffles, devouring them with sausage links and toast and jam. For dinner, he boasted that he enjoyed cooking a T-bone steak in a cast iron skillet, served with fried potatoes.

Occasionally, Roger attempted to share his home with a renter to help curb loneliness and enjoy conversation at dinnertime. Such attempts were frustrating. He concluded that the persons he selected to live in his home for companionship were too depressing. After tolerating their presence for a few weeks, he asked them to move out of the house. He derived his sparse income from his mother's estate and monthly payments from SSDI.[45] Roger did not possess a driver's license to operate an automobile, for he was labeled an epileptic because of an abnormal EEG,[46] although he had no observable seizures. A neurologist prescribed phenobarbital and Dilantin as anticonvulsant medications. Roger was not reliable for monitoring recommended Dilantin blood levels, only occasionally offering to be tested.

Although he had no driver's license, he owned a car, a shiny red Ford Mustang. The sporty car sat in the garage, where he enjoyed starting the engine on Saturday mornings and revving the motor. Once, he drove the shiny car out of the garage and headed for a nearby high school. "Yee-haw!" Roger shrieked through the open

45 Social Security Disability Income
46 Electroencephalogram, a brain wave test

car window as he drove the car wildly across the schoolyard, cutting circular swaths in the school lawn with the car's tires, terrifying the students. His antics were squelched when he was arrested by the Portland police. He was not jailed; the police recognized that he had a mental problem.

Roger never drove his sporty car out of the garage again; instead, he rode his bicycle. However, one leg was shorter than the other, and his knee would not bend. Roger was designated as learning disabled, but he was not mentally retarded. Attesting to his mental creativity was the appearance of his bicycle. He hired a welder to fashion a shortened bicycle crank on the left side of his bicycle, retaining the normal crank length on the right side, which allowed him to pedal despite one short leg with an immobile knee (plate 5). Hence, Brent thought that with Roger's innovative modified crank arm, his bicycle was really cool.

Occasionally, Roger crashed on his short-crank bicycle. Someone would discover him lying on the pavement or sidewalk. He was acquainted with a middle-aged married couple who were his friends and advocates, providing assistance whenever he needed help. When needed, Jim and Esther McAlpine would respond to an emergency call. They brought him to the hemophilia treatment center, remaining beside him while he received care after an injury. They assisted him with his household tasks, such as completing forms required for medical care. They were like parents to Roger.

Roger partially satisfied his passion for cars and motors at Portland Speedway. He rode the city bus to PIR,[47] where he volunteered to serve as traffic director in the race car pits in the center of the race track. On weekends during the summer months, Roger could be found at the race track amidst the roar of the engines, the exhaust smoke in the air, greeted by drivers and mechanics that enlightened his days and buoyed his spirits by his association with a dynamic atmosphere.

---

47   Portland International Raceway

Roger's Oldest Brother: John Berry

Roger's two older brothers' lives were complicated by residual damage from the devastation to their bodies, the effect of recurrent bleeds plaguing them during their childhood and into adult life. They were born in the 1940s and became adults before concentrates were available; therefore, they had considerable residual joint damage in adulthood.

Roger's oldest brother, John, was a businessman who operated a sewing machine and vacuum repair shop in Tillamook. When not working in his shop, he enjoyed hiking, especially on the Oregon Coast, despite his restricted joint mobility. On one of his hikes along the seashore, he jumped over a driftwood log lying on the sandy beach and landed on the other side of the log, coming down onto a large rusty nail sticking upright from an old plank lying in the sand. The nail penetrated the sole of his shoe, producing a puncture wound in the ball of his right foot. During the next few days, the wound became infected. He had no feeling in his foot as a result of nerve damage from previous bleeds. He was unaware that his foot was badly damaged from the nail puncture. Destruction of his foot was so severe that when he attended the clinic at the hemophilia center, the orthopedic surgeon declared his right foot would never heal unless the infected part of the foot was amputated. With infusions of concentrate, the orthopedic surgeon completed a Syme's amputation of John's foot during hospitalization. His clotting activity was maintained during and after surgery with infusions of concentrate. Six months after the amputation, when the stump was healed, John was fitted with a prosthesis to replace his foot. But John didn't like the artificial foot; it was uncomfortable and produced ugly sores on the skin covering the stump. He preferred walking on the stump.

John married, and he and his wife had a daughter. His daughter was aware that she inherited the mutant hemophilia gene. She was a carrier of hemophilia. All daughters of men affected by hemophilia receive the hemophilia trait from their fathers; they are obligate carriers of hemophilia. She became pregnant and gave birth to a boy named Tracy in 1992 (figure 2). The hemophilia trait of his grandfather was passed through his mother to him. Tracy has hemophilia.

Roger's Other Older Brother: Jim Berry

Roger's other older brother, Jim, married, but he and his wife had no children. When concentrates became available after he was an adult, he began to infuse himself to avoid the pain he had experienced from recurrent bleeds during his youth, when bleeds were not successfully managed. Following the introduction of concentrates into his life, he became jaundiced, attributed to hepatitis from infusions. He developed swelling of the abdomen, the result of a congested liver causing ascites, a collection of abdominal fluid. The swollen liver resulted in congestion of blood vessels in his esophagus and recurrent hemorrhages from esophageal varices, which ended in his death from liver failure.

Roger's Uncle: Joe Krostag

Joe Krostag, Roger's uncle, his mother's brother, who lived in Boise, Idaho, also inherited hemophilia (figure 2). As a youngster, he had received no clotting factor replacement for treatment of hemophilia. Joe was given transfusions of whole blood during his youth that were ineffective for the treatment of the recurrent bleeding episodes of hemophilia. He developed a great amount of painful arthritis of his joints and spine during his adult life. A married middle-aged man, he walked only with painful difficulty after slowly rising from a stuffed chair where he sat endlessly. He was a cantankerous man whose wife was very patient to live with him while he had so much pain, suffering, and disability. He had a devoted doctor who prescribed cryoprecipitate for Joe when it became available. In later years, he received concentrates for infusions.

Joe did not infuse himself. He demanded infusions of cryoprecipitate from the local hospital emergency room when pain from his bleeds became unbearable. Because of his demanding and sarcastic remarks, Joe was regarded as a difficult patient by nurses and doctors in the Boise hospital emergency room. The personnel at the hospital were stressed and alarmed whenever he showed up in agony, his pain unbearable. On one occasion prior to a trip to the emergency room for an infusion, he had read that blood from other animals, when mixed with the blood from a person with hemophilia, produces the clotting that is deficient in hemophilia. After reading the article in a magazine, on the next occasion when he had a bleed, Joe carried a large live white chicken into the hospital emergency room. When the nurse stuck a needle into Joe's arm vein for an infusion of cryoprecipitate to stop his bleed, he pulled a jackknife from his pocket, clicked open the sharp blade, and slit open the chicken's leg. Blood and feathers flew everywhere from the struggling, shrieking fowl. He demanded that the nurse suck up the free-flowing chicken blood in a syringe and infuse it into his arm vein to promote clotting. The nurse refused, and Joe became enraged. He pulled the needle from his arm and tore out of the emergency room as quickly as he could, which wasn't very quick because of his crippling deformities. He left behind a mess of chicken blood, feathers, and a dead chicken. He was never welcomed again in the emergency room of the hospital.

Roger's Cousin: Wayne Palmer

In addition to her eccentric brother who had hemophilia and lived with his patient wife in Boise, Roger's mother, Elsie, had a married sister, Arvella, who lived in Tillamook, Oregon. She and her husband had one child, a son, Wayne Palmer, who also inherited the family hemophilia trait, which affected six males in the family (figure 2). Wayne was born in 1958, one year before his cousin Roger. As a small child, Wayne received no AHF clotting factor replacement, none was available. He developed joint damage from recurrent hemorrhages, especially in his elbows and ankles. When cryoprecipitate became available in the late 1960s, when he was nine or ten years of age, his parents bundled him up, laid him on the back seat of their car, and drove from Tillamook to Portland for infusions of cryo when his pain and suffering became unbearable. The winding road through the forest over the coastal mountain range was a difficult journey in the wintertime when the mountain passes were snowy. Sometimes Wayne's father had to wait until a snowplow cleared the roadway and sanded the surface, closely following the snowplow over the summit of the mountains on the drive to Portland.

The first occasion Dr. Taillefer examined Wayne Palmer in the hemophilia clinic was in 1968, when he was almost ten years of age. At that time, the entire left side of his face was gigantically swollen and discolored black and blue. The boy had been to the dentist, who'd performed a mandibular block to anesthetize his lower jaw.[48] For two days and nights after the dental work, the young boy had bled into his jaw and left side of his face. To stop the alarming swelling and discoloration from the bleeding, cryoprecipitate was infused into his arm vein. Slowly, after the infusion, over the next few days, the extravasation of blood into his face resolved, followed by a change of skin color from deep purple, almost black, to light purple, then brownish green and yellow, finally fading after several weeks. Wayne learned to infuse himself in 1976, after concentrates became available, when he was eighteen years of age.

Brent and Wayne met when they were seated beside one another in the patient waiting room at the hemophilia treatment center.

"What on earth are you doing that for?" Brent asked Wayne.

"This helps my ankles," Wayne answered. He was wearing brown leather boots that nearly reached his knees. He had removed one of the boots and was stuffing the empty boot with handfuls of toilet paper. Wayne had an unusual build and posture. He had a very noticeable scoliosis.[49] He was tall, over six feet, and extremely thin. His joints

---

48 The mandibular nerve in the lower jaw is injected with Novocain for local anesthesia to complete a dental filling.

49 Excessive curvature of the spine, resulting in a crooked back

were dislocatable. His chest was accentuated in the middle with a keel-shaped sternum. Dr. Taillefer determined that Wayne, in addition to hemophilia, also had a disorder of his connective tissue, laxness of the tendons and ligaments that held his joints together. Although he had joint damage from recurrent bleeds from hemophilia, he easily hyperflexed his fingers and could bend his wrists backward to a position where the backs of his hands nearly touched his forearms, a trait not explainable by hemophilia.

"I have always been double-jointed," Wayne told Brent. "The doctor said I am too stretchy. He said that just because I have one condition, hemophilia, that doesn't protect me from having another medical problem. The doctor ordered insoles for my shoes, but I discovered that toilet paper is more comfortable for my ankles. My fallen arches make my feet hurt and my ankles suffer. I get ankle bleeds real often," he confided while extending his leg and holding up his thin, long, strange-looking foot with a collapsed arch for Brent to see.

Wayne was a romantic person who liked poetry, writing, and music. He married a tall attractive woman, Paula, in 1983, when he was twenty-five years of age. They had no children. After their marriage, blood tests revealed that Wayne was infected with HIV.

Roger's great-nephew, Tracy (figure 2, Individual 8000), born in 1992, also has hemophilia. He was six feet tall at sixteen years of age. He has no deformities. He was born after the advent of purified concentrate. Tracy was infused with concentrate, beginning in early infancy. Early introduction of infusions prevented the complications and deformities present in his grandfather and great uncles who did not receive infusions of concentrate in childhood. Tracy's infusions were with recombinant AHF (rFVIII), rather than concentrate derived from blood. He did not become infected with HIV or hepatitis virus. Since 1985, when heat-treated concentrate (and more recently rFVIII) became available in the United States, persons with hemophilia no longer become infected with HIV or hepatitis virus from infusions of concentrate.

Five Deaths in One Family

Other than Tracy, the five males who had hemophilia in Roger's family have died. All of them became infected with hepatitis and HIV from infusions of contaminated concentrate. Roger survived HIV infection but died at age forty-four from cancer of the liver. His brother Jim also survived HIV and died from liver failure caused by hepatitis. Roger's oldest brother, John, who developed AIDS, ended his own life. Wayne, his cousin, died of AIDS in a hospice care center in 1989. His wife, Paula, did not become infected with HIV.

Wayne composed his own epitaph, which was read at his memorial services in a Tillamook church after he died. It was written five years preceding his death:

We Remember
Seeking my own mentality,
Making sure it's really me,
But I'm not alone anymore.
One very close has come to live in me.
Who is the friend that is my honored guest?
Is He the same as all the rest?
No.
He is my God.

Written by Wayne Palmer
August 8, 1984
Inspired by God

Roger survived AIDS and lived until 2003, fourteen years longer than his cousin, Wayne Palmer, whose HIV infection resulted in his death from AIDS in 1989. Although Roger was also HIV infected from infusions of concentrate contaminated with HIV, he did not die directly from AIDS. Two lethal medical disorders, AIDS and hemophilia, affected Roger. However, he did not succumb to either. Instead, Roger died from a different cause, but it was similar in origin to the other two—given to him by the doctors who were treating the other conditions. Roger died at forty-four years of age from cancer of the liver, the effect of viral contaminant of the concentrate, with hepatitis C virus. When Roger began receiving concentrate to treat bleeds of hemophilia, hepatitis A and hepatitis B were recognized risk factors. At that time, the doctors also discussed non-A, non-B hepatitis, which subsequently was identified as hepatitis C. The hepatitis virus, which Roger received during the infusions of concentrate, resulted in the formation of a hepatoma, a tumor of the liver. The doctors prescribed infusions of concentrate for Roger for years, aware he was receiving hepatitis B and C, proclaiming that the risk to his health from the hepatitis virus was far less than the risk of dying from hemophilia. The doctors were wrong. The passage of time has revealed that those persons infused with HIV contaminated concentrate who survived AIDS have a great risk of dying from cancer of the liver, which develops after infection with hepatitis virus B and C. Over the years, the hepatitis virus remains dormant in the liver, without disappearing. Eventually, the liver reacts to the presence of the virus. The infected cells harboring the virus become malignant, resulting in cancer of the liver, an uncommon form of cancer in the general public but common in AIDS survivors who were infected with hepatitis virus.

Hemophilia Summer Camp

A meeting place where many of the boys and men with hemophilia gathered and became acquainted with one another was hemophilia summer camp. Brent knew some of those persons after sharing the waiting room in the clinic with them when he went there for checkups or to pick up supplies. Some boys with hemophilia met at summer camp, and they continued to renew their friendships year after year.

Pink Snake: John Warren's Heart Problem

"What is that weird mark on your chest? It looks like a pink snake," Brent exclaimed. He was gawking at the bare chest of John Warren, a young man, seventeen years older, who also had hemophilia, sitting on the edge of the swimming pool, shirtless and dangling his feet into the water, at Camp Tapawingo. The camp was owned by a church and rented to the Hemophilia Foundation of Oregon, which sponsored campers who have hemophilia. Located out Socialist Valley Road off Dutch Creek, west of Falls City, in the Oregon Coast Range, the camp brought together the boys and young men of the region who have hemophilia each summer for a week of camping. Most of the campers were from Oregon; some were from Idaho or Washington.

The camp included a mess hall and several bunkhouses, where the campers slept in two-level bunk beds. Campers threw their sleeping bags over the mattresses of the metal framed bunk beds. The center of the camp's expanse of land featured a large outdoor swimming pool heated by the summer sunshine. Nearby, in the camp's activity area, campers teamed up on the outdoor basketball court. Beyond the horse barn and the corral, a large expanse of forested land extended up the mountain, where trails were threaded beneath the forest canopy, allowing campers to ride horseback on beautiful brown and gray mares through the forest with a guide, after they learned how to saddle and mount a horse. Beyond the corral was a large pond filled with fresh water. It was stocked with rainbow trout so that the campers could experience the excitement of catching a fish as well as paddling a kayak and swimming in the clear springwater. Below the mess hall, the river meandered below an open field, where campers pitched horseshoes or released arrows from stretched bows, hoping for a bull's-eye in the center of a straw-stuffed target. A favorite camp activity was shooting BB guns at all the crazy targets erected by Wilbur Campbell, the hemophilia camp director. His wife, Myrna, one of the hemophilia treatment center nurses, became the camp nurse during the camp session, giving many infusions whenever guys had bleeds.

Like Brent, John attended hemophilia summer camp as a youngster. He became a counselor as an adult. He drove to the camp from his Portland home with his two daughters, ages eight and nine, in his faded dark green 1964 Oldsmobile, boasting that his old car had a 494 engine beneath the long hood, which harbored a few rust spots. John was an employee of the Oregon Department of Motor Vehicles (DMV). He used a week's vacation each summer to serve as a camp counselor (plate 6 and plate 7).

"That pink snake is a scar," John rebuffed Brent.

"A scar from what?" Brent responded. "It's right in the middle of your chest."

"You're correct," John replied good-naturedly. "It is in the middle of my chest. You may not be very good-looking, but you have good eyesight."

"But isn't that where your heart is?" Brent sheepishly grinned while staring at John's chest.

"No, my heart is beneath the scar."

"Why is there a scar over your heart?" Brent wanted to know.

John was a married man and the father of two young daughters. He had attended the hemophilia clinic since he was a young boy. He had learned to infuse himself with concentrate and had been doing so at home since 1972, when he turned thirteen. By that age, he already had damage to his joints, including his knees and a hip as well as his elbows, from bleeds during his childhood. Whenever he attended the hemophilia clinic as a youngster, he was always dressed well and appeared neat and shiningly clean, his dark brown hair carefully combed, often carrying a thick book tucked under his arm. There was a faint smile when he looked directly at someone, as if he had a secret. Sometimes the book he was bringing with him to clinic would be a large scientific encyclopedia. He spoke quietly, with confidence and seriousness, as if he wanted others to consider him a wise person. After closing time at the clinic, when the patients had returned to their homes, the doctors and nurses would amusingly remark, "Does John ever read the big book he carries under his arm? Or does he bring a serious book with him to impress people who might notice him at the clinic?"

John's father and mother had divorced when he was ten years old. He and his younger sister, Nora, moved back and forth between their parents' homes. John's father was a salesman who often sold miscellaneous goods from the trunk of his large car. John resembled his father in stature; both were tall. John's demeanor compensated for his father's relative weak station in society.

In 1974, when John was sixteen years of age, while seated in his high school classroom, the teacher called on him. In answering Mrs. Madigan respectfully, he stood upright quickly, became dizzy, and fainted. After lying on the schoolroom floor for a few minutes, John regained consciousness after the school nurse was summoned. He was all right and was able to rise up from the classroom floor. The teacher was frightened, but John was not scared. He was sent home and instructed to go see his doctor.

The staff in the treatment center was aware that John had a mild chest deformity; the left side of his chest was larger than the right side. John had a heart murmur that had not changed since birth. The doctors knew he was born with a small hole in his heart, a ventricular septal defect (VSD), that they were carefully monitoring. But they also knew John was born with hemophilia. Therefore, his congenital heart defect had not been surgically corrected because he had no symptoms of heart failure. However, as he grew to adulthood, the physiology of his body changed. Apparently, when he suddenly stood upright from a sitting position, his heart failed to provide adequate blood circulation to his brain, and he fainted. The hole in the septum of his heart was shunting blood from the left side of his heart to the right ventricle, rather than providing an adequate oxygenated blood supply to his head. Correction of John's VSD required open heart surgery, which was not possible before concentrates became available. Before correction of his blood-clotting deficiency became a reality, he would have bled to death if heart surgery would have been attempted.

The cardiologist, Dr. Byron Morrison, who was also the director of CDRC,[50] concluded that as John had grown from childhood and neared maturity—he was tall and wore size twelve shoes—he was becoming symptomatic, and further cardiovascular insufficiency was likely. The fainting spell was caused by his heart problem. He would probably have more signs of heart problems as he grew older. Already, the left side of his heart had increased in size, as indicated by the larger left side of his chest compared to the right side. After discussion and careful consideration, the hematologists and the team of cardiovascular surgeons at UOMS[51] agreed that the risk of bleeding during heart surgery, after correction of clotting activity in his blood with concentrate, was a lesser risk than the danger of impending

---

50   The name of CCD (Crippled Children's Division) was changed to CDRC (Child Development and Rehabilitation Center) in 1971.

51   University of Oregon Medical School. The name UOMS was changed to OHSU, Oregon Health Sciences University.

heart failure if no surgical intervention was implemented. John's factor VIII level in his blood was corrected to 100 percent with infusions of concentrate. He was wheeled into surgery, where the open heart procedure included splitting his sternum to gain access to his heart for repair of the small hole in his ventricular septum, while a constant infusion with concentrate was maintained. The procedure was accomplished without difficulties and without excessive bleeding. While concentrate infusions kept his factor VIII at a normal level postoperatively, John recovered well. A residual sign of the surgery was the prominent vertical scar—the pink scar noticed by Brent—extending the length of his chest in the midline, where his sternum had been split. John was one of the first persons in the United States, probably in the world, who had open heart surgery despite also having severe hemophilia. John graduated from high school, married a devoted woman named Jackie, had two daughters, and held a regular job.

"You see, it's like this," John said while running his finger along the long midline scar on his chest. "You and I are alike. We were both born with hemophilia. But we are different. I was born with a hole in my heart. The scar is where the doctors operated to fix my heart; otherwise, I wouldn't be going swimming with you."

"Holy cow!" Brent excitedly exclaimed. "You are cool, man. You are really something. I'm glad you told me. Now that I understand, I'm no longer freaked out by that pink snake in the middle of your chest."

"Yeah." John smiled. "Now you know all about me, so you must return a favor."

"Huh?" Brent quizzically wondered. "What's up?"

"You can be my helper."

"Help doing what?"

"It's shirt time. Time to hand out shirts when the dinner bell rings. Go past the guys standing in line at the door of the mess hall at dinnertime, come up to the front table, where Wilbur and Myrna Campbell sit, and help hand out shirts."

"Are those Cutter shirts? From a drug company?" Brent asked.

"Yeah," John answered. "Wear it anyway, even if it is from a drug company."

"But that's an … en … ah, encroachment, my dad said," Brent added after remembering the word. "If I wear a gift from Cutter, one of their shirts, I have to infuse with medicine sold by Cutter."

"Nah. That's not the word. The word you're thinking of is endorsement," John corrected Brent. "You do not have to use Cutter's brand of concentrate just because you were handed one of their shirts at camp."

John was referring to the shirts to be passed out to the campers, which they would take home when they returned from camp. During the weeks before camp, a contest was held, with campers submitting a design for the summer camp shirt. The selected design was printed on the shirts. Whoever submitted the winning shirt design was also honored by having that year's summer camp named after his design.

The annual shirt contest began in 1984. Rusty Harper from Pendleton submitted the winning design, Camp Radical, in 1993. Other winning designs for different years included Camp Catch'em in 1989, Camp Cowabunga in 1991, and Camp Chinook in 1988 (plates 16 and 17). Although Camp Tapawingo was owned and operated by a church, during the summer when the Hemophilia Foundation of Oregon rented and occupied the camp, the campers chose to rename the camp during their stay at that lovely place. The expense of purchasing the shirts and printing the design was paid for by Cutter, one of the drug companies who sold concentrate. The cost of renting the camp was paid by the foundation, with funds received from donations. The hemophilia foundation's camp committee worked all year raising funds to provide the opportunity for anyone with hemophilia between the ages of six years and fourteen to attend hemophilia summer camp. After age fourteen, a camper could become a junior counselor which allowed him to continue attending summer camp.

Saving Her Baby: A Silent Heroine

John was not the only one in his family who had endured remarkable events in his life as the result of hemophilia. His sister, Nora, two years younger than her brother, also experienced profound situations in her life, the effects of hemophilia, although she did not have hemophilia. The hemophilia clinic was organized to provide comprehensive care for children—not only hemophilia care, but also whatever other needs a child was lacking. In addition to doctors and nurses, the staff of the hemophilia treatment center included a social worker, psychologist, physical therapist, financial counselor, dentist, and a genetic counselor. Although John was the patient at the treatment center because of his hemophilia, services were extended to his sister since their parents were divorced. The intention of the center was to identify appropriate care and resources before problems occurred.

Although John was the only person in the family who was affected with hemophilia, it was possible that his mother was a carrier of hemophilia and had transmitted the bleeding disorder to her son and her daughter.[52] If the mother of the two children was a carrier of hemophilia, the likelihood that John's sister, Nora, was also a carrier of the mutant hemophilia gene, was 50 percent. As a result of the significant risk of being a hemophilia carrier who could have a son affected with hemophilia, the clinic staff concluded that Nora should be informed of the possible risk of hemophilia if she were to marry and have children. It was further concluded that sixteen-year-old Nora should know the methods of birth control to avoid becoming pregnant.

She attended the clinic and was interviewed by the clinic director, Dr. Taillefer, a pediatrician. He was comfortable discussing such issues as acne, obesity, hygiene, diet, smoking, and sex education with sixteen-year-old males and females. He was shocked when Nora suddenly rose

---

52 Results of modern genetic tests reveal that when an infant male is discovered to have hemophilia, where no previous males have been affected in the family, the mother is nearly always a carrier of hemophilia.

from her chair during the counseling session with the doctor and angrily stomped out of the clinic as soon as he began questioning her regarding her knowledge of methods of avoiding pregnancy. She thought he was a dirty old man. He had never previously experienced a young person walking out of his office when discussing sex with him or her. Dr. Taillefer was baffled. Disappointed. Concerned. What had he done wrong? Why was Nora insulted by him? He thought he had been gentle, discrete, and appropriate. He lamented to Nurse Myrna that he had totally failed in his attempt to reach out to the sixteen-year-old girl.

A few weeks passed. Then Myrna provided information that explained Dr. Taillefer's dilemma. "Did you know that when you saw Nora in your office, intending to provide sex education to her, that she was already pregnant? I just found that out. Nora telephoned here for help."

During the next weeks and months, Nora returned to the clinic for information and advice for prenatal care. She wasn't angry at anyone, including Dr. Taillefer. She had walked out of the clinic because she was already pregnant when she was offered counseling, and she was angry at herself. She felt hurt. Independently, Nora arrived at a remarkable decision. She decided to continue her pregnancy, but she would not keep her baby after it was born. She asked the clinic staff to locate a married couple, a suitable married man and woman, who would agree to adopt her baby. She carefully stipulated that the couple must legally adopt the baby before its birth. She wanted no prenatal sex determination and no tests to determine if she was carrying a child affected with hemophilia. The married couple must adopt the unborn infant without knowing if the child was a boy or girl, not knowing if the infant would have hemophilia.

A married man and woman—both schoolteachers, childless after ten years of marriage and desiring a baby—were chosen. They attended the hemophilia clinic for counseling, without meeting or contacting Nora. They were informed of the nature of hemophilia in preparation for the infant's birth, realizing the chance was fifty-fifty that a boy would be born, and if so, there was a fifty-fifty chance that he would have hemophilia. The overall risk of hemophilia for the unborn child was 25 percent, one in four. Through their attorney, adoption of the child before birth was finalized in court. The adoptive parents anxiously waited for the day their child would be born.

Nora gave birth to a healthy, vigorous baby boy without complications. Swiftly and sadly, Nora left the hospital immediately after the birth without seeing her baby. A blood sample was collected from the umbilical cord at birth. The beautiful baby boy was examined in the nursery and found to be a perfectly healthy infant. Test results from the umbilical blood sample revealed that the baby boy had normal blood clotting. He did not have hemophilia. The parents were ecstatic. Nora had requested that no one tell her whether her baby was a boy or a girl, nor did she want to be informed of the test results for hemophilia.

Two years later, Nora again became pregnant. This time, she decided to keep the baby. She gave birth to a baby boy. Nora's second baby boy had hemophilia. Nora was a real hero, an unacknowledged hero. She'd given a beautiful normal baby boy to a couple, filling their desire for a child, in a caring home. She kept a son with hemophilia, one who would be confronted by all the problems of hemophilia and HIV, bearing up under the stress despite adverse circumstances.

Death of John Warren

John is no longer dangling his bare feet in the swimming pool at Camp Tapawingo while basking under the summer sunshine in the Oregon Coast Range. He became weak while continuing to work at the DMV, issuing driver's licenses and automobile permits. He tired easily and became exhausted at his job. Eventually, he was not strong enough to go to work. Despite his confrontation with a hopeless fatal outcome, caused by conditions in his life that he was helpless to overcome, John was not depressed. John was innocent. He had followed the doctors' recommendation, which unsuspectingly sealed his fate. He remained at peace in the world, for he had discovered the meaning of his existence, which allowed him to suppress his suffering. His existence, he rationalized, brought happiness to Jackie, his loving wife, his two daughters, and to his sister, Nora. He recognized that he did not exist in isolation within this world. John died March 21, 1996, at thirty-eight years of age. He died of AIDS from the HIV infection he received from the concentrates infused to treat his hemophilia to make his life more bearable.

John left his wife and his two daughters mourning for him. John's sister mourns for him and endures the agony of hemophilia and HIV in her son. John's daughters, who are obligate carriers,[53] must face the risks of hemophilia and its treatment when they marry and have sons. If they have sons affected with hemophilia, those who treat hemophilia will tell them that the medicine is safe, that if their sons are infused with new safe concentrates, they will not bleed; instead, they will enjoy near-normal lives, the same information John received a generation earlier. Will the doctors provide correct information to the new generation of patients this second time or will the doctors be wrong again?

In addition to John, other counselors from hemophilia summer camp would not return—their lives ended prematurely from AIDS, including Joe Kennedy, Bruce Dessellier, Doug McAllister, Mike Charles, and Joe Singler.

---

53   All females born of a father who has hemophilia are obligate carriers of the hemophilia mutant gene because they receive their fathers' X chromosomes. Therefore, they are obligated to inherit his X-linked genes, including hemophilia.

1987: Brent Faces a New Test

Test for HIV

Brent was well, without signs of illness of the new disease. Neither he nor his father favored withholding infusions because of fear of becoming stricken with the new disease, a disease that was threatening but seemed remote to him and his parents. They reasoned that compared to the risk of the unknown disease, his fate was more threatened from the risk of life-threatening bleeds if infusions were withheld. Brent was not interested in being tested to determine if he harbored an agent that would subsequently progress to illness.

In 1987, the name of the infectious virus causing the new mysterious disease affecting persons who had been infused with concentrate was changed from HTLV to HIV.[54] A test became available for discovering who had become infected with HIV from infusions of concentrates. The new test, an HIV antibody test, an ELISA assay, could be completed on a blood sample. A positive HIV test result indicated that a person had been exposed to HIV. A negative HIV (ELISA) test result indicated the person had not been exposed to HIV. The HIV antibody test is a useful screening test. Confirmation of an HIV-positive person is confirmed with the Western Blot test, which directly detects the presence of the

---

54 HTLV, human T lymphotropic virus, discovered in Japan, was the first identified human retrovirus. HTLV is implicated in T-cell leukemia. HIV, human immunodeficiency virus, was first identified December 1, 1981. Previously it was known as HTLV-III. Dr. Luc Montagnier discovered HIV as the cause of AIDS in 1983.

virus.[55] Most persons who had been infused with concentrate, the individuals to be tested for HIV infection, were not ill. Records were examined; a rapid process was mobilized for HIV testing of at-risk persons. Everyone who had received concentrate dispensed from the hemophilia treatment center was contacted by telephone and notified that the treatment center recommended HIV testing.

HIV Test Recommendation

The hemophilia treatment center staff advised the Perrys that it was in Brent's best interest to be tested. If he had become infected with HIV, treatment could begin before he became ill, although treatment for HIV was not optimal in 1987. Nurse Myrna Campbell conferred with his mother and recommended to her that Brent should be tested. A dilemma exists when a person is presented with testing for a devastating or fatal disease when the person at risk, especially a youth, is without signs or symptoms of the disorder. Is it best to know or wait until the disease strikes? Often the doctors, nurses, and social workers recommend presymptomatic testing. But what do the persons who are at risk prefer?

Dilemma of HIV Testing

In response to the distress and frustration confronting Gwyn, posed by the dilemma of whether to test her son for HIV, she went on an outing for a few days to reflect and meditate. With some of her friends, Gwyn traveled to a remote area in eastern Oregon, to the small hamlet of French Glen and the Steens Mountains. The Steens gently and smoothly rise to nine thousand feet, sloping upward from the West. After the ascent

---

55 HIV screening with an ELISA (enzyme-linked immunoassay) requires confirmation of an HIV-positive test result with the Western Blot test. A person could be recently HIV infected before antibodies have been produced, as revealed with the Western Blot test (ELISA/Western Blot test, 2009).

to the summit of these uninhabited mountains, there is an abrupt drop down a steep, nearly vertical escarpment on the east side to the flat Alvord Desert below. The wide smooth-packed white sand of the level desert is bordered by hot springs, where cowboys soak in the soothing waters after dismounting from their steeds following a long day in the saddle. She told her family the high desert air and the sweeping panoramic landscapes cleared her thinking, helping her overcome her confusion. She said that sometimes when a person is confronted with a burdensome, difficult decision, whose choices offer little chance of a pleasant conclusion, it's best to go away, to a place where there are few people and few distractions, and look back, viewing the circumstances from afar.

"Is it best to wait until the ugly disease strikes?" Gwyn asked herself. "If the test results reveal that my son is infected with the mysterious disease, should I tell him he is infected with HIV?" She struggled, frustrated, trying to decide what to do.

"Of course Brent knows why he is being tested," Nurse Myrna told Gwyn after she returned from the desert. "Brent is twelve years old. He knows what's going on. Kids of that age always know what's going on."

Brent was well. He had no signs of the disease everyone seemed to be talking about, not directly to him but hush-hush to one another, as if they were afraid to talk to him about it. He wanted nothing to do with AIDS. Why should he be tested for an ugly disease he did not have? But his mom was uptight, and to make her feel better, he followed her advice, reasoning that he could ease her tension with a simple blood test. What the heck? Why not? HIV testing would help his beautiful mother keep from worrying about him so much. Myrna collected a blood sample from Brent. It was sent to the State Public Health Laboratory for HIV testing.

An ELISA antibody test was completed on a blood sample from Brent. If a person has been infected with a virus, his body responds by making antibodies to the virus. The presence of antibodies indicates that the tested person has been infected. Antibody testing is not a direct test. It's not the same as trapping the virus that causes an illness. It's only a test to let you know the virus has been present. Doctors who treat persons who become ill from infections with a variety of infectious diseases, like the ones kids get when they are young, know that if a person has antibodies to a specific virus, he was infected sometime during his childhood. If a child gets measles or mumps, the immune system in his body makes antibodies to measles or mumps. That is good, protective. If they are around another child who has measles or mumps, they will not break out with those contagious infectious diseases. Their antibodies are recalled from their white blood cells, their small lymphocytes, which fight off the virus. The diseases of childhood last about a week, while the body musters up its defense, its immune system, which fights off the virus to end the disease. Each virus makes a specific antibody. Measles antibodies fight measles; mumps antibodies attack only the mumps virus if the virus comes around again after a child had mumps previously. These antibodies last the entire life of the child, protecting him forever. Once a child has measles, he will never be sick again with measles, for he is immune to infection from the measles virus. The same is true for chicken pox—if a child is infected once during childhood, he will never get chicken pox as an adult, although as an older adult, he might become ill with shingles if his immune system is weak.

HIV is a different kind of germ. A person infected with HIV develops antibodies, becoming HIV-positive. But unlike other viral infections, the virus is not destroyed in his body by his immune system. Despite the presence of HIV antibodies, the virus lives—and it lives forever. When a child is exposed to another person who has chicken pox, he becomes sick with chicken pox right away, within two weeks, if he doesn't have antibodies. A person who is infected with HIV doesn't become ill even when he receives a large dose of the virus directly into his bloodstream during an intravenous infusion. At the time of infection, he is not aware of the virus. Signs of the presence of the virus do not develop until later, usually five to ten years later. Some HIV infected persons never become ill. A person who has been infected with HIV, discovered with HIV antibody testing, who has neither signs nor symptoms of illness is said to be HIV-positive. After months or years pass, an HIV-positive person may become very ill with all the signs of AIDS. The presence of HIV antibodies does not protect a person who has been infected with HIV from progressing to AIDS, the disease caused by HIV. HIV is a different kind of infectious disease than those disorders that doctors have known about in the past. Persons who become infected with HIV develop antibodies to HIV—they become HIV-positive—but the disease is progressive despite antibodies. HIV-positive persons are infectious, but they are not contagious. One person cannot catch HIV from another person by just being near him.[56]

> HIV is different from most other human infectious diseases. Although a person develops antibodies to HIV, the disease can continue to progress, leading to AIDS months or years after infection.

In addition to becoming infected with HIV, Brent was also hepatitis B antibody positive and hepatitis C antibody positive. When he was born in 1975, there was no immunization against hepatitis B.[57] He had become infected with hepatitis B and hepatitis C from his past concentrate infusions. Like HIV, the viruses that cause hepatitis B and hepatitis C may provoke the development of antibodies without destroying the viruses; the virus may not be cleared from their bodies. Hepatitis B and hepatitis C viruses can live forever in the liver of a person who has been

---

56 Infection with HIV can occur by the transfer, from one person to another, of blood, semen, vaginal fluid, pre-ejaculate, or breast milk. The four major routes of infection are sexual intercourse, intravenous needles, breast milk, and during the birth of a baby from an infected mother.

57 Immunization against hepatitis B became available in 1982. No vaccine exists to prevent hepatitis C. Experimental hepatitis C vaccines offer hope, possibly in 2010 or later, that a vaccine will become effective.

infected, despite the presence of antibodies. Hepatitis B and hepatitis C are similar to HIV with respect to development of antibodies. Hepatitis A is different from hepatitis B and hepatitis C. Hepatitis A is an acute illness. Signs and symptoms of hepatitis A—jaundice, nausea, and weakness—develop within two weeks after infection, which occurs sometimes after eating a contaminated hamburger that was not well cooked. After recovering from hepatitis A, the person is well, without developing continuing chronic illness. Hepatitis B and hepatitis C differ from hepatitis A; they can become chronic illnesses with liver damage, unlike hepatitis A.[58]

Brent Discovers That He Is HIV-positive

HIV is a reportable infectious disease. Whenever a doctor discovers that his patient has been infected with HIV, the doctor is required to report the name of the person to the health department. The Oregon State Health Department requires HIV reporting to prevent the transmission of the virus through sexual contact.

The hemophilia treatment center and the health department reached an agreement that the treatment center would conduct appropriate follow-up and provide counseling to HIV-positive adult men to assure adequate protection of their sexual partners. A goal of the hemophilia treatment center was to prevent HIV infection in wives or any sexual partner of HIV infected hemophilia men. The hemophilia center had been informed by the CDC[59] that sexual partners of HIV infected men

---

58 Of adults who become infected with hepatitis B, 10 percent become chronic carriers; the frequency is increased if the infection occurs in children. Of persons who are infected with hepatitis C, 10 to 20 percent become chronic carriers. Individuals who do not clear hepatitis B or C may develop cirrhosis of the liver and hepatocellular carcinomas (liver cancer).

59 Centers for Disease Control, Atlanta, Georgia. In 1987, CDC proclaimed that anyone infected with HIV would develop AIDS, a fatal illness. Since the 1980s, not everyone who has become HIV infected has died. Not all women who were married to HIV infected men have become infected with HIV.

were likely to become infected. The CDC told the center that HIV infection leads to AIDS, a fatal disease.

Brent said that he didn't want all his friends to know if he was HIV-positive. They might think he had AIDS, and AIDS was a bad word. Myrna told his mother that she would keep his name secret. When she collected his sample of blood for HIV tests, Myrna said that his name would not appear on the label affixed to the glass test tube containing his blood sample. A number, not a name, would be placed on the test tube label, a secret code for which only Myrna knew the identity. When the tests were completed, the health department would report the number and the test results to Myrna, who would then inform Gwyn of the results. No one else would know whom the number belonged to.

Brent's mother held out hope, not giving up until she received the disheartening report of the HIV test result. There was reason to hope infection had bypassed her son, spared him from the dreaded infection, for HIV is mysterious in some ways. Not everyone who was infused with HIV contaminated AHF became ill from AIDS. The two Singer brothers who had been infused many times did not develop AIDS or liver failure from hepatitis. Some men who were infused with concentrates that produced HIV infection in other persons did not become HIV infected. Even when persons infused from the same batch of medicine, the same lot number, not all of them became HIV infected.

After the test results of 1987 were received, Myrna told Gwyn that Brent was HIV infected. Gwyn told his two sisters and his father that Brent was HIV-positive, however she did not tell him right away.

Finally, after the two weeks of agony, Brent's family decided to meet with him in the living room of their house. His parents and his two sisters wanted to be present when the dreadful result of the HIV test, which they knew but he didn't, was revealed to him. Brent silently sat back into the soft brown leather couch. His light brown hair, which was trimmed neatly in the back, was combed over to the side in front. He was wearing his favorite loose-fitting short pants and a loosely fitting white shirt with long sleeves, shirttail not tucked in. Most of the time, Brent managed a deceptive smile when faced with a decision or anticipation—but not that day. He was somber. Everyone looked at one another. Gwyn leaned over her son and softly said without crying, "Brent, the test result have been completed. You are HIV-positive. You have been infected with HIV. We don't know what will happen. None of us know what to do next."[60] The expression on Gwyn's face was one of suffering. Those in the room were somber and quiet.

Gwyn's words made Brent terribly upset. He thought a brick had fallen onto his head. Red color rose up in Brent's face. He went into a furious rage.

His mother intended to console him, saying, "Options exist; medical treatment is available if you become sick and need treatment."

He wasn't sick. "There is something sinister, something rotten here!" Brent shouted at everyone in the room. He leaped up from the sofa, half sobbing, tears running down his cheeks. He quickly grabbed a ceramic pottery bowl and flung it as hard as he could across the room. The bowl, one of his mother's favorites, crashed to the floor, bits of pottery going everywhere. He swiftly turned around and shoved open the back door, immediately running out of the house like a speeding bullet. Brent crossed the terrace and vaulted over the creek to the other forested stream bank. He sat motionless and alone on the ground—among the green sword-leaf ferns, beneath the canopy of the towering cedars, Douglas firs, and alders—his tears falling. Brent didn't move for two hours. After a while, he felt a little less upset, but he was still angry; he was hurt. Like a wounded animal, he returned to the house.

His parents and his two sisters looked anxiously at him; they were tormented by his pain. Without looking at anyone, Brent rapidly tromped straight to his room. He slammed shut the door of his room and locked it from the inside. Lee and Gwyn knocked on the door. Brent made no response. His sister Paula banged on the door loudly.

---

60   Related by Gwyn McCann, Brent's mother, August 31, 2007.

"Brent, open the door. We want to be with you. Let us in, Brent." He didn't open the door. He was sulking inside, filled with rage. Their pleading with him to open the bedroom door was ignored.

The next day, Brent emerged from his room. Gwyn remembered that he remained quiet and upset. He was outraged. He felt like a weirdo and a leper. He thought it was unfair. He wondered what kind of person he was now. He had changed. He was different than he was a few days ago.

Life for Brent completely changed after he discovered that he was HIV infected. Hemophilia wasn't so bad. With hemophilia, he could handle the shots, visit with his friends. and enjoy a good life. It may not be normal for most people to bleed so much, but hemophilia was normal for him. But HIV was not normal; it was weird. At age twelve, he was depressed. Brent understood the significance of HIV. He knew that HIV was a fatal illness. He was not sick, but that had all changed. Being told he was HIV-positive gave him a death sentence.

Besides information provided by the Oregon Hemophilia Treatment Center, Brent's mother received facts about HIV and AIDS from his uncle, his mother's sister's husband, who was an employee of the Georgia State Communicable Disease Department in Atlanta. The nation's Centers for Disease Control, CDC, was located in Atlanta; therefore, his uncle had access to the latest, most up-to-date information about HIV and AIDS

What about hemophilia? All the shots Brent had received for treating his bleeds with concentrates were derived from plasma obtained from the blood of paid donors. The threat of contaminated concentrate was intensely discussed by hemophilia families. Is it safe to use concentrate if it is polluted? Brent didn't have a shot unless he was certain he had a bleed. He didn't infuse concentrate prophylactically. His parents were a little more conservative about giving him shots for infusions than they had been before they heard of the ugly disease that might come from concentrate. But they did not discontinue infusions or withhold concentrate. Lee and Gwyn discussed HIV and AIDS with the doctors and nurses at the hemophilia treatment center. Gwyn read everything she could find about HIV. They received information from the Medical Advisory Committee of NHF (National Hemophilia Foundation) and several other sources describing the effects of HIV infection.[61] The recommendations of the committee were passed on to hemophilia families. Brent's parents were advised that the risk of dying from a head bleed, an intracranial hemorrhage, if concentrate was withheld, exceeded the risk of dying from AIDS from infusing with contaminated concentrate. The doctors and nurses who treat hemophilia, based upon the advice of the NHF, recommended that infusions of concentrate for treatment of bleeds in hemophilia continue rather than be withheld for fear of AIDS.

There was skepticism concerning the influence of the drug companies who made the medicine. They financially supported NHF. They were anxious to sell their medicine for a profit. Did they influence the recommendation to continue infusions rather than improve safety of concentrate?

---

61   MAC, the Medical Advisory Committee, was comprised of experts who had the most recent HIV and AIDS information available.

Providing a Safer Product in the Wake of HIV

Improvement in the Safety of Concentrates with Heat Treatment

Efforts to assure the safety of concentrates were discussed, but what changes were actually implemented by the pharmaceutical manufacturers of AHF? Before successful treatment of the plasma, pooled from hundreds of donors, to eradicate harmful viruses was completed in the United States, concentrate was already prepared with a method that included heat to destroy viruses in plasma-derived concentrate in Germany. Scientists and doctors in the United States were concerned that heat would inactivate the factor VIII clotting activity. Factor VIII was regarded as an unstable clotting factor, a delicate protein, present in miniscule amounts in plasma, one that required low temperatures for isolation and preservation. They were cautious about losing AHF activity if heat was included in the production of concentrate from plasma. A further concern was the fear that heat might alter the composition of the clotting factor, resulting in the induction of inhibitors to AHF that would reduce clotting activity. After a number of hemophilia patients had been infused with heat-treated (HT) concentrate and the effect of treating bleeds was not diminished, without inactivation of the clotting factor from heat exposure and without appearance of inhibitors, HT concentrate[62] was released and became available for distribution to U.S. hemophilia families in 1985,

---

62 Heat treatment (HT) of the dry composition of powder derived from plasma at sixty degrees Celsius for a predetermined amount of time eliminates HIV as well as hepatitis viruses, cytomegalovirus, and Epstein-Barr virus.

several years after its use began in Germany. The good news was that heat treatment effectively removed viruses from concentrate. But requirements demanded of the producers of HT concentrate before approval by the government delayed the introduction of an effective antiviral treatment in the United States. Persons who were infused with HT concentrate were protected from infection with hepatitis and HIV. Hepatitis virus and HIV are destroyed by heat treatment when they are present in the plasma obtained from donors.

The stored bottles of non-HT concentrate in the homes of hemophilia families were recalled and exchanged for HT concentrate. This process was completed by 1986. Beginning in 1985, Brent and all the other hemophilia patients who were enrolled at the Oregon Hemophilia Treatment Center received only HT concentrate to prevent infection with hepatitis and HIV. His concentrate was changed to HT concentrate in1985 when he was ten years of age. It was 1987 before he found out he was HIV infected. The change to HT concentrate was too late. Brent was already infected with HIV by the time he began infusions with HT concentrate, the deviralized clotting factor.

Brent's treatment became complicated. It was difficult for a twelve-year-old to understand. The complexity was apparent in the change in concentrates being dispensed from the hemophilia treatment center. He had been receiving Koate HP[63] from the center for his infusions. However, the center instructed his mother to return all the Koate HP and exchange it for Koate HT.

The hemophilia caregivers across the country were informing the hemophilia families that they would be safe from HIV if they infused with heat-treated concentrate. Brent's family had heard that before. His family, like the other hemophilia families, mistrusted the medical community. The doctors had told his parents to give him a shot at the earliest sign of a bleed so that he wouldn't have a stiff, painful ankle. The

---

63 Koate HP (high purity) was marketed by Cutter Biological, a division of Miles Laboratories. Koate HP was replaced with Koate HT (heat-treated), also produced by Cutter, at the hemophilia treatment center in 1985.

doctors had said he wouldn't have destruction of his joints from bleeds. They were wrong. They said to infuse with concentrate, and he would live to become an old man. Later those same good doctors said that because he infused with concentrate, he had HIV. They said to use heat-treated concentrate, and he wouldn't get sick. But infection with HIV leads to AIDS, and AIDS means death. When concentrate dispensed from the hemophilia center was suspected of being polluted, the bottles of medicine were exchanged for a different batch of concentrate. Frequently switching medicine quickly became confusing. The Perry family didn't trust the doctors. Why should they trust the doctors?

Brent wanted to know why the drug companies didn't stop making concentrate if the medicine was suspected of being polluted. His father replied that the drug companies exist to make a profit. They didn't deliberately intend to harm anyone by allowing an infectious germ to exist in the medicine they made, but more importantly to them, and to their stockholders, they wanted to make money. They were not reckless, but the major effort of drug companies who made concentrate was focused on marketing, not research and development.

Years ago, drug companies actively conducted research to discover new drugs for treating disease. That is no longer correct. Nowadays, new discoveries of medicines for treatment are made at universities and scientific companies, not drug companies. The drug companies obtain patents on the drugs developed in research laboratories at the universities. They manufacture and market such medicines as concentrates.

The hemophilia families had been instructed to infuse at the earliest sign of bleeding to prevent deformity and to prolong life. The adage "When in doubt, infuse!" was often cited, referring to the decision of whether to infuse or not to infuse concentrate for a suspected bleed. Such a promotion was beneficial for the pharmaceutical manufacturers of concentrate—the more concentrate infused, the greater the profit. Persons who had hemophilia would be free of pain and suffering, they were told. They could lead near-normal lives as a result of the benefit of the miracle-like concentrates.

Brent acknowledged that hemophilia prevented him from making the football or wrestling team, but he could attend school and be like the other regular guys in lots of ways. When thinking about the help he received from the concentrate, he realized that it made his life a lot better. Without concentrate, his life would have been miserable. He concluded that during all the past years he'd received the benefits from infusions of concentrate, he was also was being infused with a deadly virus.

When heat-treated concentrate was approved and released in the United States for infusions to stop bleeds in persons who have hemophilia, it was in short supply; availability was limited. Cutter, the company that made Koate HT, the new concentrate free of HIV and hepatitis, sold the medicine in Germany. In that country, concentrate was paid for by the government. The German government was willing to pay the price Cutter requested. The higher the price, the greater the profit for Cutter. Cutter could make more money selling Koate HT in Germany than they could make selling the medicine in the United States.[64]

When Brent asked his father what the drug companies did with the recalled concentrate, he was told they dumped it. He assumed they dumped it down a sink drain. Lee assured his son that the drug company didn't dump the polluted medicine down the drain. They dumped it overseas. Cutter exchanged the old concentrate, regular Koate HP, which was polluted with viruses, for the new stuff, Koate HT, which was free of HIV and hepatitis, and brought Koate HP back to their drug company where it had been made.

Cutter took the old non-heat-treated concentrate, Koate HP, the stuff returned from patients as well as the concentrate stored on shelves in their warehouse, and sent the supply to other countries—including Japan, other parts of Asia, and Argentina—where Cutter sold it inexpensively (Bogdanich and Koli 2003).

---

64 Cutter, a division of Miles Laboratories of Elkhart, Indiana, was purchased by Bayer AG, of Germany, in 1978.

Slowly, over months, sufficient sources of heat-treated concentrate became available to assure an adequate supply without the frequent, inconvenient, confusing switching of the lots of recalled medicine. With the passage of time, months, families in Oregon and across the United States became confident of the safety of the heat-treated concentrate.

Part III

HIV and Hepatitis in Persons Attending the Clinic

System Failures

Hurricane

"Hurricane!"

"Remember to take Hurricane with you!" Pearl shouted at Dr. Taillefer.

"My goodness, what's happening?" Brent demanded of his mother. "A hurricane? What do they mean telling Dr. Taillefer to take a hurricane with him?" He noted Dr. Taillefer rushing past him and his mother, who were sitting in the waiting room. He was clutching the handles of his black leather doctor's bag in his right hand, quickly heading out the door. "He must be leaving to go see someone. Wow!" Brent exclaimed. "I didn't know Dr. Taillefer could move so fast. He's in a hurry!"

Dr. Taillefer was on his way to the north Portland home of Davy Jarrard, a twenty-three-year-old married man. He'd first met Davy when he was a little fellow. Davy's father was a logger. In 1973, at ten years of age, Davy was helping his father in the forest of the Oregon Coast Range on a sunny afternoon. Using an orange Husqvarna chainsaw, his father was preparing to fell a medium-sized straight-trunked Douglas fir tree. Davy didn't notice the plastic fuel bottle filled with gasoline, used to refuel the chain saw, lying in some sawdust on the ground next to a tree trunk. The tightly closed container exploded from the impact when Davy unintentionally stepped on it. He yelled with fright and pain as the leg of his blue jeans caught fire.

His father threw him to the ground and covered his leg with dirt and sawdust to smother the flames. After the fire was out, he picked

Davy up in his arms and rushed him to the hospital with a badly burned leg. Davy was taken to surgery the day after he was hospitalized. He had hemophilia type B, which was mild, without bleeds unless he was injured. He had been infused with plasma only once previously. For the present injury, he was infused with concentrate to restore his blood-clotting activity to normal to prepare him for surgery. A thin piece of skin, the size of a slice of bread, was surgically removed from the outside of his upper thigh and transferred to his lower leg to cover the burned area, a skin graft. During the postoperative recovery, he was infused each day with concentrate to prevent bleeding into the grafted skin, which was protected with a sterile white Kerlix bandage. After two weeks of healing, when the skin graft was secure, concentrate infusions were discontinued.

The graft to the burned leg was a success. The doctor said the young boy's skin graft had a good take. Because of his age, his skin attached quickly. Davy required few infusions during the next years. Once he was infused for dental work. Another infusion was after a cow stepped on his bare foot. He was infused only five or six times during the late 1970s and early 1980s. He had no deformities. His physical condition was excellent, robust; he was active. Hemophilia was not a big problem for Davy; he did not think about it on a daily basis.

He married Julie in 1983, when he was twenty years of age. After he was married, he began to lose weight. He was tested and discovered to be HIV-positive. He had become HIV infected from the infusions he'd received, even though he was seldom infused. Julie, his attractive young wife was tested. She had avoided infection; she was HIV-negative.

Davy developed one of the complications that occur in some persons who become ill from AIDS. When he attended the clinic at the center, white patches were discovered inside his mouth; he had thrush. The cause of thrush is a fungus, *Candida albicans*. Dr. Porter, the hemophilia treatment center dentist, dispensed lozenges of ketoconazole in an attempt to eliminate the fungal growth in Davy's mouth. He was instructed to suck on one of the thin wafers several times each day. Davy's HIV infection progressed to AIDS despite therapy with AZT.[65] He became weaker, and his mouth pain became excruciating. Unrelenting tormenting pain prevented him from sleeping and eating. He was miserable. He had attempted pain relief using Tylenol and codeine, without success.

In 1993, when Dr. Taillefer arrived at his home, he found Davy lying on the sofa in agony, suffering from unbearable pain in his mouth. The Hurricane Dr. Taillefer brought with him was an aerosol canister containing a topical anesthetic for spraying into Davy's mouth. A couple of puffs from the canister brought relief. However, the relief persisted for only fifteen minutes, followed by return of the severe pain. Dr. Taillefer also brought with him, in addition to the Hurricane, a small white jar containing topical lidocaine, a local anesthetic in a gel form. After swabbing the inside of Davy's mouth with the gel, applied with a cotton swab, some relief from pain was noted, but pain returned and persisted. Finally, after only a little success in relieving Davy's mouth pain, Dr. Taillefer returned, frustrated and feeling helpless, to the clinic. He had been defeated in his attempt to bring relief from pain to a suffering person.

As a doctor, Dr. Taillefer knew that patients expected him to relieve their pain. But sometimes doctors do not know how to make pain go away. After returning to the clinic, he recognized that the next step in discovering a way to relieve Davy's mouth pain should include a consultation with specialists who are knowledgeable about the inside of the mouth: dentists. In comparison, medical doctors know very little about the mouth. He recalled the previous experience with Jason Cobb in Alaska. He asked the dentist at the center, Don Porter, for his suggestions. Several other hemophilia patients who'd developed AIDS had thrush and were treated with ketoconazole, but they did not have the severe mouth pain that plagued Davy.

Dr. Porter recommended making a telephone call to Dr. Isaiah Burgstein—a dentist who directed a dental clinic on the North Side

---

65   AZT, zidovudine or azidothymidine, also known as Retrovir and Retrovis, has been used to treat AIDS since 1987.

of Portland, where AIDS patients could receive an examination and treatment. Most dentists would not accept an AIDS person for care in their practice. They were fearful that if word spread that a person with AIDS was sitting in their dental chair, other patients would not return for dental care. However, Dr. Burgstein provided dental treatment for anyone who needed care, regardless of his HIV status. HIV infection was not a reason for denying treatment to a suffering person, Dr. Burgstein reasoned. Dr. Porter said he was not aware that Dr. Burgstein had hemophilia patients attending his clinic. But Dr. Porter was certain Dr. Burgstein had the most knowledge of any dentist when the subject was AIDS in the mouth.

Describing Davy's painful mouth, Dr. Taillefer informed Dr. Burgstein by telephone that the young man had hemophilia, and he was HIV-positive and had AIDS, which had caused the thrush in his mouth and terrible mouth pain.

Dr. Burgstein quickly suggested that Dr. Taillefer's patient had dry mouth. He related that dry mouth occurs in AIDS patients when the HIV virus knocks out the salivary glands that normally provide lubricant and cleansing inside the mouth. Without saliva, bacterial infections set in, inflaming the mouth and leading to pain. He said that the suffering patient needs replacement of saliva with artificial saliva.

Dr. Taillefer was amazed. He hadn't previously heard of dry mouth in AIDS patients. He learned that dry mouth is not a common condition in AIDS victims, but Dr. Burgstein had seen several cases of it. It is extremely painful and debilitating. He said that with the artificial saliva, the young man's pain should abate.

Davy's wife rushed to the pharmacy near their home after Dr. Taillefer telephoned a prescription to the drugstore. She returned to their home with a small bottle of Salivart, a lemon-flavored artificial saliva. During the next few days, by gently swabbing the inside of her ill husband's mouth, she was able to relieve Davy's pain. He began to drink more fluids; however, he had no appetite. Although he no longer suffered the pain of dry mouth, Davy became more and more inactive.

His wife took a furlough from her job to be at his side in their home. A hospice care worker came to their small home daily to assist her. Julie realized that the end of her husband's life was near. Davy died from AIDS at home on February 7, 1994. His wife was at his bedside, as were his mother, father, and brother. They said good-bye to him when he closed his eyes for the last time.

Following Davy's death, Julie returned the supplies used for Davy's concentrate infusions in their home to the hemophilia treatment center. She was sad, but she also related to Myrna and Pearl, the nurses, and Hanna Whitman, the social worker, that she had achieved an elevation to a peaceful plateau in her young life by serving her husband until he died in their home. She said she couldn't understand why her husband's life had detoured from the happiness that prevailed at the beginning of their marriage to one of suffering illness relieved only by death. Despite the inability to understand why the man she loved was picked from the crowd of men inhabiting the earth to suffer and die so young, she professed that serving him during his life brought meaning to her life. She would not have understood that meaning without him.

The young recently widowed woman recounted while sobbing that Davy had been such a happy, positive, and innocent person. Her husband had assured her, she tearfully professed, that hemophilia could be managed, allowing them to enjoy a normal life without fear of bleeds, thanks to concentrates. But the medicine that he had seldom used harbored an unsuspecting threat, unaware to her husband. Despite the opportunities created by advanced medicine and health care, medical disaster struck a fatal blow to an innocent person. Davy had done everything the doctors had told him to do. He had followed the recommendation of Dr. Ned Strong, the hemophilia treatment center's oncologist, who specialized in AIDS treatment, by taking AZT when his T-helper cells became depressed and he became ill. And yet he wasted away and died. She wondered why. Why her husband? What went wrong?

After Davy's wife left the clinic, the treatment center staff talked with one another. They were grateful that Julie was HIV-negative; she had not become infected with the virus that claimed her husband's life. Somberly, almost helplessly, painfully wounded, Hanna, the social worker; Arnold, the physical therapist; Dr. Watson, the hematologist; Pearl and Myrna, the nurses; and Isabella, Josephine, and Katrina, the office staff, consoled one another. When they had tried with great dedication to create a facility that could offer relief from suffering and disability, replacing the threat of a short life with a possibility of a normal life expectancy, what went wrong? What had they done to violate the trust of Davy, who had depended on them? He had been a happy guy whom they had known since he was a little boy. He seldom infused with concentrate, yet it caused his death. He had not asked for much from them. He only wanted to have a normal life.

The burden of losing patients who were close to them, one after another, was heavy. They were weary. When would the loss of life within a medical center designed to save lives ever end? Who would be next? They felt devastated, helpless.

Airplane Mechanic from the Land of Chief Joseph

On the afternoon of September 8, 1989, silence was broken by the sound of *whup, whup, whup*—the flapping of helicopter blades beating the air above the hemophilia treatment center in the Southwest Hills of Portland. On a flattened hilltop in the clearing among the tall fir trees beside Gaines Road, a paved round pad was marked with a large white cross in the center of the black pad surrounded by a waist-high chain-link fence. Located across from the clinic, the fifty-foot-wide pad was the landing area for helicopters that brought critically ill patients to the university hospital from across the region—over the mountains, from the seashore, through the Columbia Gorge, up the Willamette Valley.

An ambulance waited beyond the fenced pad. A driver and two attendants stood beside a wheeled stretcher near the fence as the helicopter circled the pad, nose lowered, and then dipped over the landing pad. Dust and leaves whirled across the ground as the helicopter slowly descended, the sun glistening on its long metal fuselage. The side door of the craft opened, and a figure wearing a helmet and earphones stood in the doorway. After the black rubber-tired wheels hanging below the fuselage touched down onto the white cross, the revolutions of the engine diminished, and the turning of the overhead rotor decreased, then ceased, the long blades limply sagging. Quickly, the stretcher was wheeled through the fence gate to the open door of the resting aircraft.

A motionless, recumbent Randy Gibson—strapped to a stretcher, connected to IV tubing, his face covered with an oxygen mask—was gently handed from the helicopter personnel to the attendants beside the waiting stretcher. Randy was transferred by Life Flight from the La Grande hospital three hundred miles away, where he had been admitted after his condition had deteriorated in his home. He was quickly transported in the ambulance the short distance to the university hospital on the north hill, where a team of doctors intensely treated him for AIDS.

Randy recovered and returned home.

One year later, Randy again developed generalized system failure, the effect of AIDS. He was readmitted to the university hospital. His father rushed to the hospital from their home on Hurricane Creek. His mother said that while she was at home near Joseph, the nurses at the hospital told her on the telephone that Randy was responding to treatment. Other relatives drove to Portland to be at his bedside. The medical report indicated that Randy would be discharged the next day to return home. But prior to the next day, and before the relatives arrived, Randy quietly died in the hospital on October 5, 1990, at age twenty-five years.

Two years after Randy died, in 1992, his wife, Cindy, also died of AIDS. They are buried beside each other three miles east of Joseph, in the Joseph cemetery, where Cemetery Road turns off Imnaha Road.

The valley where the two small towns of Wallowa County—Enterprise and Joseph—are nestled in northeastern Oregon is pristine, enchanted, a heavenly kingdom. Wallowa County is the only county in Oregon without a traffic light. The gentle, wide valley is intensely green, guarded by sharp mountain peaks of the Wallowas, rising like sentries, hooded with snow, beneath a blue clear sky. The Wallowas, once the land of Chief Joseph and the Nez Perce, accessible only on foot or by horseback, is a roadless wilderness, where the fresh, cool mountain air is inspirational.

On the way to visit Randy's surviving parents in their country home south of Enterprise, off Hurricane Creek Road, during the long daylight of a June evening in 2008, we drove down a narrow lane with wire fencing stretched between wooden fence posts on both sides of the roadway. After crossing Hurricane creek on a small one-lane bridge with a planked driving surface, without guardrails, the Gibsons' house appeared. Hurricane Creek is aptly named—it was bursting with energy, full of clear, cold mountain water from the spring runoff of the melting snow in the nearby mountains, producing a soft tumbling sound.

David and Sharon Gibson live in the single-story home they built in 1973, the home where Randy and his brother spent their boyhoods. The threshold of the Gibson home directly faces the Wallowas viewed to the south, a short distance away, across a level green pasture where a few horses graze with two cows that will become the Gibsons' supply of beef for their dinner table when the calendar indicates that autumn has arrived. The Gibsons greeted Dr. Taillefer and his wife, Pierrette, warmly at the front door.[66] They had not seen one another for eighteen years, when Dave was fifty years of age.

Dave, now sixty-eight years of age, and a suntanned Sharon, both revealing healthy, fit appearances, were casually dressed in Wranglers and Western-style shirts, their cowboy boots sitting inside the front door. They said they were pleased that the doctor and his wife had

---

66 Interview with Dave and Sharon Gibson in their home on Hurricane Creek, June 17, 2008

driven all the way from Portland to see them. "I wasn't sure I would recognize you," Dave confessed. "It's been a long time."

Dr. Taillefer responded by acknowledging the great distance the Gibsons had traveled numerous times when their son Randy attended the hemophilia center in Portland, three hundred miles to the west, across the state of Oregon. How little the persons in the center in Portland realized the distance and effort the parents had made to bring their son to the clinic, Dr. Taillefer indicated after his arrival at the Gibsons' home.

"Oh my goodness, yes," Dave replied. "The doctor in the clinic would see Randy, prescribe a medicine or treatment, and say, 'Come back in two days if you're not better,' not appreciating the hardship of returning to the clinic from such a distance."

"I'm sure the doctors and nurses didn't appreciate the amount of effort required to bring Randy to the clinic. This visit is revealing, very rewarding," Dr. Taillefer replied.

"Come on in," Sharon said, smiling, holding the front door open for Pierrette. "Did you have any difficulty finding our house?"

"Not at all. Dave gave us good directions on the telephone. I have been along Hurricane Creek Road, although it was years ago."

"I remember in the years gone by, when we came to Portland to attend the clinic, and you told us you had camped with your family in the Wallowas along Hurricane Creek, at the campground between Chief Joseph Mountain and Ruby Peak," Dave replied.

"That's right," Dr. Taillefer said. "That was when my children were young, in the sixties. They could all be stuffed into a station wagon in those days—not anymore. They are grown-ups now. And now I have a different wife. This is my wife, Pierrette. She has a bit of an accent; she's from France."

Sharon and Dave were pleased to meet Pierrette. "Would you like to sit at the table?" Dave asked, suggesting that they have a seat at the dining room table. "You probably want to take some notes."

Sharon directed the conversation to Pierrette, whom she was meeting for the first time. "We don't know much about France except that it's a long way away. Not much around here to make us think of France. Would you like some water or some lemonade?"

"No, thanks. We had dinner in Joseph before coming to your house," Pierrette responded. "But you do have a reminder of France with you all the time."

"We do?" Sharon exclaimed with delight. "My goodness, I can't imagine what you're talking about."

"You are both wearing Wranglers, which are blue jeans made of denim," Pierrette responded. "The first cloth that was used to make blue jeans came from Nimes, a Roman town in the south of France. De Nimes translates to 'of Nimes' in French. The word denim in America comes from de Nimes in France. The word 'jeans' comes from the French word 'Genes,' for Genoa, a city in Northern Italy. Denim from Nimes was stained blue with indigo dye from Genoa to make blue jeans that have become Wranglers."

"Before we begin, I want to say how sorry I am that Randy died," Dr. Taillefer said with respect. "Everyone at the hemophilia center is sorry for the tragic death of Randy and Cindy. Randy is not here, but at any moment, I keep thinking he will come walking through the doorway. His death is so sad. It is unfair."

"Thank you," Sharon said. "It is sad."

"How long has it been since Randy died?"

"Eighteen years," Dave replied. "Randy died October fifth, nineteen ninety."

"He died of AIDS up at OHSU," Sharon said. "He had become ill and was admitted to the hospital. But I was told that he was getting better. In fact, the doctors said he would be coming home the next day. Suddenly, we had an unexpected telephone call telling us that he had turned for the worse."

"I rushed there as fast as I could, but it's a long way and requires hours to drive there," Dave said. "Others from the family also drove there, including Johnny, Randy's older brother. "But it was too late. Randy slipped away before we could get there."

"How old was Randy when he died?"

"Randy was born in Enterprise just before Christmas, December twenty-first, nineteen sixty-five. He was twenty-five years of age when he died in nineteen ninety."

"Was there anyone else in the family who had hemophilia before it was discovered in Randy? Did you know about hemophilia before Randy was born?"

"We didn't know about hemophilia until Randy was born," Sharon stated. "My sister and I are twins. No one else had hemophilia, and no else has since been born with hemophilia. I had a blood test done after hemophilia was discovered in Randy. They said I'm a carrier of hemophilia, but my sister isn't."

"How was hemophilia discovered in Randy?"

Sharon said, "Dr. Blackburn, the doctor in Enterprise, told us that after Randy was circumcised, he thought there might be something wrong. Randy bled more after his circumcision than he should have. But no tests were done at that time. The doctor didn't tell us of his suspicion until later."

"When was the first sign of bleeding that indicated he had hemophilia?"

"When Randy was learning to walk in nineteen sixty-six. He was just nine months of age. He stumbled and fell forward, bumping his mouth. He began bleeding from that little thing between his two upper teeth, inside his lip.[67] The bleeding wouldn't stop. Blood was all over the bedding … everywhere. I held my hand in his mouth to try to stop the bleeding. We called Dr. Blackburn. He said something was wrong and transferred Randy to the medical center in Lewiston, Idaho, a larger clinic with several doctors."

"That's a treacherous drive, after leaving Joseph, from Enterprise to Lewiston," Dr. Taillefer exclaimed. Oregon Road Number 3, which becomes Washington 129 at the Washington/Oregon border, covers the ninety-five miles distance between Enterprise and Lewiston.

---

67 Labial frenum

"We successfully completed the drive across the bridge over the Grande Ronde at the bottom of the canyon into Washington from Oregon, then to Idaho with a bloody, crying child," Dave recalled. "The doctors in Lewiston stuck a needle into his vein, collected a blood sample for later testing, and then hooked him up to the new medicine, cryoprecipitate, assuming Randy was a bleeder, that he had hemophilia. The doctor had telephoned the hemophilia center in Seattle, who advised giving the cryo without waiting for the results of the test for hemophilia. The doctors at the hospital quickly completed a prothrombin assay that was greatly prolonged, indicating that Randy had hemophilia. Cryo had only been discovered in 1964, just two years earlier, and it was successfully delivered by airplane to the Lewiston hospital. The bleeding stopped after cryoprecipitate was infused into a small vein on the top of Randy's forehead at the hairline. The doctor stuck a small needle right into the middle of his head."

After Randy was identified as affected with hemophilia, his parents bundled him into the car and drove to Lewiston for additional infusions with cryo for stopping his bleeds. Dave and Sharon sometimes made the treacherous drive in the darkness of night, despite the sharp curves. Randy's older brother, Johnny, once tossed a rock that unintentionally struck his little brother in the middle of his forehead. A huge, frightening swelling developed, prompting another trip for an infusion, this time a trip up Highway 195 to Spokane. At home, Randy would cry at night in his bedroom from pain, especially from bleeds into his elbows. His parents would attempt to comfort him, and then they would call Dr. Blackburn, in Enterprise, who would telephone the doctors in Lewiston or Spokane. Before Randy's arrival, they thawed and prepared frozen cryo to be ready upon arrival of the suffering child from the hurried trip to the doctor. Dave said that the infusions brought great relief and the end of pain.

As a young boy, Randy was always active, despite hemophilia and damage to his knees and elbows from recurrent bleeds. He enjoyed being outdoors with his father. At age eleven, he was hunting elk with his father, riding horseback, when he had a painful bleed into his leg.

The hunting party was down in a canyon along the Imnaha River, near the Nee-Me-Poo Trail when Randy began to suffer. But he didn't give up. Despite the agony, Randy rode his horse out of the canyon, returned home, and finally received an infusion to arrest his painful bleed.

In 1977, when Randy was twelve years of age, Dr. Blackburn in Joseph telephoned the treatment center, requesting help for Randy. Two nurses from the center drove the long distance to the Gibsons' home. Abby Hinckley and Sue Underwood instructed Randy's father how to infuse his twelve-year-old son with concentrates, which had become available by that time. David remembered that his son's veins were difficult to find. He had a vein on his left biceps that his father could poke pretty well. The Gibsons began keeping the medicine at home and infusing Randy whenever he had a bleed, avoiding the trip to the doctor in the middle of the night, which made a big change for the better in the family's daily life. After Randy began receiving infusions at home at the earliest sign of a bleed, his painful suffering was greatly reduced. By age fifteen, he had learned to infuse himself when he had a bleed.

"Being able to provide his own treatment for hemophilia enabled Randy to control his life; he was empowered," his mother offered. "He could do so many things. He suffered consequences as a result of the active life he desired, the life he chose."

While skiing, Randy had crashed into a tree and broken both legs. He spent six weeks with his legs enclosed in casts, spending his days on the davenport in the living room, but he didn't complain. He was always cheerful. Life for Randy had great meaning. Later, after the broken bones in his legs healed, he tripped and stumbled while walking across the floor of the high school gymnasium, breaking his femur and requiring yet another leg cast.

Randy continued to explore adventure in his youth. After the fractured leg bones were healed, he became a scuba diver. His mother recalled her alarm when she discovered that Randy and his friends had been scuba diving in the wintertime, wearing wet suits, in a frozen lake a few miles from their home. Wallowa Lake, at an elevation of 5,004 feet, develops a thick ice covering in the winter. Randy and his friends cut a hole through the ice, which allowed him entrance to the frigid water below the thick ice covering. She was especially alarmed when she learned that her son was not tethered with a line to the entrance hole in the ice. One of his friends stood atop the ice, whose silhouette was visible to Randy below the ice. Randy looked upward for the figure as it walked on the ice to guide him back to the entryway, where he could emerge from the icy waters to safety.

Who would imagine there was a person with hemophilia below the ice covering the remote frozen lake? Dr. Taillefer wondered.

Randy completed high school and enrolled as a student at Lane Community College in Eugene, quite a distance from his home. He finished the required instruction courses and passed the examinations to become a licensed aircraft mechanic. He was able to attend all his classes, not missing any, because he could infuse himself with concentrate whenever he had a bleed. Although his elbows were limited in motion, the result of recurrent hemorrhages as a child, he was capable of performing the necessary motions required to complete repairs on airplanes and airplane engines. Randy also proudly completed flying lessons and training to become a licensed private airplane pilot. After successfully completing training and required courses, he secured a job as an airplane mechanic at the Baker City airport in eastern Oregon. To improve ambulation by correcting the loss of motion in his knee, he was infused with concentrate, allowing surgery to be performed, a synovectomy, on his knee, which had been damaged from recurrent hemorrhages during childhood.

Randy married Cindy, a beautiful young woman from his high school, in 1985. He and Cindy enjoyed a good life together, a life free of pain and suffering by infusing concentrate to control bleeds. Prior to their marriage, Randy and Cindy were not tested for HIV. When Randy was tested for HIV after he and Cindy were married, unfortunately, he discovered he was HIV infected from the concentrate he had infused during the previous years. Although he was unaware of HIV infection, he probably had been infected for several years.[68] Randy informed his father that he was HIV infected. They did not tell Randy's mother until a year later. Cindy, Randy's wife, was tested for HIV, and she discovered that she was also HIV infected.

In 1988, at age twenty-three, Randy became ill. Weakness sapped his strength, which prevented him from continuing working at the Baker City airport. Despite his strong character, which had always sustained him from backing away from a challenge, he was forced to acquiesce to his illness. He and Cindy moved back to Hurricane Creek from Baker City. They made their home in a small house adjacent to his parents' property, where they quietly lived during the last two years, while Randy's life relentlessly slipped away. After Randy's HIV infection was discovered, an attempt to prevent progression to AIDS with AZT was unsuccessful. The combination of medicines, antiviral drugs, was not developed, which might have saved his life and Cindy's life, until several years later (HAART 2009).

Approved in 1987, AZT, zidovudine, also known as Retrovir, was the first drug to treat HIV infection. It was used alone in the 1980s, but resistance developed with progression of HIV infection to AIDS. With combination of antiviral drugs, AZT, as of 1996, is nearly always used as part of "highly active antiretroviral therapy" (HAART). This form of treatment has been designed to prevent mutation of HIV to a resistant form. Since then, AIDS has become regarded as a chronic illness rather than always fatal.

---

68 HIV tests completed on blood samples collected from hemophilia persons earlier and then stored, revealed that most persons who were infusing concentrate became infected between 1979 and 1982, before 1985.

"My, how things turn out differently than expected," Sharon remarked.

Dave continued, "Randy suffered from pain and agony from bleeds caused by his hemophilia. Nothing helped much when he was a small child. Then the sunshine appeared. Cryo became available to treat his bleeds. After cryo in the nineteen sixties, concentrate in the nineteen seventies brought good changes to his life."

Sharon emphasized her husband's remarks, saying, "He was able to treat himself at home. Randy finished high school, went to college, got a job, and married. His future seemed so bright."

"I never get tired of looking at those mountains and hearing the rush of Hurricane Creek," Dave said, looking out the window at the nearby Wallowas. "This tranquil setting of country living in such a magic area was always a delight to Randy. If he had lived, he could have continued enjoying it today. Randy was only twenty-five years of age when he died. But he lived fifty years in those twenty-five," Dave proudly quipped. "There was nothing he couldn't do. He tried everything."

"How do you explain the meaning of Randy's life?" Dr. Taillefer asked. "His life was cut so short. He was innocent. He was faced with death from conditions intended to improve the quality of his life, the result of concentrates, which were beyond his control. Was he desperate as he suffered while facing a fatal outcome, realizing there was no escape from certain death?"

"Oh, no, Randy was never depressed." Sharon spoke with enthusiasm while reflecting upon her son's life. "His cheerfulness despite suffering and an irreversible outcome demonstrated that Randy was capable of defying and braving even the worst conditions. He did not just exist as those cows do in front of our house. He made decisions based upon his freedom to choose, as a young man, and live an active life, bringing happiness to his wife, Cindy, and to us, his parents. The potential for overcoming harshness with endurance and bravery resides within all of us. But our choices for overcoming suffering are unpredictable. Those who discover meaning in their lives can endure great hardship, as demonstrated in my son. Now Randy and Cindy are resting together for eternity," Sharon sadly remarked.

On the mantelpiece of the living room, Randy and his beautiful wife, Cindy, are together in a photograph with Chuck, Randy's dog, lying at their feet (plate 9). Their pet was named in honor of a man whom Randy, as an airplane mechanic and pilot, admired: General Chuck Yeager. On October 14, 1947, General Yeager, as a test pilot flying the experimental Bell X-1 at an altitude of forty-five thousand feet, was the first man to break the sound barrier.

David and Sharon were asked, "When Randy was a little fellow, if he had a bleed and was suffering in pain and agony, would you have used the medicine even if you had known it was contaminated?"

"That's a tough question," David solemnly answered after thinking for a few moments. "You had to do something. He hurt so badly. You couldn't do nothing. Randy had to be helped somehow. I can't answer your question."

"Are your lives destroyed? Do you sit and think about *what if*? What if Randy had not died?"

"No, we are busy," they both replied.

"I rode in the saddle for three hours today," Sharon enthusiastically proclaimed with a big smile.

"Where did you ride to?" she was asked.

"I helped in a cattle drive," she proudly stated. "I'm a cowgirl."

The sixty-year-old Sharon rides her horse every day in the summertime. She recounted how she helps neighbors move cattle from one pasture to another. The summer pastures at higher elevations in the nearby Wallowa Mountains provide excellent grazing grounds, with abundant mountain meadows not accessible in the wintertime.

Dave continues hunting elk in the land of Chief Joseph. When she is not riding in the saddle on a cattle drive, Sharon keeps the large lawn in front of their home mowed twice weekly in the summertime, as the green grass grows to the edge of Hurricane Creek, a stream in a hurry to get down off the mountain. The beautiful rolling lawn extends down to the water's edge of the rapidly moving creek. On the bank of the creek grows a tree that was planted eighteen years ago in memory of Randy by his uncle and aunt, David and Leona Gridley. As they look out from the front of their home across the green pasture where they keep some cattle, and as they ride by Randy's tree in their front yard, they are reminded of their son and what might have been. What happened?

The pristine magical land of the Wallowas, the land of Chief Joseph and the Nez Perce people, witnessed a great amount of suffering when the white man invoked great tragedy, displacing the innocent people in 1875. This enchanted land again, one hundred years later, is the seat of another tragedy, the death of two innocent young people, the effect of the white man's behavior, the pollution of the blood supply by HIV and hepatitis, lethal viruses. Pretty places are not spared from the ravages of human aggression.

"Doctors are supposed to make people better," Dr. Taillefer said. "They are supposed to provide medicine that heals people. The doctors told Randy to take the medicine and he would have a good life. Instead, the medicine they gave to your son was polluted with a virus that killed him. Do you think the doctors are guilty for giving your son bad medicine?"

"We don't know," David replied. "If the doctors aren't guilty, they surely were wrong."

Sharon agreed with her husband.

"How do you think this happened—that the medicine for giving Randy a good life became contaminated with HIV, which killed him and his wife, causing them to die so young of AIDS?" they were asked by Dr. Taillefer.

"Oh, I don't know," Sharon replied. "They were innocent. They had nothing to do with the cause of getting AIDS."

"As far as I am concerned," Dave quietly stated, "both of them were murdered."

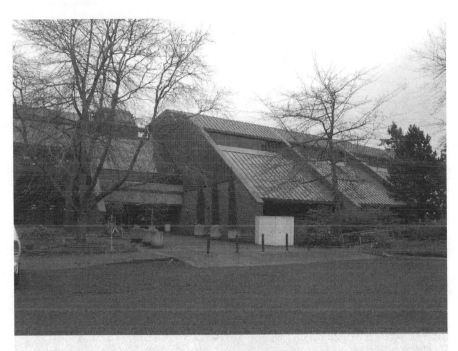

PLATE 1. HEMOPHILIA TREATMENT CENTER
CDRC BUILDING PORTLAND

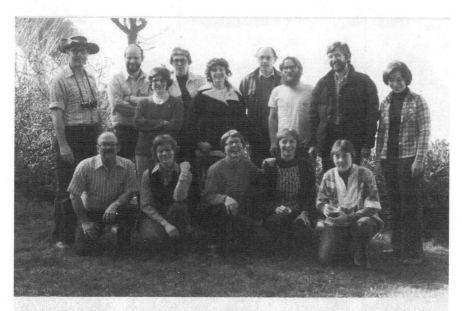

PLATE 2. GRANT WRITING RETREAT 1976

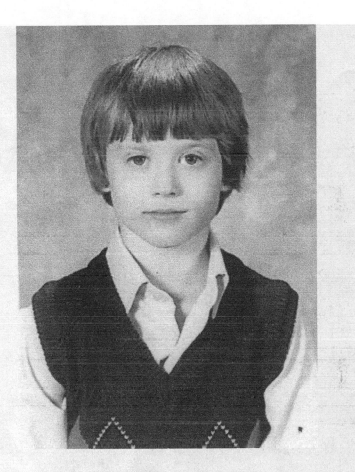

PLATE 3. JASON COBB
1975 - 1987
MOVED TO ALASKA
AHF INFUSIONS RESULTED
IN ILLNESS   DIED FROM AIDS
AGE ELEVEN YEARS.

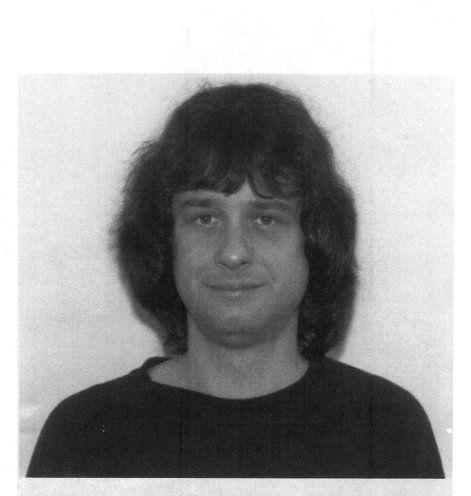

PLATE 4. ROGER NORMAN 1959 - 2003
HEAD BLEED AGE 5 YEARS
SURVIVED BRAIN SURGERY
DIED AGE 44 YEARS OF LIVER CANCER

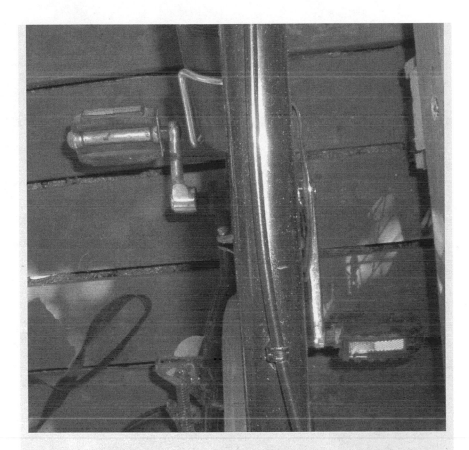

**PLATE 5. ROGER NORMAN'S BICYCLE
SHORT LEFT CRANK ARM
COMPENSATION FOR LACK
OF KNEE MOBILITY**

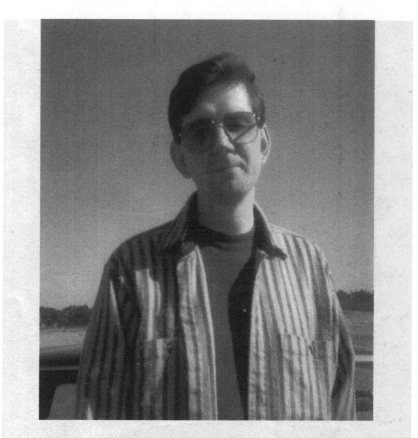

PLATE 6. JOHN WARREN 1958 - 1996
HEART SURGERY AGE SIXTEEN
DIED FROM AIDS
AGE THIRTY-EIGHT

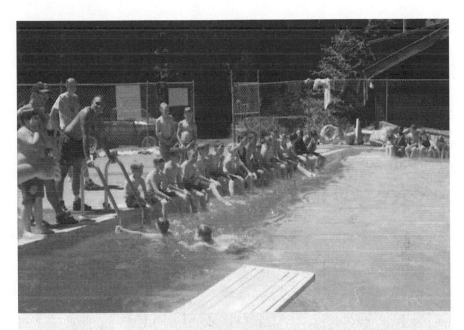

**PLATE 7. POOLSIDE CAMP TAPAWINGO
HEMOPHILIA SUMMER CAMP**

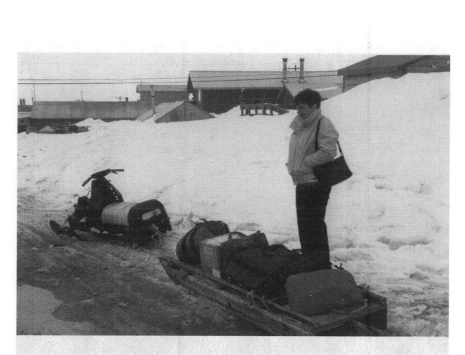

PLATE 8. HEMOPHILIA TREATEMENT CENTER NURSE MOVING SUPPLIES ON A SNOW SLED CHEVAK, ALASKA

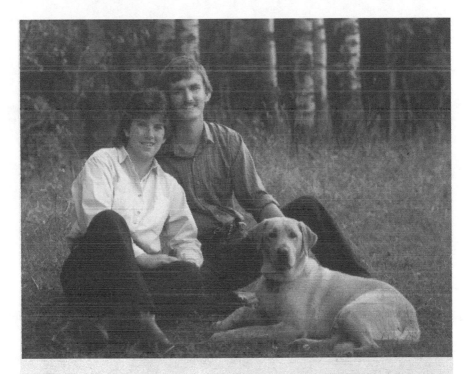

PLATE 9. RANDY GIBSON 1965 - 1990
OUTDOORSMAN, AIRPLANE MECHANIC
AIRPLANE PILOT
MARRIED CINDY 1985
RANDY DIED AGE TWENTY FIVE
FOLLOWED BY THE DEATH OF CINDY
THEIR DOG, CHUCK, WAS NAMED
AFTER GENERAL CHUCK YEAGER

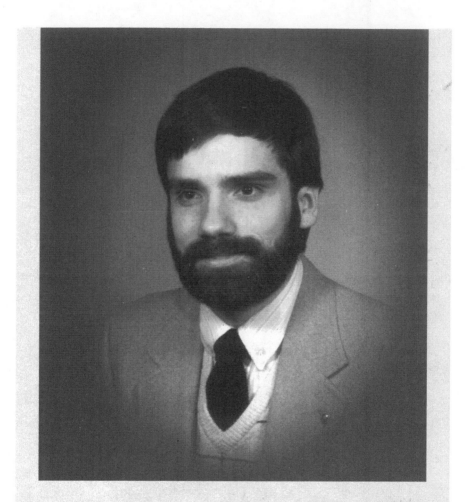

PLATE 10. DOUG MCALLISTER 1960-1991
SUMMER CAMP COORDINATOR
OREGON STATE UNIVERSITY DEBATER
CHILDREN'S SHOE STORE PARTNER
MARRIED 1990
DIED FROM AIDS AGE THIRTY ONE

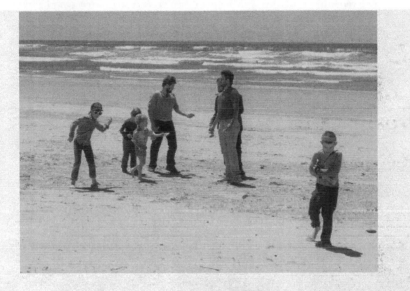

**PLATE 11. SUMMER CAMP
PACIFIC SEASHORE
COUNSELORS   BRUCE DESSELLIER
JOE KENNEDY, JOE SINGLER
SUMMER CAMPERS**

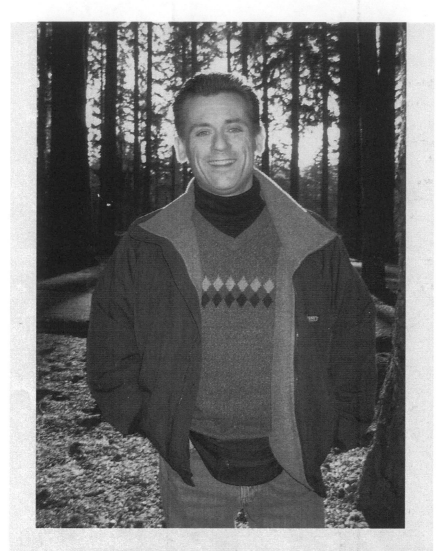

PLATE 12. MIKE CHARLES 1961 - 2005
DRUM AND BUGLE CORPS
SNARE DRUMS - CHOPS
DIED LIVER FAILURE AGE 44

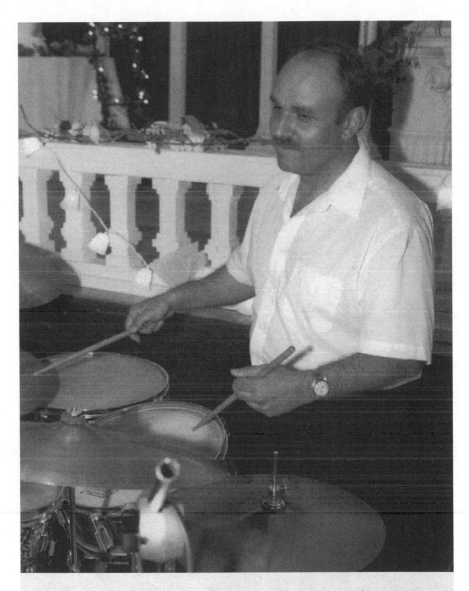

PLATE 13. DICK WAGNER 1957 - 2004
DRUMMER, MUSICIAN, FISHERMAN
PIANO REBUILDER
DIED OF LIVER FAILURE BEFORE
BLOWING UP OLD HOSPITAL CLOCK

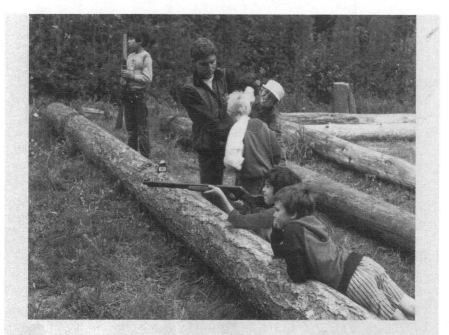

PLATE 14. DAVID WITBECK 1975 -1992
PETER WITBECK 1978 - 1992
BB GUNS AT SUMMER CAMP
BROTHERS DIED ONE DAY APART
AGES 17 AND 14 DAY AFTER CHRISTMAS

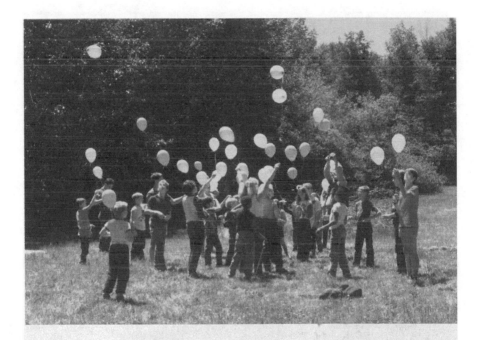

PLATE 15.   RELEASE OF BALLOONS
LIFTING MESSAGE HEAVENWARD
TO CAMPERS WHO DID NOT RETURN

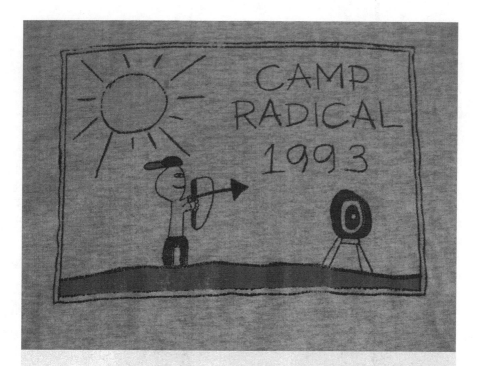

PLATE 16. CAMP RADICAL 1993 SUMMER CAMP SHIRT DESIGN BY RUSTY HARPER

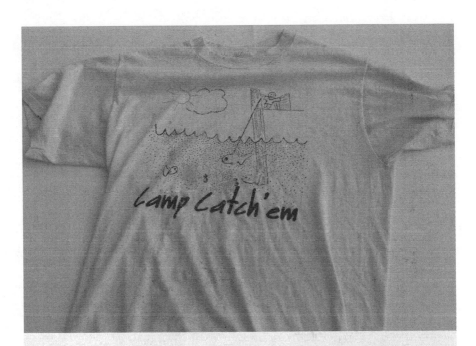

**PLATE 17. CAMP CATCH'EM
1990 SUMMER CAMP SHIRT**

Death of a Shoe Salesman

Marjorie and Jim McAllister were dismayed and unprepared when they discovered that both of their children, two sons, were affected with hemophilia. Their first son, Doug, was a Halloween baby, born October 31, 1960. He lived only to his thirtieth year, dying from AIDS in 1991. Their second son, Greg, was born in January 1964, four years after Doug. Five years after his birth, Greg died on Easter Sunday in 1969, not from AIDS but from hemophilia.

Doug was born in Gresham Hospital, a hospital that no longer exists. He was a large baby at birth, weighing ten pounds. When he cried and opened his eyes after coming into the world, a swelling was noted on his head. He had a hemorrhage into his scalp, a scalp hematoma. A blood transfusion was completed, followed by an increase in his active movements. The experienced doctor who delivered the infant recognized that a scalp hematoma was extraordinary, and circumcision was withheld. The anxious parents could not dismiss the unusual appearance of the prominent black and blue swelling on the head of their otherwise beautiful baby boy. They demanded an explanation. Was the discolored lump an ominous sign? Should the concerned parents be worried? By the time the infant was four months of age, the lump had disappeared. Without a doctor's referral, the parents carried their infant son to the university hospital for tests. Results of tests completed on a blood sample revealed grim information. Their son was affected with hemophilia. The McAllisters were surprised; no children with hemophilia had been born into their families in the past generations.

"The doctor laid out before us a negative course; he was not encouraging," Jim McAllister related.[69] After their four-month-old son was diagnosed with hemophilia, the McAllisters moved away from Oregon when Jim was awarded a scholarship to study at the University of Illinois. While living in Illinois, further tests were completed by a

---

69   Interview with Jim and Marjorie McAllister in their apartment, October 24, 2005.

branch of the Mayo Clinic, which confirmed the diagnosis of severe hemophilia. Following the completion of his training in public education, Jim McAllister, in 1962, accepted an appointment in Brookings, Oregon, a long distance from Illinois, but closer to the McAllisters' roots. Both parents, Jim and Marjorie McAllister, had completed training in special and public education. Brookings, a small community on the seacoast of southern Oregon, where the Chetco River opens into the Pacific Ocean fifteen miles north of the California border, was a remote place to live without adequate treatment for a child who has hemophilia. Cryoprecipitate was not discovered until two years later, and AHF concentrates had not been developed. Whenever Doug had a bleed after they moved to Brookings, local blood donors were summoned from the community, and whole blood was transfused into the infant. The blood transfusions were given slowly to avoid overloading the small infant's circulatory system, which could lead to heart failure.[70]

One wintry day in January 1963, after a bleed developed, Marjorie and her son were flown from Brookings, in Josephine County, in a small airplane over the Siskiyou Mountains, inland to Medford in Jackson County, a larger town with a regional hospital.

"I hope you will like your flight trip with me," the pilot, wearing a brown leather bomber jacket with sheep's wool lining, said. "The ride should be smooth. In the winter, the air is cold and dense; it is not bumpy as it is in the summertime. During the hot months of July and August, updrafts bounce the plane around when passing over a clearing in the forest," he continued.

The pilot walked around the airplane, inspecting the movable parts of the wings and tail section, also kicking the tires to make sure they were inflated properly. He advised Marjorie to keep her seat belt fastened, just in case they hit a bump. And to keep the child's belt tight

---

70   The concentration of clotting factor (AHF) present in whole blood is insufficient to restore blood clotting in a person who has hemophilia. Replacement requires isolation of AHF from multiple units of plasma that are pooled together into a small volume for an infusion. Blood transfusions are ineffective in treatment of hemophilia.

too. He gently informed her not to hold her son in her lap. Instead, he showed Marjorie how to strap the little fellow into his infant seat.

Thoughtfully, the friendly pilot cautioned, "And it may be a little chilly in this old airplane when we're up there. The heater ... sometimes she don't put out much heat."

After they were airborne, Marjorie discovered the pilot was correct. The interior of the four-place red and white high-wing Cessna airplane was cold. The cabin heater wasn't heating the cold air. Marjorie could see her breath from where she sat directly behind the pilot. As the airplane gained altitude to pass over the snowy mountain peaks of the Kalmiopsis Wilderness below, the cup of water that she was holding in her lap froze during the flight. Her small son remained safely strapped into his infant seat, bundled into a thick snowsuit to protect him from the cold. The dazzling snowy expanse visible below made her realize how isolated she and her family were from a medical center.

"It's gonna take us a little longer than I'd like," she heard the pilot say. "We're bucking a pretty strong headwind. In the summertime, the prevailing wind is from the coast, directed inland. But in the winter, the wind blows seaward from the land. We'll burn up a lot of fuel before we reach Medford." The drone of the engine seemed to lull the infant into an undisturbed sleep. Forty-five minutes after takeoff, the pilot shouted back to Marjorie, the worried mother, "That's a good sign," his voice muffled by the sound of the engine. "The Medford airport east-west runway is clear of snow. Be sure your seat belt is fastened tightly. We are going to set her down for a landing. It may be bumpy going down. And check your kid's belt too."

After that wintry flight to the hospital, the McAllisters concluded that they could not continue living in Brookings, a long way from medical help, if their son was to survive. They moved from Brookings to Medford, where better medical care was available. Dr. Allison, a pediatrician in Medford, assumed medical care of Doug.

In 1964, following the birth of their second son, Greg, while he was still in the newborn nursery of the Medford hospital, the newborn infant's heel was pricked to obtain a small blood sample, just a few drops, for completion of the required newborn blood tests. Soon after the heel prick, his parents were frightened when they observed that his heel began to ooze blood from the puncture site. They were shocked when they discovered that their second son also had hemophilia. For the second time, they thoroughly searched their family history. Neither preceding the two sons' birth nor since then have any other males been born into the family who had hemophilia. Marjorie's older sister has two daughters who have sons, and none are bleeders. Her mother had two brothers who were not bleeders. She discovered that her maternal great-great-grandmother had been a lady-in-waiting for Queen Victoria. Marjorie thinks her mother had some form of a bleeding tendency, and she has wondered if she had a Von Willebrand type of coagulopathy, which, unlike hemophilia, affects females as well as males.

At the time of the birth of their second son, Jim decided a change of careers would be best for his family. He accepted an appointment in the Oregon Department of Education and moved his family 250 miles north, from Medford to Salem, the state capital, a small city with good doctors and a modern hospital in Marion County, in the Willamette Valley.

On a Saturday in 1969, the youngest son, Greg, age five years, became very ill. He was hospitalized at Salem Memorial Hospital when his skin color turned to a sickening yellow, and the white sclera of his eyes also changed to yellow. The doctor thought he became jaundiced after contracting a hepatitis infection from a blood transfusion. He died on Monday, two days after he was admitted to the hospital. The cause of his death was from internal bleeding into his abdomen rather than from liver failure resulting from an acute hepatitis infection. Before Greg died, he had not suffered from recurrent joint bleeds like his older brother, Doug. He had no joint deformities. At the time of the youngest son's death, Doug was nine years of age. He had complications from hemophilia, damage to his joints and destruction of his hip. Doug's doctor, Dr. Birchman, a Salem pediatrician, advised the McAllisters to take their surviving son to the hematology department at the university hospital in Portland.

During their appointment at the university hospital in 1970, their second visit to that hospital, Jim and Marjorie were advised that the outlook for their son was not encouraging. They were reminded that life expectancy of boys with hemophilia was not favorable. They were discouraged after recently losing one son and then receiving bleak information about their surviving son. The hematology department recommended a get-acquainted visit at the hemophilia clinic. There, they met a compassionate nurse, Sue Underwood. Doug had recurrent joint bleeds and suffered from hip, knee, and ankle joint pain and deformity. He had Legg-Calvé-Perthes disease[71] of his hip, which began when he was six years of age. For one year, he had worn a leg sling to relieve weight bearing on the deformed right hip while walking with crutches or hopping on the left leg. At the time of Doug's hemophilia clinic visit, cryoprecipitate was available at the hospital and in the Clinic for treating joint bleeds in hemophilia, but was seldom utilized with infusions in the home by the parents.

The following year, Humafac, a concentrate manufactured by Parke-Davis pharmaceutical company, became available, which promoted infusions at home as a welcome reality. Previously, Hyland pharmaceutical company produced a freeze-dried concentrate, but it was not always available for uninterrupted home infusions. The Oregon hemophilia clinic adopted Humafac and began teaching families home infusion in 1971, as soon as the clinic was assured of an uninterrupted supply of concentrate. Marjorie quickly acquired the skill and knowledge for infusing her son at home with the welcome concentrate.

---

71 Legg-Calvé-Perthes disease occurs in childhood, when pressure on the blood supply to the head of the growing femur is compromised, resulting in avascular necrosis, characterized by destruction of cartilage and bone loss.

The Oregon Hemophilia Treatment Center began teaching families home infusion in 1971, when Parke-Davis produced Humafac. Each dose of this concentrate was provided in a small volume. Its availability was reliable.

Jim McAllister had maintained a residence in Salem while he was employed by the State of Oregon. He had been writing educational grant proposals. He and Marjorie decided it was time to return to their roots. They moved back to Gresham, where their lives had begun, and the town where Jim's father had been the Gresham city attorney. Jim opened a shop in Gresham, McAllister's Children's Shoes, with his son Doug. Marjorie capitalized on her educational background and accepted a position with the Reynolds School District as a facilitator for students who need special education.

With home infusion to treat bleeds, Doug attended school without missing classes. Whenever a bleed occurred, at the earliest sign, before severe pain developed, he was infused with concentrate at home. In 1978, he graduated from Gresham High School at age eighteen. After his graduation, Doug was accepted as a freshman student at Oregon State University in Corvallis. In his dormitory room, he infused himself with concentrate whenever a bleed occurred. Previously, Doug had been reluctant to infuse himself, preferring infusions by his mother. He abandoned his hesitation for self-infusion when he went off to college.

He became an active member of the Oregon State debate team. The team traveled to California for a debate. The team members crowded together into a van for the trip. During the night, when Doug was selected to drive the van filled with students, an unexpected treacherous icy patch was suddenly encountered on the highway in northern California. The van skidded off the road and flipped over in the ditch.

Although the van was not badly damaged, Doug was admitted to the hospital in Yreka for treatment of a bleed. His parents did not learn of the accident until later. Doug had his infusion kit with him in the van. He was able to be infused with the concentrate that he furnished to the hospital. He recounted the accident and the hospitalization later with an adventurous spirit and sense of humor.

Doug was a positive, upbeat person who had suffered a great amount of pain from recurrent joint bleeds and internal hemorrhages without ever complaining. Recalling his past suffering was not part of his conversation. His mother suspects that her cheerful son sometimes mismatched the color selection of the clothes because of his color blindness. He was tall and lanky, and he walked with an unusual gait because of his stiff leg. His legs were of unequal length. But that did not prevent him from standing in the kitchen before the stove, where he enthusiastically created one of his favorite dishes—pork pot roast garnished with delightful herbs, which he prepared with his characteristic smile. Doug had flashing dark brown eyes; he was delighted with his accomplishments. He was lighthearted, amusing, and recognized humor in otherwise challenging situations.

Doug received supplies for his infusions at home from the hemophilia treatment center, where he scheduled regular appointments for evaluations, always accompanied by cheerfulness and good humor. In 1984, when he was twenty-four, checkups at the clinic included HIV testing. One of the lots of concentrate Doug had used for infusions at home had been recalled; it was regarded as unsafe because of viral contamination. By the time of the concentrate recall, Doug's test results revealed he was HIV infected. He also had antibodies to non-A, non-B hepatitis, later known as hepatitis C. Doug and his parents were counseled at the hemophilia treatment center. Dr. Bercher, the center psychologist, informed them that he had been infected with HIV, the virus that causes AIDS, and that it would just be a matter of time before Doug's life would be over. Such a proclamation was very sobering, unwelcome information.

In 1984, AIDS was regarded as a universally fatal disease by CDC; however, Doug had no signs or symptoms of AIDS. He was well. A neat, well-dressed appearance was characteristic of Doug's presentation, reinforcing his positive image of himself. His dark hair was well styled, and he had a full beard and a moustache that he kept neatly trimmed (plate 10). Within the next two years, he began to lose weight and strength. He developed the features of slim disease, with weight loss and a wasted appearance. Relentlessly, HIV began exerting its unwelcome toll. Although he had lost a great amount of his physical reserve, Doug attempted to remain as active as his body would allow. Though his face became thin and his cheeks hollow, his brown eyes remained bright. Although his smile was often present, it seemed less spontaneous, as if smiling was a conscious effort.

One of Doug's passions, administered through the hemophilia foundation, was hemophilia summer camp. Although he had to struggle to overcome weakness, he attended Camp Tapawingo and interacted with Brent and the other young campers during their activities. Brent met Doug at Camp Tapawingo before Doug became ill, before he developed signs of AIDS, such as slim disease. When Doug returned to summer camp, the changes in his appearance were profound. An activity at the summer camp, arranged by Doug, Bruce Dessellier, and Joe Singler with the help of Arnold Deaton, the physical therapist and Wilbur Campbell, the camp director, was the AIDS memorial. The campers gathered in the grassy meadow by the riverbank, where colorful balloons were inflated with helium from a tall green cylinder and tied with a long string. Each camper wrote a note to a camper who had not returned from the previous year—the campers who had died of AIDS. Each message was fastened to a separate balloon with the long string. The inflated balloons were released together all at once, bearing the messages written on the papers tied by the string, rising to heaven (plate 15).

As the colorful balloons were released, Rusty Harper, a young camper from Pendleton, exclaimed with a flashing smile, "Look. See where my balloon is going. Now I know where heaven is. It's up there—that's where God lives." His red balloon glided upward through an opening in a white cloud, into the blue sky above, bearing the message he had written to a friend who had not returned, a friend who had gone to heaven. When Doug heard Rusty's remarks, he smiled, realizing that some pleasant moments could be achieved despite the unpleasant features of AIDS.

After Doug died in 1991, the camp AIDS memorial has continued each summer in memory of those who did not return to camp from the previous year. One of those not returning was Paul Aina, born January 4, 1982. He was infused beginning in infancy, prior to the introduction of heat-treated medicine in 1985. His first infusions preceded safe concentrate by only two years. If he had begun infusions just two years later, he would not have died from AIDS. When Paul was at camp in 1992, he was determined to ride a horse. The child was too small and too ill to be on a horse. Despite his illness and size, he was lifted up into the saddle by Arnold and Wilbur. The horse had taken only a few steps when Paul began to sob. His swollen belly was too painful to endure a horseback ride. Sadly, the young boy was gently lifted from the saddle, from his last horse ride. Paul had an enlarged spleen and a swollen liver, which caused great discomfort during the last days of his life, preceding his death from AIDS on August 3, 1993.

In addition to hemophilia summer camp, which provided great peace and respite from his illness, another encompassing passion for Doug was a lovely young woman named Kim, whom he had met at his church. Kim became his constant companion and supported him despite his illness. They were married in their church and lived together for one year and three months. Death from AIDS separated Kim and Doug in 1991, when Doug was thirty years of age. Kim did not become HIV infected.

After Doug's death, Jim and Marjorie McAllister recounted the impact their son had had on their lives, the rich experiences he'd contributed.[72] They also recalled the stigma associated with their son's AIDS. He not only suffered the unpleasantness of the illness and all of its effects, but he also suffered when people regarded AIDS as an affliction affecting gay persons. Doug was not homosexual. People were afraid to come near Doug for fear he would infect them with HIV.

Following Doug's death from AIDS, his parents were not angry—despite the premature deaths of both of their sons. However, they were disappointed by the slow response of the U.S. government and the pharmaceutical industry in addressing the threat of viral contamination of the medicine utilized by Doug and the rest of the persons affected with hemophilia. They do not blame their son's death on the doctors who prescribed the medicine that was contaminated with deadly HIV. They do blame the doctors and scientists who worked closely with the manufacturers of the AHF medicine.

"There was too much financial incentive," Jim McAllister professed when he explained why he was disturbed by doctors who served the pharmaceutical manufacturers in return for financial support, often disguised as grants for the doctors' research. "Research grants, cost of publications, travel to seminars, and attendance at meetings across the United States and in Europe were funded by the drug companies who produced the concentrate the doctors prescribed."

"Drug companies contributed funds for hemophilia summer camps, and their representatives served on the boards of hemophilia foundations," he continued. "The distance between the manufacturers of the expensive concentrates and the recipients was too narrow. The intimate contact of the drug company representatives created a compassionate image of the pharmaceutical manufacturers, whose real motive, to make a profit by selling costly concentrate, was masked by their friendly salesmanship tactics. Competition between drug companies was intense. Drug companies sought to be selected as the supplier of concentrates over their competitors. By serving on the local

72 Remarks from Jim and Marjorie McAllister in their apartment on October 24, 2005

hemophilia foundation boards, the representatives became acquainted with the clients and attempted to influence their choice of products by recommending their products over other brands of concentrate. The energy of the drug companies was directed toward marketing rather than improving the safety of their products."

Jim and Marjorie continued expounding in agreement with each other. "Free marketing and capitalism dynamically promote the development of desirable new drugs," Jim said. "However, when the primary goal of drug manufacturers is marketing for a profit, enterprise is sometimes tarnished by recklessness. Therefore, private enterprise that serves the public requires regulation and governance because of human nature. In the case of producing concentrates for treatment of hemophilia, there was not enough caution; instead, there was too much greed. The doctors and the government should have been more cautious. More regulation should have been implemented."

"America was left far behind compared to Europe in prevention of viral contamination in the plasma collected from blood donors," Jim continued. "Heat treatment of concentrate for viral deactivation was implemented for several years in Germany before acceptance in the United States."

Marjorie and Jim McAllister alleged that during the 1980s and 1990s, Europe lost fewer young men who were affected with hemophilia to AIDS than the United States did.

The McAllisters solemnly proclaimed that American drug companies who manufactured the concentrate Doug required to treat his bleeds were careless in procuring blood from paid donors, including some who were IV drug users, which resulted in contamination of the pooled plasma supply. They were greedy, driven by a profit motive to satisfy their shareholders and CEOs at the expense of a few but important numbers of persons who had hemophilia.

The pharmaceutical manufacturers have recently introduced concentrate produced by genetic methods utilizing molecular and recombinant techniques that are regarded as safe without risk to humans of viral contamination.

"For every action, there follows a reaction," Jim cautioned. "What will happen to the present generation of persons who have hemophilia? We have concerns. Marjorie and I hope and pray to God that nothing ominous happens. But the present treatment of hemophilia must include the necessary wisdom to stay ahead of developments and be cautious to assure lives of quality. The medical doctors must remain diligent and scrutinize the production of medications. The doctors must not take for granted that a profit-motivated pharmaceutical manufacturer will always incorporate all of the necessary safety procedures."

> Just as there is separation of church and state in America, there must be separation of medical practitioners and drug companies.

Jim and Marjorie McAllister lost two sons. The first son they lost, the doctor said, had hepatitis and became jaundiced and died of liver failure. The doctor was wrong; their son bled into his belly and died from internal bleeding. As for the second son they lost, the doctors said he would live to be an old man if he took his medicine, concentrate. The doctors were wrong. The concentrate he infused was contaminated with HIV, which killed him.

Doctors can be wrong.

I Am Free

Most married men who became HIV infected from the concentrate they infused to treat their hemophilia had wives who did not become HIV infected. One of the young men whose wife did become HIV infected was Randy Gibson. His wife, Cindy Gibson, died of AIDS after her husband's death. At the time of Brent's death in 1993, many men who had been infused with concentrate prior to 1985, when heat treatment was included in its production, were dying. Some had married, leaving a widow and children to mourn their loss. When HIV infection became a recognized threat to the men who had hemophilia in the 1980s, the CDC cautioned hemophilia treaters that all the wives of HIV infected men would, or already had, become HIV infected. The passage of time has revealed that the outcome of the marriages has been different. Most wives of HIV infected men who had hemophilia did not become infected with the virus.

Joe Singler was eleven years older than Brent. Joe, like Doug McAllister and Joe Kennedy, was a counselor at hemophilia camp, where he and Brent met during summer camp. He enjoyed supervising the activities of the young campers, especially when they were on an outing to explore the Pacific seashore (plate 11). Unlike Brent, who died at seventeen, Joe lived until he was thirty-nine years of age. He died November 15, 2003, ten years after Brent died. Joe married. He and his wife, Tammy, had two children, a girl and a boy, Tasha and Joe III. Although Joe was HIV infected, Tammy did not become HIV infected. She did not become ill. Despite their father's infection, two children were conceived; their mother escaped infection, and the children did not become HIV infected. They are both well. Joe's son was a casket bearer at his father's funeral. Joe's father, who is also named Joe, was also a casket bearer. At the funeral, Joe I and Joe III, son and father of Joe II, were two of the eight casket bearers. The three generations of Joe Singlers are referred to as Big Joe, Joe, and Little Joe. Only Little Joe and Big Joe remain.

Joe is now free. Free of the burden of hemophilia and AIDS. His freedom was reflected in his eulogy at the memorial service for him at Hillside Chapel in Oregon City:

I'M Free

Don't grieve for me now, I'm free,
I'm following the path God laid for me.
I took his hand when I heard him call,
I turned my back and left it all.
I could not stay another day
To laugh, to live, to work or play.
Tasks left undone must stay that way.
I've found my peace at the close of day.

If parting has left a void,
Then fill it with remembered joy,
A friendship shared, a laugh, a kiss.
Ah yes, these things I too shall miss.
Be not burdened with times of sorrow.
I wish you the sunshine of tomorrow.
My life's been full, I savored much,
Good friends, good times, a loved one's touch.

Perhaps my time seemed all too brief.
Don't lengthen it now with undue grief.
Lift up your heart and share with me,
God wanted me now, He set me free.

Joe's brother, Tim, also was born with hemophilia and developed AIDS following HIV infection from contaminated concentrates. No other persons were born with hemophilia in the family—only the two brothers, offspring of Mary—despite her large sib ship. Her mother, Joe's grandmother, had fourteen pregnancies, giving birth to eighteen children, including four sets of twins.

Although Joe Singler, Randy Gibson, and Doug McAllister became infected with HIV at nearly the same time, in the early 1980s, Randy died in 1990, and Doug died in 1991. Joe died in 2003, thirteen years later. All died of AIDS, and all three of the HIV infected men married. Not all three wives became HIV infected—only Randy's wife did. She died of AIDS two years after Randy died. Neither Joe's nor Doug's wife became HIV infected. They have remained well.

Part IV

Differing Effects of HIV and Hepatitis

Treating AIDS

Rhythm from the Drum and Bugle Corps

Present at the memorial services for Joe Singler on November 20, 2003, were several of his friends who also had hemophilia, whose lives had not been claimed by hepatitis or AIDS. Gatherings in the past years for boys, men, and their families who had hemophilia had been at meetings and events of the Oregon Hemophilia Foundation, hemophilia summer camp, and at the hemophilia treatment center. The occasion for gathering changed with the effects of HIV and AIDS. Funerals and memorial services became frequent meeting places.

Mike Charles was one of the friends who came to say good-bye to Joe Singler that November day in Oregon City. Mike had known Brent at hemophilia summer camp. He also knew Brent's family through the Hemophilia Foundation of Oregon, where he had once served as president. Brent had died ten years earlier, in 1993, from AIDS. Mike and Brent became infected with HIV from infusions to treat recurrent bleeds of hemophilia during the same years, before 1985, the era when concentrate contained HIV and hepatitis viruses. If Brent and Mike were infected at the same time, why did Mike live ten more years than Brent? A suggestion has been offered that the length of time between HIV infection and the onset of AIDS may be related to the age of the person at the time of HIV infection. A young child who becomes infected from infusions with HIV-contaminated concentrate may develop AIDS sooner than an adult who becomes HV infected. Many examples of death in infants from AIDS have been noted in children born of HIV infected mothers in Africa.

Mike was born October 11, 1961, fourteen years before the birth of Brent. He received his first infusion of concentrate in 1975, at age fourteen. Brent received his first infusion of concentrate in 1976, when he was six months of age. For the next ten years, Brent and Mike both received multiple infusions of concentrate to treat their recurrent bleeds, prior to introduction of deviralization by heat treatment.

In 1998, at age thirty-seven, Mike married Linda. They moved into their home together in Vancouver, Washington, in 1999. When they purchased their home, they inherited a cat named Tweet-Tweet. The previous owner of the home related that the cat was happy only in that house and refused to move to a new residence. Mike and Linda agreed to accept the cat with the house. They changed the cat's name to Jar-Jar, which the cat didn't seem to mind.

Excessive bleeding following circumcision was the first sign of hemophilia for Mike. Although there was considerable loss of blood, he was not transfused; hemophilia was not suspected then. Bruises appeared on his body as a small infant. After he was lifted from his infant crib and held, a large bruise, the shape of a handprint, was discovered on his small back. The family, who lived in Gresham, Oregon, received medical care from Kaiser Hospital, who referred them to Dr. Rutherford Skyles at the university hospital. At age six months, a blood sample was successfully collected. Test results revealed severe hemophilia, type A, factor VIII deficiency.

Mike's bleeding episodes in the 1960s were neatly recorded by his mother during infancy and childhood, listing the sites of his bleeds, the intensity of pain he suffered, the amount of swelling and discoloration. He suffered a bleed beneath his tongue from an injured frenum. He bled into his arms and legs as well as his face. The recurrent hemorrhages, before concentrates became available, were treated by applying ice packs to the bleeding area of his small body and immobilization with splints, slings, and bandages. When he suffered from the worst bleeds, he was admitted to Kaiser Hospital and infused with thawed-out fresh frozen plasma, without noticeable improvement. Plasma is not effective for persons who have hemophilia type A. He cried, having such severe pain that he would not eat and could not sleep. He would not move for days, until finally the swelling in the leg or arm diminished and returned to normal, followed by the next painful episode. Usually, it was several weeks before another bleed ravaged him, sometimes only days. When Mike was four years old, in 1965, cryoprecipitate became available for infusions to treat the painful bleeds. When cryo was infused at the hospital, a big difference was noticed within a few hours after the infusions. Bleeding subsided, swelling diminished, and pain relented   in contrast to the experience after infusions with plasma, when little improvement was noticed. Mike's mother emphasized that cryo was a great advance in treating hemophilia, bringing relief from suffering.

At eight years of age, Mike suffered from the worst bleed he'd ever experienced. An intense headache, sensitivity to light, and a painful neck were signs that directed the doctors to perform a spinal tap, a lumbar puncture, which revealed bloody spinal fluid. He had a bleed somewhere in his brain. The source of bleeding was never identified during the one month of hospitalization in the medical school hospital at OHSU. After daily infusions with cryo, he gradually improved, recovered, and went home. By age ten years, the location of bleeds no longer randomly involved his body. He developed target joints, which were his ankles. The doctors instructed him to stick his foot into a bucket of crushed ice to treat ankle bleeds. With his foot in a bucket of ice, he couldn't elevate his leg; therefore, swelling ensued.

The new "miracle medicine," Humafac concentrate, became available from the treatment center in 1971. Mike began receiving infusions with Humafac in 1972. In 1973, when he was twelve years of age, Mike was selected as the poster boy for the magazine published by the National Hemophilia Foundation, which promoted the new magic medicine.

In 1975, at age fourteen, sufficient commercially prepared concentrate was available, which allowed Mike to learn the procedure for infusing himself at home to treat recurrent bleeds. "Concentrate at home was a miracle, like magic," Mike professed.[73] No longer was it necessary to telephone the doctor, drive to the hospital emergency room, and wait while frozen cryo was thawed for the infusion before he experienced relief from a bleed. With infusions at home, he could treat bleeds at the earliest signs, before he was laid up. He no longer missed classes in school while suffering for days, as he had before he began infusing himself at home. Enabled by concentrates, he went backpacking for the first time and had a great adventure discovering the out-of-doors, seeing nature as he had never seen it before.

Mike attended Gresham High School, the same school Doug McAllister had attended. He developed a passion for music that sustained him during his high school years, a passion he carried with him when he attended Mt. Hood Community College following high school. As a musician, he became a percussionist with a love for snare drums. He became involved in music ministry, attending a large nondenominational church that featured an orchestra. His music horizon expanded as he began playing drums in a Portland drum and bugle corps. Mike graduated from Gresham High School in 1979, a year after Doug McAllister's graduation. He was selected to present the graduating seniors' commencement speech. He said it was a hard act to follow after U.S. Senator Packwood's commencement address.

One year later, he made trips north to Seattle and became a member of The Imperials, a Seattle drum and bugle corps. During the summer of 1980, at age nineteen, Mike traveled to thirty-eight different states in a bus with The Imperials, completing a seven-week U.S. circuit of drum and bugle corps competitions. They performed in Casper, Wyoming, one day, traveled at night in their bus, and performed the next day in Denver, Colorado. The bus left Denver and traveled all night to Texas for a performance the next day. "Every day," Mike recalled, "was practice and more practice, whenever we were not on the road." Mike developed his favorite style—his musical chops. The

---

73 Comments from an interview with Mike Charles and his wife, Linda, in their home January 19, 2004

bus bearing Mike and The Imperials continued on to the National Drum and Bugle Corps Championships at the University of Alabama in Birmingham. As a member of the music team, a long, circuitous route was completed, extending from the Northwest to the South, through the Midwest, to the East Coast of the United States, arriving in Birmingham seven weeks after The Imperials began their overland bus tour. He packed concentrate and supplies for infusions on the bus, which he used whenever he had a bleed. He was able to keep active, participating in all the events without any downtime from a bleed.

"The travel and the performances with the Seattle Imperials was a great experience, a highlight of my life," Mike proudly proclaimed.

When Mike passed his twenty-first birthday, he was forced to retire from the drum and bugle corps. "It's called 'aging out.' It's like the Cub Scouts; you have to give it up," he related with regret. He followed his musical career after the drum and bugle corps travels by attending the annual drum and bugle corps contests as a spectator. After he first met Linda, one of the activities they shared was attending the drum and bugle corps performances in San Francisco. "Linda liked it. The performance turned her on. She really got into it." Mike beamed. After Mike and Linda were married, he realized that he couldn't keep his drums—they required too much space, made too much noise, and demanded too many hours of practice for a married man. "Who needs a drum set in the house?" Mike offered. He continued playing drums from time to time and wanted to continue his music as long as his elbows allowed him to play.

After Mike had turned twenty, in the early 1980s, he wasn't infusing as often as he had in the preceding years. He infused about once every ten days, usually for an orthopedic problem, especially an ankle bleed. He heard discussion within the hemophilia community concerning the possible threat of a contaminant in the blood supply, which perhaps was polluting the concentrate he was infusing to treat his bleeds. Mike regularly attended the hemophilia treatment center. He was well except for his orthopedic problems. The center offered a blood test to discover if a person had become infected with an infectious substance, which subsequently became known as HIV, even if he was not ill. At the clinic, he also learned that the blood test was not completely reliable.[74]

Mike reasoned that if he was destined to become infected with the mysterious disease from an infusion of tainted concentrate, he was probably already infected. He had been infused many times. Mike was well informed and knew that transmission of the virus that causes the disease occurred through sexual contact, but he was not sexually active at that time; therefore, he knew he would not spread the disease to anyone else. Although he assumed he was already infected with whatever the disease was, he did not lie awake at night worrying about it. "Knowing whether I was HIV-positive or HIV-negative was not necessarily useful information that would make my life better," Mike concluded when he thought about HIV. He knew some other hemophilia persons who were HIV infected, but despite their infection, they were well, not ill. Some of those persons were infusing with the same medicine he was using, and they were HIV-negative. He was surprised and wondered why some guys became HIV-positive, while others remained HIV-negative. "Why the difference? Someday, someone will tell me the reason. Until then, why worry about it?" he stated. Mike did not withhold infusions because of fear of the medicine. Some persons, he knew, were changing their infusions because they feared the threat from the new mysterious disease, but Mike did not feel threatened.

But there was a change of life for Mike. He became interested in a pretty young woman from his church and began dating her. He thought about marriage, thinking that someday he would like to marry. If he were to marry, he should know if he had been HIV infected. Although, at twenty-five years of age, he was well, without symptoms suggestive of AIDS, he reasoned that it would be best if he were tested, and he

---

74 The initial screening blood tests to establish HIV infection detected antibodies to HIV, an indirect test. If a person was infected within the past few days, an antibody response might not have occurred. Later, a more accurate test, the Western Blot test, directly detected the presence of HIV.

assumed he was HIV-positive. In 1986, a blood sample was collected from Mike for HIV testing. [75]

He waited until Myrna Campbell, the hemophilia treatment center nurse, and Dr. Taillefer called him back to the clinic to inform him of his HIV test results. He was HIV-positive. "I was not surprised to discover I was HIV infected," Mike emphasized. "There's a lot more to be discovered."[76] He left the clinic after being informed he was HIV infected and enjoyed a nice dinner at a restaurant with some friends. He wasn't worried about becoming ill from his HIV infection, about developing AIDS.

His biggest concern, the most troublesome, was ankle pain. Although he was HIV-positive, Mike requested orthopedic surgery to fuse one of his ankles. Ankle fusion was completed in 1987, after his clotting activity was restored to normal with infusions of concentrates. The surgical procedure did not result in improvement. The fusion of Mike's ankle bones was unsuccessful; it didn't take. Following the postoperative infusions of concentrate during healing after surgery, he continued to infuse concentrate once every ten days. He became president of the Hemophilia Foundation of Oregon, remaining active despite his disabling joints.

In 1989, at age twenty-seven, Mike utilized his college training. He had graduated in broadcasting and communications from Mt. Hood Community College, where he received excellent instruction in a highly rated curriculum. He became employed as a monitor of television stations. After his marriage to Linda, he changed procedures and began monitoring radio stations from his home. Using equipment in the office in his home, Mike was capable of listening to ten or twelve radio stations simultaneously, which occupied him until he retired in 2002 at age forty-one.

75 In 1986, the Western Blot test for HIV became available at the Hemophilia Treatment Center. The improved test is not an antibody test but a test that directly detects the presence of the coat of the HIV virus.
76 January 19, 2004, interview with Mike Charles

By age thirty, in 1991, Mike's hemophilia was under control. His joints, damaged from bleeds during his youth, no longer bled. They were only stiff and painful. He rarely had a full-blown bleed anywhere in his body. He felt well, without signs of illness (plate 12). He continued to attend the treatment center for scheduled periodic checkups. New tests were adopted by the clinic as more experience was gained from providing care for HIV infected persons—tests that monitored the medical condition of a person at risk of becoming ill—so that guided intervention treatment could begin. Dr. Ned Strong, the center's hematologist, who specialized in oncology, directed Mike's HIV medical management. Mike felt well, without signs suggestive of impending AIDS illness, despite his HIV infection. He had been infused with concentrates for twenty years. Blood test results revealed that his T4-helper cells were diminished. Low T4-helper cells are an indication of damage to the immune system.

In his midthirties, Mike was enrolled in a double-blind research study designed to evaluate the effectiveness of AZT in preventing progression of HIV infection to AIDS. At the beginning of the study, Mike's T4-helper cells measured $238/mm^3$, compared to a normal range of $500–1,500/mm^3$. He began receiving 1,500 milligrams of AZT each day, intended to keep him well by preventing progression of HIV infection to AIDS. After beginning the study, he became ill. "I felt terrible after the AZT study began," Mike confessed. Mike was in the real drug arm of the study, not the placebo group. Other research investigators determined that the proper dose of AZT is only one-fifth the amount of the drug Mike was receiving. His AZT was reduced to 200 milligrams daily. His T4-helper cells reached a plateau of $200–250/mm^3$ but subsequently declined to $50/mm^3$, a dangerously low level, an indication of a badly damaged immune system.

Medical problems other than bleeds from hemophilia confronted Mike. A blood test revealed a low platelet count: $8,000/mm^3$, compared to a normal platelet count of $250,000/mm^3$. With such low platelets, he was at risk of a hemorrhage, not from deficient clotting factor from hemophilia but from a leaking blood vessel, especially in his brain. To discover the cause of Mike's low platelets, the doctors performed a bone marrow aspiration—three different times. His body was making platelets in his bone marrow normally, but his spleen was destroying the new platelets.[77] He was transfused with platelets, but they were quickly destroyed in his spleen. The platelets he needed to prevent leaks from his blood vessels were not surviving. The doctors discussed surgically removing his spleen. However, the spleen is necessary to prevent infections. He already had a compromised immune system. A splenectomy would have created new risks; his spleen was not removed. Gradually Mike's platelet count increased to 50,000 /mm^3, low but not dangerous.

He became fatigued and noticed that his leg had become swollen. He could no longer work. He had pains everywhere in his body. Because his painful leg continued to swell, he was hospitalized. He became gravely ill and almost died before the doctors discovered he had a staphylococcal infection of his hip.[78] After intense intravenous antibiotics, his blood- clotting activity was restored to normal to allow hip surgery to clear the infection from his hip socket. He survived the surgery, recovered, and went home with most of his right hip dissolved by the infection.

Following recovery from the hip infection, Mike became jaundiced and constipated. "I was confronted with what became ninety percent

---

77   The spleen is the organ in the body where old red blood cells are destroyed to allow the contents, the iron, to be recycled to make new hemoglobin, which transports oxygen in the blood. When the spleen becomes congested and overactive, hypersplenism results. Usually the cause of hypersplenism is a swollen liver, resulting in a backup of blood flow from the spleen to the liver. Platelets passing through the circuitous route of the congested spleen are trapped and destroyed. Removal of the spleen may help prevent destruction of platelets, but removing the spleen is risky and places the person at increased risk of infections.

78   Life threatening infections are common in HIV infected persons whose immune systems are damaged.

of my health problem—hepatitis," Mike related. "I had never been jaundiced before. I knew I had liver damage; my liver function enzymes were abnormal. That was something my doctors and I took for granted from the number of infusions of concentrate I received during my life." Mike then said, "I don't know how many times I have been infused, probably two or three thousand times in my lifetime. Before 1985, when I turned twenty-four, most of my infusions were with Cutter's Koate, which was polluted with hepatitis viruses and HIV. After 1985, I was infused with Koate HT, which no longer contained live viruses."

Mike was asked if the number of infusions he had received could be tallied from the bleed sheets. He was required to fill out a bleed sheet, each time he was infused, and he was supposed to submit accumulated bleed sheets to the hemophilia treatment center whenever he was issued a supply of concentrates. The results on the bleed sheets were entered into a database. By inspecting the results compiled from the bleed sheets, the information could alert the treatment center when problems such as a target joint developed. Prophylactic infusions could be used to prevent frequent bleeds and avoid further joint damage. Mike smiled and said, "Bleed sheets were a big joke." He laughed. "I became tired of filling out bleed sheets, hundreds of them ... or even thousands. I knew that I would be required to turn in bleed sheets whenever a clinic appointment was scheduled. If I didn't turn them in, I was threatened with refusal for a continued supply of concentrate. 'No ticky, no juicy' the saying went. The clinic told me that accountability was necessary for the expensive medicine I had used since the previous clinic visit." Mike continued, recounting that the times when a scheduled clinic visit approached, he would fill out all the forms at once. Instead of completing the form at the time of infusion, providing accurate information listing the site of his bleed and the amount of concentrate infused, he "batched them," filling out twenty or thirty bleed sheets at one time. "Bleed sheets were the subject of countless discussions among my friends at hemophilia summer camp," he said. "They were all doing the same thing—'Garbage in, garbage out.' If the doctors wanted to know if I had a target joint, all they needed to do was ask me."[79]

After Mike's skin turned yellow with jaundice and the odor of his breath became foul, he became delirious, as if he were in a coma. When he was rehospitalized, tests revealed high amounts of ammonia in Mike's blood. Ammonia is a sign that the liver is damaged and cannot provide the necessary enzymes to digest proteins. Mike recalled being told that the general anesthesia for his hip surgery and the staphylococcal infection had added further damage to his already sick liver, which had previously been damaged by hepatitis.

Mike's wife, Linda, said, "At the hospital, I was cautioned that Mike was dying. He wouldn't live another week. I was told to get his affairs in order." But Mike did live. He survived to be sent home, where Linda cared for him.

"The pain I have in my hip nearly sends me through the roof. I don't know if the infection in my destroyed hip is gone or if it is still smoldering. So I am directed to continue taking dicloxacillin, which makes me sick to my stomach. I don't feel well. My hip hurts, and I feel sick all over my body, even though I am taking many medications to fight AIDS." Mike discussed his complicated medical treatment directed by the treatment center. Doctors discovered that AZT by itself did not prevent progression to AIDS in HIV infected persons. The virus mutated and became resistant to AZT. Since that realization, survival of persons who developed AIDS has been extended by HAART therapy (HAART 2009). AIDS is no longer regarded as a universally fatal illness; it has become a chronic illness from improved treatment using multiple drugs. Mike's HAART regimen and the other medicines he was prescribed—twelve different medicines, seven different pills to swallow two times each day, four different pills once daily, and one each week—required full time attention.

---

79 This comment and the following quotes in this section are from the continued conversation with Mike Charles and his wife, Linda, in their home on January 19, 2004.

Mike Charles's HAART medicines and his other medicines			
Zerit (stavudine)	40 mg	twice daily	HIV cocktail
Epivir (lamivudine)	150 mg	twice daily	HIV cocktail
Viread (tenovir)	300 mg	once daily	HIV cocktail
Norvir (ritonavir)	100 mg	twice daily	HIV cocktail
Angernase (amprenavir)	400 mg	twice daily	HIV cocktail
acyclovir	800 mg	twice daily	prevent herpes zoster
SMZ/TMP	400/80 mg	once daily	prevent pneumocystis
spironolactone	50–100 mg	once daily	for leg edema
Zithromax (azithromycin)	1200 mg	once weekly	prevent toxoplasmosis
dicloxacillin	500 mg	twice daily	staphylococcus
Oxycontin (oxycodone)	140 mg	twice daily	joint pain
Celexia (citalopram)	20 mg	once daily	depression

"I do not know the origin of HIV, which causes AIDS. But I do know how I became HIV infected. It was from concentrate." Mike said he distinguished between the drug companies, the pharmaceutical manufacturers who produced concentrate and the doctors and clinics who treat hemophilia patients. "Hemophilia treaters were not just new, young doctors fresh out of medical school. They were doctors who devoted their lives to taking care of guys with hemophilia. They could not have treated their patients for so many years, getting to know them well, to not care if they became infected with hepatitis virus or HIV." Mike went on to offer, "Those doctors were so encouraged, so excited to see a change for the better when concentrates became available. It was only human nature to see the good side and not see the downside."

He lowered his voice, saying, "But I know the pharmaceutical companies were making lots of money, huge profits, from selling their concentrates. Rightly, or wrongly, left to their own independence, they were unlikely to be vigilante and demand safety first in the production of the medicine, which was selling so well everywhere, not only in America. The makers of the medicine solicited persons who lived in undesirable parts of cities as donors for their source of blood plasma to make concentrate. Included were homeless people and drug users who sold their blood to the drug companies. Walk-in plasma centers accommodated the donors who walked in from the street when they needed money. The drug companies pooled all the plasma together, from hundreds of donors. One infected donor would contaminate the whole batch. America had a source of plasma that was quickly made into concentrate for supplying other countries, almost the whole world, as well as the USA.

"There should have been more regulation of the drug companies. Those of us who have hemophilia turned to the National Hemophilia Foundation for advice. What should we do, we asked, when we heard that the medicine might be polluted? Is the medicine safe? If not, how can it be made safe?" Mike said persons with hemophilia were "innocent, not aware that Cutter, a manufacturer of concentrate, was providing half of NHF's funding.[80] Cutter sent representatives to the NHF board meetings, requesting the board to pass a resolution issuing a statement proclaiming that there is far more danger of bleeding to death than there is danger of becoming ill from HIV infection."

"We—that is, those of us in the hemophilia community—requested a safer concentrate. The drug companies argued that concentrate would become too expensive if they were required to include manufacturing methods to make it safer. We should have put pressure on them. You can't put the price of a person's life on the line of a budget sheet. We should have had the safer heat-treated concentrate sooner for our infusions rather than continuing to infuse ourselves with polluted concentrate. It was a year and a half after heat-treated concentrate became available before I was notified of its existence. Why? I don't know why. Once we did find out that heat-treated concentrate was available, the drug companies were worried how they could sell the supply of contaminated concentrate they still had on their shelves. The drug companies knew the FDA would not let them sell the old polluted

---

80 National Hemophilia Foundation

concentrate in the USA, so they dumped it into other countries, such as Costa Rica and Japan."

Mike continued, saying that when he was fourteen, he began infusing with concentrates. He wished he could have made better decisions. Everyone has freedom of choice when making decisions to react to his or her conditions. But when you are young, your decisions depend upon your past experiences, he said. He thought he was indestructible. He said he was like a bullet. Mike's father was not involved in his medical care. Mike was an only child whose parents divorced when he was three.[81] His mother had such guilt feelings for giving him hemophilia that she only wanted to hear good news. Mike said that he should have been more vigilante, but the treatment of hemophilia upon the introduction of concentrates became such a success story that he was distracted and failed to be critical. Mike said he wished someone would have sat down with him and told him more about the risks of hepatitis from concentrate. He knew guys ten or fifteen years older than he was who asked questions about concentrate. They asked about risks and concluded that the medicine was such an improvement that the risks were worth taking. They got caught just as he did. Mike said he regarded hepatitis as a long-term thing, something that seemed far away.

Mike recalled that when he was young, none of his friends had hepatitis. Since then, some who had hepatitis died from liver failure. They were just as dead from liver disease as those who died from HIV. Hepatitis and HIV are parallel; they are part of the same problem. Mike hoped the friends he knew didn't die just because he and others in the hemophilia community didn't demand enough. He believed they should have learned a lesson from hepatitis. A person gets hepatitis, he is well for years, and then liver failure sneaks up on him and he dies. The same is true of HIV infection. A person becomes unknowingly HIV infected, often followed by years of wellness. The illness of AIDS

---

81 Before concentrates became available, fathers who had a son with hemophilia were frustrated by feeling helpless without a means to provide treatment to relive their son's suffering.

creeps into a person's life and is followed by death. If hepatitis infection from concentrate would have been knocked out, AIDS would have been prevented. Hepatitis and AIDS are terrible, unfortunate situations that could have been prevented.

The people in the hemophilia community began talking among themselves. Was HIV and hepatitis infection in hemophilia "an unavoidable tragedy," a phrase Cutter used to characterize the status of hemophilia infusions in the 1980s? Mike agreed that it was a tragedy, but it was preventable.

Mike related recently discovering an old photograph of the first summer camp for boys with hemophilia in his region. The camp was at Orchards, Washington, in 1972, when he was eleven years old. He said he was in that photograph. There were thirty guys in that photo, and only three were still alive. Included in the photo were Joe Kennedy, Mike's counselor at camp; Cary Carlstrom, his junior counselor; and Doug McAllister. All three had hemophilia, infused themselves with concentrate contaminated with HIV, and died of AIDS. Did the new concentrate, the miracle medicine, prolong life as predicted?

Mike said that some persons confronted with the dilemma in hemophilia were angry and wanted to sue everyone, including the doctors and the center where they got their concentrate. He said he never felt that the hemophilia treatment center or the doctors were where he wanted to vent his anger. He continued vocalizing his feelings and offering information, saying that with a couple of hundred other persons who had hemophilia, he'd joined in filing a lawsuit in Louisiana against one of the producers of concentrate. But he dropped the lawsuit in exchange for payment of one hundred thousand dollars. That money enabled Linda and Mike to purchase their home. He said he would make the same decision again. Receipt of the money lessened the sting somewhat. Still, if he could go backward and bring back some of those guys who'd died of AIDS—Joe Kennedy, Cary Carlstrom, Doug McAllister, Joe Singler, and other guys he got to know at hemophilia summer camp—he would do so in a hurry.

The days seemed to become longer for Mike. He attempted to keep busy with activities other than the great amount of time required for monitoring and consuming his medicines. He remained cheerful despite pain and illness.

"What meaning is there for a life filled with constant suffering and misery with a hopeless fatal outcome?" Mike was asked by Dr. Taillefer. He responded cheerfully, despite not feeling well, by saying, "I have found meaning for my life in two ways. I discovered love in my life for my wife, Linda, and I received love back from her. It's as if the good Lord intended to keep me alive long enough to allow me to experience her love rather than bury me earlier, before I met this wonderful woman in my life. Without her, I would never have known the level of affection I experienced, which resulted in the cessation of suffering in my life. My suffering was traded for affection. Secondly, I discovered the meaning of life by the experiences I have had and the friends I have known, especially my mother. I recall those past events as if I was assigned to complete tasks by a Supreme Being, to bring happiness into the lives of my mother and my friends. My mother gave me so much when I was a youngster, and now I can give a little happiness back to her, which translates into a meaning for my life. I freely chose actions without yielding to circumstances, which could have numbed my contribution to the lives of others. I believe my existence has enriched the lives of a number of persons over my short life span, when I chose to be upbeat rather than downbeat."

Finally, Mike's liver failed, as he predicted. Mike was like his friends who died before him. Although Mike had AIDS, that is not what ended his life. He died from liver failure caused by hepatitis. The doctors knew that the concentrate he used for infusions contained hepatitis viruses. But they continued to recommend infusions with concentrate, despite the viral contamination, to prolong his life. Were the doctors wrong? Mike closed his eyes for the last time with his wife, Linda, nearby on May 2, 2005. She composed a poem as a tribute to his life:

Leap of Faith

Take a leap of faith,
Cast away all doubt.
Darlin' come what may we can work it out.
A love that's real will always find a way.
I will trust in you,
Like you trust in me.
There'll be no rain or fire that we can't go through.
The first step's always the hardest one to take,
It's a leap of faith.
"I love you with all my heart."

Linda Charles 2005

Many of the men who had hemophilia—and became infected with HIV and developed AIDS—married. Their surviving wives, left to mourn them, did not all become HIV infected. Of nine HIV infected men, John Warren, Davy Jarrard, Wayne Palmer, Gary Morgan, Randy Gibson, Doug McAllister, Joe Singler, Mike Charles, and Cary Carlstrom, only one wife became HIV infected. She died of AIDS. Five children were born to three different HIV infected fathers. None of the children became HIV infected.

A Safer AHF Concentrate

Attempts during the 1980s and 1990s were directed toward producing a better and safer concentrate for the fifteen thousand persons who had hemophilia in the United States. Methods for producing a safer concentrate had been developed in other countries, including Italy, France, and Germany.[82] Two principal sources of producing safer AHF concentrate were pursued, one as a derivative of human plasma, the other as a man-made concentrate produced by genetic molecular methods (recombinant FVIII). In addition to depleting viruses such as hepatitis and HIV in plasma with heat treatment, a purification method was introduced using monoclonal antibodies. This method removed viruses from the plasma, leading to the manufacture of Monoclate[83] and Hemophilia M.[84]

The welcome announcement of a new concentrate, Monoclate, came by the back door. Armour, the drug company that marketed the new safe concentrate, contacted the hemophilia patients directly. Face-to-face contact between drug company representatives and clients was foreign to Dr. Taillefer. During his career, he had been trained to believe that the doctor—not a drug company salesperson—knew which medicine was best for his patient. Direct contact with hemophilia persons became

---

82 World Hemophilia Federation (WHF) and scientific journals reported progress for producing safe, effective AHF internationally.

83 Monoclate was marketed as Monoclate-P (derived from plasma and pasteurized and purified), manufactured using pasteurization and immunoaffinity chromatography purification.

84 Monoclate was introduced by Armour Pharmaceuticals in 1987. Hemophilia M was introduced in 1988 by Baxter Pharmaceutical.

possible whenever a pharmaceutical representative became a member of the Oregon Hemophilia Foundation, attended the meetings where hemophilia persons gathered, and met affected persons who were potential customers for the drug company's new monoclonal concentrate. The salesman introduced himself to individuals and families who had hemophilia. He approached them by offering to provide patients with a starter supply of free Monoclate for their infusions at home. After their trial infusion with Monoclate, they were expected to request a supply from the hemophilia treatment center.

After exhausting his supply of free Monoclate, Barry Kurath, an adult man who had hemophilia, requested a supply of Monoclate from the hemophilia center. His request was refused.[85] The hemophilia center did not maintain an inventory of Monoclate. Barry Kurath angrily called the newspapers, including Portland's *Willamette Weekly* and the *San Francisco Chronicle* in California, complaining that the hemophilia center director, Dr. Taillefer, was obstinate, unreasonable, and refused to prescribe a supply of Monoclate for his infusions. Within a few days, journalists from the newspapers descended upon Dr. Taillefer to report the story. Randy Shilts, an author and a journalist for the *San Francisco Chronicle,* flew to Portland from San Francisco. He arrived at the hemophilia treatment center and requested an interview with Dr. Taillefer at four o'clock in the afternoon on Monday October 16, 1989.

Dr. Taillefer informed the newspapers of the reasons the hemophilia treatment center declined to comply with Barry Kurath's request for new concentrate, including the foremost one—that the treatment center did not have any Monoclate. He acknowledged that Monoclate (Philipp 2001) was a reputable concentrate. But rather than the drug company directly contacting Mr. Kurath, they should have approached the prescribing physician. The treatment center maintained a sizable concentrate inventory. Changing or replacing one brand of concentrate for another was a major task. The choice of concentrates to dispense to patients depended upon several factors. The hemophilia treatment center did not have the funds to switch everyone to Monoclate. Previously, the cost of concentrates had been ten cents per unit of AHF. Infusing with ten units per pound of body weight, a one-hundred-pound person required one thousand units, which cost one hundred dollars. Moncoclate cost one dollar for each unit, amounting to one thousand dollars for an infusion, a tenfold increase in cost.[86] The higher the cost, the greater the profit for the drug company. The safety profile of Monoclate, which incorporated a viral inactivation system utilizing immunoaffinity chromatography and pasteurization, portrayed a desirable concentrate to be offered in hemophilia treatment. However, the spiraling cost of Monoclate compared to older products was alarming.

Drug companies that manufacture concentrates have little competition. Their noncompetitive pricing strategy is intended to maximize their profit, as a result of their limited competition in the market (Guirguis and Rogoff 2004). Within the pharmaceutical manufacturing industry, product costs have risen each year. The increase in cost of medications is not apparent in existing products. Instead, the main cause of rising costs of pharmaceuticals is the introduction of those new products, without competition, on the market. Newer products increased the cost of concentrates nearly 50 percent compared to existing products (Rogoff et al. 2002). Government price controls and public health policies have had minimal effect on the prices demanded by the drug companies that manufacture concentrates. The United States, unlike most other developed countries, has not implemented pharmaceutical cost controls (Chen 2008). The U.S. pharmaceutical manufacturers have financially benefited from the free marketing system that prevails. As far as treatment options, the threat of escalating prices affects doctors and patients. When their pricing policies are directed more toward maximizing profit rather than emphasizing availability of

---

86 A $1,000 infusion cost in 1989 is equivalent to $1,740 in 2009. The cost of an infusion has increased in addition to changes in the value of the dollar; the cost per unit of AHF activity has increased (RE: *Dollar Times* 1990).

concentrates at an affordable cost to as many patients as possible, the drug companies are serving the interests of their stockholders instead of the hemophilia patients.

Randy Shilts' authored report of his interview with Dr. Taillefer appeared in the *San Francisco Chronicle* on Tuesday, December 5, 1989 (Shilts 1989):[87]

"Portland doctor withholding new version of clotting factor"

Portland, Ore. — Barry Kurath was ecstatic when he learned that researchers had devised a pure new version of the clotting factor he needs to treat his hemophilia.

The new factor VIII product, he knew, would drastically reduce his exposure to hepatitis viruses — a major development, given that liver disease is the second-highest cause of death among hemophiliacs.

But when Kurath went to ask for the new treatment, his doctor told him he would not give him a prescription.

The physician, Dr. Anton Taillefer, medical director of the treatment center at the Oregon Health Sciences University, concedes that the product is "a very fine medicine" but refuses to give it to Kurath, in part because he does not like the company that makes it.

The company, Armour Pharmaceuticals, has been contacting patients directly to sell the factor VIII. To discourage such direct marketing, Taillefer is simply refusing to prescribe much of the product.

"We don't want to lose control of our patients," he says bluntly.

Complicating the issue is the high cost of factor VIII and other treatments in general. Taillefer says he will not give expensive new treatments to patients who, like Kurath, are HIV infected.

"If you take some patient who's HIV-positive and put [him] on a medication that costs $50,000 a year — and the reason to do it is that

---

87   Permission granted by Copyright Clearance Center to republish Randy Shilts' article (confirmation number 2093452).

it's safer, but [he already has] HIV — that doesn't make sense to me," he says. Taillefer controls financing for Oregon's Hemophilia Assistance Program, which is what pays for Kurath's factor VIII treatments.

As for the treatment's effect on protecting immune-deficient patients from further liver disease, he says such benefits are yet to be definitely proved.

Jonathan Botelho, a man who has hemophilia and a staff member with the office of civil rights of the Department of Health and Human Services, said such decisions violate federal laws banning discrimination against people with disabilities, such as HIV infection.

But Taillefer says, "I don't pay attention to the law. I try to do what's logical — sometimes that's illegal."

At the U.S. Department of Health and Human Services in Washington, Sharon Barrett, who administers the federal program that finances the Portland center, says she is "a little disturbed" by the problems patients face in obtaining monoclonal factor VIII. "It is definitely an area I'm looking into this year," she said last week.

Many hemophilia persons say they feel restricted in their ability to protest, because they worry about their access to treatment altogether. Kurath is reluctant to pressure Taillefer because he is chief of the only hemophilia treatment center within six hundred miles of Kurath's Portland home.

"You don't want to sue your doctor when he's the only one who's got the medicine you need," says the computer programmer.

Taillefer's apparently capricious ill will toward Armour Pharmaceuticals has denied patients millions of dollars in free factor VIII. He refused the company's offer of free monoclonally produced factor VIII for his patients, saying he "doesn't believe in rebates." Patients who wanted the factor were simply refused a prescription.

To make matters worse, patients who have already obtained prescriptions from other doctors often find themselves thwarted later when they ask insurance companies for reimbursement. Third-party payers often seek the advice of the region's foremost hemophilia expert before paying for the product. That expert is Dr. Taillefer, who advises them not to pay for the factor.

"You end up feeling like you're hitting your head against a brick wall," Kurath says.

Questions rose regarding who should receive the next generation of concentrates. Soon after Monoclate became available, a man-made concentrate, Kogenate,[88] was released. This concentrate was not derived from human plasma. Instead, it is made by molecular genetics methods using recombinant technology. The revolutionary new rFVIII[89] has no risk of infecting recipients with viruses. No human viruses were present in the manufacturing process. When first released, the new medicine was expensive and in short supply. Who should receive the new medicine intended to prevent viral infection? The new generation of concentrates, Monoclate and Kogenate, were designed to prevent recipients from becoming infected with HIV and hepatitis viruses. If a person was already infected, should he receive these new man-made medicines manufactured by molecular genetics technology? Or should the available supply of rFVIII be reserved for HIV-negative individuals and persons who have never been previously infused with concentrate?[90] The supply of rFVIII was not sufficient to change all hemophilia persons to this new medicine. Brent was already HIV-positive. Should he be switched from plasma-derived concentrate to rFVIII? During the first months after rFVIII became available, some of the available supply was shipped to Europe, especially Germany, where there was no objection to its high cost, in contrast to the United States. Initially, within the USA, rFVIII was reserved for newly diagnosed hemophilia patients who

---

88 Kogenate, produced by Bayer, a German pharmaceutical manufacturer, became a reality in 1987.

89 Recombinant factor VIII antihemophilia factor (rFVIII), manufactured using recombinant genetic techniques, for treatment of bleeding in persons who are deficient in factor VIII

90 Newborn hemophilia infants and previously un-infused persons were referred to as PUPS.

had never been previously infused with concentrate. Brent, already HIV infected, waited before discontinuing infusions with HT concentrate and changing to infusions with rFVIII. Although he was already infected with HIV, rFVIII would eliminate any further exposure that would be harmful to his damaged immune system.

Please Help Me!

It was 1983. Gwyn parked her car in front of the hemophilia treatment center, and Brent scrambled out the passenger side door. Gwyn opened the car door.

"Help! Please help me. I'm over here!" a voice cried.

Quickly responding, she moved around the cars and came upon an alarming scene. David Jones lay on the cement sidewalk beside his overturned wheelchair. He was a forty-two-year-old man who had no legs. Both of his legs had been amputated, the result of pelvic pseudotumors, a complication of hemophilia.

David arrived at the center in a van with a side door ramp that allowed him to exit and enter his van while seated in his electric-powered wheelchair. He had been carrying the infusion supplies dispensed from the center in his lap, the necessary materials for his infusions at home, while steering the electric wheelchair as he returned to his van. He related later that after his clinic appointment, he'd guided his wheelchair through the automatic doors while leaving the building. The paved entryway to the building leads to a gentle downward slope. Rather than maintain a steady, normal course on the sidewalk to his van, he daringly attempted a shortcut across the front lawn. As he was crossing the grassy area, he reversed direction, turning his wheelchair around in order to back up onto the sidewalk in front of his van. He had given his motor-driven wheelchair full power in order to rise up onto the sidewalk. With a burst of power, the wheelchair flipped over backward. The device had a large heavy black battery mounted low in the rear. It is susceptible to overturning backward, which is prevented with extension wheels in the rear. David had removed the extension wheels.

With alarm, Gwyn and eight-year-old Brent rushed to where David was lying on the cement sidewalk. Although he was crying loudly for help, he was laughing at the same time, amused by his own stupidity. Gwyn and Brent couldn't lift the grown man from the sidewalk to his wheelchair. After a moment, a doctor passing by on the sidewalk assisted Gwyn and Brent by lifting David from the pavement to the open door of his van. He could not rise up to a standing position to return to the chair, for he had nothing to stand on.

A bleed into David's hip when he was twenty years of age, in 1961, before concentrates were available, became a pseudotumor. A pseudotumor in hemophilia occurs when a massive untreated blood clot forms, which becomes differentiated into anatomical structures, including small blood vessels that extend beneath the periosteum, the covering of bone. When an unchecked pelvic pseudotumor enlarges, there is danger that it may erode through the body wall to the outside, which creates a draining fistula, exposing the inside of the body to the outside. Although the tumors are not malignant, they are a threat to life when they enlarge to the size of a football. When cryoprecipitate became available in 1964, allowing surgery to be performed after his blood-clotting factor was restored to normal with infusions, the orthopedic doctors disarticulated his leg. His right leg was removed from the hip socket. After recovering from the surgery, David was able to stand on his left leg, which allowed him to vault from his wheelchair to a dinner table, chair, or the sofa. He could sit on the toilet and stand before the mirror in the bathroom to brush his teeth. Before sufficient supplies of the new concentrates became available for home infusion in 1971, David had another hip bleed on the opposite side of his body. He bled into his remaining left hip in 1970. Another pseudotumor developed. The doctors believed the progressive nature of this pathological process was threatening to David's life, and they followed the advice available in the hemophilia literature, which recommended disarticulation. After restoring his blood clotting activity to normal with concentrates in 1971, he was returned to surgery where his left leg was disarticulated at the hip, leaving him with no legs. David ambulated in a wheelchair and drove a van fitted with hand controls, which is far different from his ambitions in his younger life. At one time, despite hemophilia, David drove a race car.

After 1971, David was able to infuse himself at home. He survived his bilateral disarticulations of his legs while living at home with his mother for a few years. He overcame his adversarial challenges of suffering and physical disability to participate in a meaningful social life. His wheelchair is empty now. It no longer tips over backward. It no longer moves. He no longer laughs at his own mistakes. His laughter, his warm smile, his friendliness—they are gone. David developed liver failure and pneumonia and died of AIDS in February 1988, at age forty-seven. The medicine that had saved him from the havoc of pseudotumors of the pelvis unsuspectingly infected him with HIV, followed by AIDS and death.

Pentamidine: I Hate That Stuff!

B rent did not tell anyone at his school that he had HIV. He was not ill. He did not miss school because of illness. When he discovered he was HIV-positive in 1987, at age twelve, he did not begin taking antiviral medicine to prevent illness. In the 1980s, doctors at the hemophilia treatment center were not familiar with the new virus that infected Brent. Although HIV infection was regarded as ominous and fatal, the doctors could not predict the course of the viral infection in any one person. They believed that the duration between the time of the infection by HIV and the onset of AIDS[91] was slow—that it would be months or years before the signs of AIDS became noticeable. Research for treatment of HIV included reexamining previously discovered medicines to select one that would combat HIV. One of the drugs that had been synthesized to fight cancer, twenty years previously, was azidothymidine, which had been investigated in 1964. It was not approved for cancer treatment because of its adverse side effects and its ineffectiveness in preventing cancer in mice. In 1984, it was discovered that this compound inhibited HIV. It became known as AZT and Retrovir as well as Zidovudine.[92]

Brent questioned why he should take AZT. The doctor told him he should swallow sixteen pills a day, four pills four times each day. But

---

91 The Public Health Department introduced the name AIDS (Acquired Immunodeficiency Disease) in 1982. The cause of AIDS, a virus, was discovered in 1983 by Dr. Luc Montagnier and named HIV in 1987.
92 Burroughs Welcome patented AZT in 1985 to use against HIV to prevent AIDS. AZT was approved by the FDA for use in treating HIV in 1987 and for the prevention of AIDS in 1990.

he didn't think he could do that, especially because he wasn't ill. No other antiviral treatment of HIV was known in 1987. The doctors began using the name AIDS, the name of the disease caused by HIV. Could AIDS be prevented in an HIV infected person by taking AZT before he became ill? Should the doctors wait before beginning treatment until symptoms of illness, the signs of AIDS, appeared? Could the course of AIDS be altered by AZT? Could death be prevented with AZT? The hemophilia treater doctors did not know the answers to the questions they were asked about AIDS prevention by their patients and families. They relied on information provided to them by the Medical Advisory Committee of the National Hemophilia Foundation and from statements provided by infectious disease experts at the Centers for Disease Control, located in Atlanta, Georgia.

When tests in 1987 confirmed that Brent was HIV-positive, he was only twelve years of age. He was not started on AZT. At that time, HIV-positive children less than fourteen years of age were not given AZT. When he turned sixteen, in 1991, he was enrolled in a study program at the hemophilia treatment center that was intended to determine the benefits of AZT for young individuals. Half the people in the group of HIV infected youths in the double-blind study were given AZT. The other half of the individuals in the study group were given a placebo. Brent did not know which arm of the study claimed his enrollment. Individuals in both halves of the study had health examinations and laboratory tests, including measurements of different kinds of white blood cells and T4-helper cells. While he was still enrolled in the AZT study, he was started on pentamidine by inhalation. Although he wasn't ill, the treatment was an attempt to prevent the development of pneumonia,[93] which commonly develops

---

93 Pneumocystis pneumonia (PCP) is the result of depletion of the immune system, which cannot prevent overwhelming the lungs with *Pneumocystis jiroveccii*, a fungus that is harmless ordinarily. The agent is not spread from person to person. By the age of four, 75 percent of children become seropositive for this ubiquitous fungus. When T4 cells become less than 200/μl, PCP develops.

in HIV infected individuals and is one of the leading causes of death in persons who die from AIDS.

Brent proclaimed that he hated pentamidine. It made him nauseated. He felt like throwing up when he breathed that yucky stuff. But if the doctor recommended it, he said he would inhale it anyway, although he was skeptical that it would do him any good.

Since he was twelve years old, he'd known that he was HIV-positive. Hemophilia didn't bother him much. HIV had not made him sick. He didn't even know it was there.

Five years passed from the time Brent was discovered to be HIV infected without signs or symptoms of AIDS. Exposed to HIV since he was six months of age, when he was first infused with concentrate, he was repeatedly further exposed from the infusions with polluted concentrates. Brent was a student at Oswego High School where his school attendance record was not tarnished with absences caused by bleeds from hemophilia. Even when he knew he was HIV infected, he seldom missed school. He liked school. Art class was his favorite subject. He had a 3.5 grade point average.

Brent had to make a decision between treatment with a drug with objectionable side effects and the risk of developing an illness that would probably be fatal. When does the effect of the drug exceed the risk of the illness the drug is intended to prevent?

An Old Blue Piano

Brent, age thirteen, and his mother, on the morning of Friday, August 11, 1989, sat in brown wooden chairs in the clinic before picking up supplies to take home for infusions.

In the hemophilia treatment center waiting room, the stacks of magazines piled on the low tables for the patients to examine while they waited for the nurse or doctor were always old and out-of-date; sometimes pages had been torn from them, evidence they had passed through many hands. "Yikes! That is a really ugly piano," Brent exclaimed as he stood up from his seat, and walked over to an old upright piano that had been painted a light blue color. "I wonder if it can make a tune. Is it playable?"[94]

"No. You can bang on the keys and make some noise, but that old piano is no longer tunable," a young man proclaimed, slowly rising from his chair with difficulty and walking almost straight-legged over to Brent.

"How do you know that?" Brent replied. "How come you know about that piano?"

The young man smiled and replied, "Pianos are my trade. I am a piano rebuilder."

"Oh, you mean if the piano lid is cracked, you can repair the woodwork? Can you fix those broken piano keys?" Brent asked with interest. "I once met a guy who was a piano tuner, but I don't know any piano rebuilders."

"I can fix a broken piano cabinet, and I can tune a piano," the man remarked. "But I specialize in rebuilding the insides, the works of the piano."

---

94 Extracted from notes recorded during an interview with Gwyn McCann on August 31, 2007

"I guess you must have hemophilia or else you wouldn't be here," Brent said. "I see you can't straighten your arms. I bet you have bad elbows. How can you work on the inside of a piano if you can't reach out straight, down inside into the works?"

"That is a problem. The way I solve that challenge is by removing the piano's inner works and setting them on a workbench," the man confided.

Gwyn walked over to the piano. "Hello, my name is Gwyn Perry. I'm Brent's mother."

The young man turned to Gwyn, smiled and said, "It's a pleasure to meet you. My name is Dick Wagner. I have hemophilia. I work for myself as a piano rebuilder with a shop in Moe's Pianos on Foster Road in southeast Portland."

Brent was meeting a remarkable man who also had hemophilia. Dick Wagner was born in 1957, before concentrate became available. He had hemophilia type B, which had affected another man in his family. His mother's father died from a nosebleed when the hemorrhage couldn't be stopped. Dick had three brothers and two sisters. Born the fifth of the six children, he was the only one of the children among his brothers and sisters who had hemophilia. His hemophilia was discovered after he bled when he was circumcised after birth. The type of hemophilia that affected Dick, type B, the result of a deficiency of factor IX, was treated with infusions of plasma during his childhood. The plasma was collected from donors, frozen, and stored until used. However, he became jaundiced when he was infected with hepatitis from the infusions of plasma. After receiving plasma infusions for several bleeds, he became sensitized, allergic to plasma. He became very ill if an infusion with plasma was attempted. Most of his recurrent bleeds during childhood were managed by lying, without moving, in bed, waiting for the pain to disappear. In his mid twenties, in the early 1980s, he began infusions with concentrate, Konyne.

The nurse from the hemophilia treatment center, Sue Underwood, instructed Dick how to infuse himself during the month of October 1980, when he was twenty-three years of age. The new concentrate was a miracle for him. He no longer needed to go to the hospital for an infusion. His painful bleeds could be stopped at the earliest sign before intense pain developed. By the time Konyne became available for infusions, he already had irreversibly damaged joints. But when he learned to infuse himself and kept concentrate at home, he could plan his activities without downtime from the pain of a bleed. Soon after Dick began the new innovational treatment of infusing himself, Sue Underwood retired from nursing. He was dismayed, his sister, Jan Crider, recalled. Why would Sue, his favorite nurse, leave him? He thought he had lost his angel.[95]

Dick's home infusions were implemented at an important time in his life. A lump was discovered in his throat. Dick underwent surgical removal of a thyroglossal duct cyst November 12, 1980.[96] Following the surgery, he was able to infuse himself at home during healing. Dick's sentiment was expressed in his journal entry of November 7, 1980:[97]

---

95 Conversation with Jan Crider on December 1, 2005, at AIDS Remembrance Day, Doernbecher Children's Hospital, Portland, OR

96 Thyroglossal duct cysts are a congenital remnant. Occasionally they become malignant; therefore, they are surgically removed.

97 Journal entry, Dick Wagner, November 7, 1980, provided by his sister, Jan Crider, November 21, 2008

My life has really changed. First, I'm to have surgery on my throat Nov. 12. Right now, I'm not too scared. I sort of have the feeling "let's get it over with so I can get on with my life." More important and most likely to change my life, in the last two weeks, I've learned home infusion therapy for my hemophilia.

I'm qualified and well stocked to inject myself with factor IX concentrate to stop bleeds. No more weeks in agony. And yet I'm almost sad. I have a sense that I'm leaving behind so much of my childhood ... so much of what makes me, me. I'm even sad that I won't be seeing a lot of people at U of O HTC [hemophilia treatment center] anymore ... the people that I was scared to death to meet a month ago. The nurse that taught me the bulk of home program in the past two weeks told me today that she was quitting in a few weeks. My heart sunk at the thought of not seeing her again. I feel so grateful to her for giving me this gift that I feel I would do practically anything for her if she were in need. I just pray that God totally blesses her just for teaching me, let alone all the others she has helped. I just hope I never forget the gifts I've been handed lately. I feel so humbled, scared, lonely, insecure, and joyful ... all mixed together.

As a child, Dick spent many hours, weeks, in bed at Doernbecher Children's Hospital for treatment of his recurrent bleeds. He was often alone (Stark 2004). During afternoon hospital visiting hours, he waited, hoping for a visit by his parents, but with a large family at home, they could not go to the hospital often. Lying in bed motionless, he watched the slow movement of the black hands of the large mechanical clock on the wall. He thought a lot as the old clock ticked away the hours of his young life. At age ten, in 1967, in bed, while listening to the clock tick, Dick wrote a poem:

a little boy—alone

A little boy sits in an overstuffed rocking chair,
Gazing outside at children playing—alone,
While the radio sings a mellow, sweet song.
The boy reads about pirates
And adventures in the days of yore—alone.
Soon, fantasy replaces reality,
And he is sailing, fighting, and killing.
The music dies down,
And he finds himself again in a room,
Rocking in his chair, and living—alone.
He sighs, picks up his book along with his hopes
Of running and playing with other children,
And slowly and quietly makes his way with his cane
To his bedroom to sleep and dream—alone.

Richard Wagner 1967

Dick dreaded the loneliness of the hospital. Loneliness was a prominent part of his life before concentrates became available—similar to the life experienced by young Leopold of Queen Victoria's royal family (appendix II). Sometimes Dick relieved his despair by constructing model airplanes from balsa wood and paper. Once, on his birthday, Jan, his sister, recalls that he had a bleed, and rather than going to the hospital, she helped him construct a model airplane at home. They doused the airplane with gasoline, set it on fire, and then sent it flying.

Although he preferred being outside tossing Frisbees like the other boys, he was aware that he must be careful, realizing he could die from something simple like falling from his bike. If he bit his tongue, he would end up in the hospital for a month. If he stumbled when he stepped off the school bus, he could end up with a knee or ankle bleed. The joint bleeds kept him out of school for weeks. He developed permanent damage to his elbows, knees and ankles. Healing from a joint bleed required a long time, and he had to hold still for hours, for days.

Despite the threat to his body, his mind was active, limitless. Jan recalled that Dick thought about both the big things and small things in life—the orbits of carbon atoms, electron forces, relativity, chaos theory—and the work of Stephen Hawkins, a brilliant man with a broken body, and of Richard Feynman, who received the Nobel Prize in Physics in 1965. Feynman was known for his path of integral formulation in quantum mechanics. Dick had an enlightened spirit that simulated Feynman's intellectual lightheartedness. Dick was motivated by Feynman's popularization of physics, including his top-down nanotechnology when he wrote *There's Plenty of Room at the Bottom* and another popular philosophy on science: *What Do You Care What Other People Think?* Dick and Feynman shared similar traits, revealing their love of life. Feynman was a prankster, a juggler, a painter, and a bongo player. Dick was always anxious to open the pages of the latest copy of *Scientific American*. While he was receiving infusions of concentrate, he thought about atomic configurations, sometimes reading *In Search of Schroderinger's Cat: Quantum Physics and Reality*. And this was a young man who had often been absent from school.

Energy and entropy fascinated Dick. He liked to break things down to examine them, but since childhood, he also liked to blow things up, a release of anger, a way to achieve an adrenaline rush the way other guys become exhilarated from playing sports. As a child, he would scrape the gunpowder off toy caps that other boys used in their pistols. Dick rigged up concoctions with pop bottles, Drano, and balloons—the more smoke and noise during an explosion, the better. He had a prized possession—a lidded tin box full of gunpowder he had meticulously removed from firecrackers and saved. He had enough, his sister said, to send a cannonball halfway across town. On average, Dick suffered a joint bleed once each week.

When he was able to, he attended Our Lady of the Lake School and then Lake Oswego High School, where he began playing the banjo and the drums. He was rhythmical and developed a lifelong passion for Buddy Rich and Gene Krupa. Following high school, he served a three-year apprenticeship as a piano rebuilder, followed by a career at Moe's Pianos, where he was recognized as superb in piano restoration. Dick invented a method of restoring broken piano keys, utilizing a formula he invented, composed of acrylic and pigments. He shipped his product all over the world. In addition to music, Dick had a passion for fly-fishing, although the casting motion was difficult because of his damaged elbows. He played the drums for religious services at St. Ignatius Catholic Church and for the Madeline Parish in Portland.

Selectively, Dick tuned pianos for special clients. When Dr. Taillefer's house burned down in 1990, his mother's piano was destroyed by the fire. Dr. Taillefer purchased an old upright cabinet grand, manufactured by the Schubert Piano Company of New York. Dr. Taillefer asked Dick to come and take a look at the piano. Dick came to the house and inspected the piano, which had been painted an antique bronze by the former owner, locating the serial number inside the cabinet. After looking up the number in a catalogue that listed piano serial numbers, he remarked, "This piano is more than one hundred years old. Most of these old uprights aren't tunable. The wooden sounding board will break if the high tune strings are tightened enough for tuning."

To please the doctor, Dick removed the interior works of the piano for transfer to his workshop at Moe's Pianos. After he loaded the parts of the piano into his van, he said, "Remember, the piano may not be tunable, but I will give it a try." Two months later, Dick returned to Dr. Taillefer's home with the piano works. "Guess what?" he cheerfully remarked with a grin. "Your piano had been rebuilt as a student project at a piano rebuilding workshop. The students did only a C-plus job. I have completely replaced all the felts and pads and liberated all the movement. I discovered that it's tunable." Dick replaced the works of the piano and tuned the strings on the soundboard in the living room of the old wooden house. During tuning, he demanded complete silence. After the piano tuning was completed, which required several hours, he played "Linus and Lucy," the *Peanuts* song composed by Vince Guaraldi. Dick and the doctor were both delighted with Dick's amazing piano restoration success.

Despite pain in his elbows when reaching down into old upright pianos and lugging around a box containing fifty pounds of tools, Dick kept working. He did not like being alone, a reminder of his lonely childhood. When Dick moved into a condominium, he had a girlfriend and a cat named B minor. His interests included nostalgia for old music. He loved old tapes and comedy shows with Jack Benny and Fibber McGee and Molly. He had watched old movies from his hospital bed. He knew their contents by heart. When Dick was having a bad day, he prepared comfort foods, which included a baked casserole combining rice, a can of cream of tomato soup, cut-up hot dogs, Wheaties, and cheddar cheese.

Although Dick played drums, the banjo, and the piano at a Catholic church, he had no use for organized religion (plate 13). He wrestled with the big questions: How does the universe work? How did he fit into it? What is the soul? Is the soul immortal? Do all of us have individual souls, or is there one big soul for everyone? As a child, Dick was raised in a Catholic family. He had asked God to make his hemophilia disappear. It didn't go away, yet he still believed there was a God. He believed he had gotten a bum rap, and he questioned that if there is a God, why him?

Dick was a good example of a person who has a fatal illness that is struggling with religion. People with fatal medical conditions often contemplate the concepts of God and the universe. It is common for them to ask questions like, If there is a God, why did this happen to me?

In his forties, his elbows no longer moved much. He knew that before long he wouldn't be able to play his drums, his banjo, or the piano. Dick had a difficult time going up and down the stairs. His bleeding sites shifted from his joints to internal bleeding. His liver, damaged from hepatitis, the effect of hepatitis C virus he received in the concentrates used for infusions to treat recurrent bleeds, became swollen. The effects of hepatitis on Dick's liver had been quiescent, but slowly, over the years, progressive damage led to liver failure. As his liver swelled, pressure increased within the liver's portal vein, resulting in bleeding from distended blood vessels in his esophagus and stomach. Recurrent gastrointestinal bleeding sapped his strength.

In November 2003, Dick telephoned his sister, Jan, telling her that he was very ill. She said that she would call an ambulance to bring him to the hospital. He said he wanted her to take him to the hospital. She understood his request and brought him to the ER. He was vomiting bright red blood. She stayed with him while the doctors and nurses hovered over him. Although he was ill and the scene was intense with activity, Jan and her brother had some conversation. She assumed he would choose DNR,[98] but instead he requested "Do everything." Dick indicated that he was not resigned to giving up hope. He understood that he could not alter the conditions affecting his body. But he could make decisions that determined his reaction to those conditions. He was not nihilistic, although he realized that humans are a finite thing; instead, he recognized a meaning for existence, and for him life had a precious meaning.

He was moved from the ER to surgery after he was infused with concentrate to elevate his clotting activity to normal. A shunt was surgically placed in his liver to relieve the pressure that produced congestion in the veins of his esophagus and stomach, a procedure that the doctors optimistically asserted might allow him to live another year. For two weeks following surgery, Dick was on life support. His life was touch-and-go. Finally, he was disconnected from the ventilator; however, he was confused afterward. Dick's medical insurance had capped, reached its limit, so he went to his father's home to recover. Jan and their father took care of Dick. He treasured those days.

---

98 Do not resuscitate.

Exactly one year to the day after the intrahepatic portosystemic shunt procedure, Dick was rehospitalized when another gastrointestinal bleed struck an additional blow to his life. His sister held his hand in the ER. This time, as she wept, he said to her, "Sister, if this is it, thank you for everything. This is no way to live. I am a walking time bomb, waiting to blow up." The bleed that reoccurred was soon accompanied by pressure building up inside his head. This beautiful person could no longer talk or move his face normally. The doctors reported that the pressure inside Dick's head had shoved the base of his brain downward through the foramen magnum, the spinal canal opening in the bottom of his skull. His brain stem had herniated. Dick was conscious and aware he was dying. He could not speak or move. Dick's friends came to his bedside and played guitar music. Jan remained by his side at night, sleeping by his bedside on the floor of the ICU. Dying was peaceful for him as long as he didn't die alone. Although he'd felt alone many times in his life when he was hospitalized, when he died, he wasn't alone. He died November 17, 2004, surrounded by his friends and his sister. Dick is no longer here, but the sound of the pianos he tuned will emulate his melodies forever.

During his life, Dick frequently talked about the big old clock in Doernbecher Hospital, relentlessly ticking away minutes while he lay motionless. The building where the clock hung on the wall was eventually demolished. Before he died, Dick gained possession of that merciless old clock. While lying in bed, recovering from a bleed, Dick pondered a long time, trying to figure out the best way to blow up that old clock. Dick's surviving family and friends have sworn in an oath to someday, somehow, someplace get their hands on some dynamite and blow up that old clock. Dick isn't here to tell them how to find the dynamite.

The old blue piano in the hemophilia treatment center waiting room is not the only piano that is silent. Dick and Jan's grandparents, their mother's parents, were both musicians. Each evening, together, their grandmother played the piano, and their grandfather played his violin. Their grandfather died from a nose bleed. After he bled to death, their grandmother covered the piano with a bedsheet. She refused to play the piano again or to let anyone touch the piano. It has stood silently ever since the night their grandfather died. Jan confessed that she was fascinated that her brother became a piano rebuilder after their grandfather's death. She said, "Most people can only play middle C. Dick played the whole keyboard."

"There are two sides to the story of my brother," Jan attests. "On one hand, there is great sorrow. On the other hand, there is great joy and appreciation for all he was given. The concentrates that took my brother's life also gave him life … in more ways than one. You only need to look at my brother's journal to know how he felt. Hemophilia is much more agonizing and painful than hepatitis C."

As a child Dick suffered immensely from painful deforming joint bleeds. As an adult, he benefited from pain relief after he began infusions with concentrate to prevent bleeds. The concentrate seemed like a miracle medicine. The doctors told him to take the medicine and he would have a more normal life and live many more years to become an old man. The doctors were aware that the medicine Dick received contained hepatitis virus. However, they maintained that the risk of developing complications from hepatitis was less than the risk of dying from hemophilia. The doctors were wrong.

On Trial in Alaska

During the springtime of 1991, Brent went to the hemophilia treatment center with Gwyn to pick up a supply of concentrate. When he was greeted by the two nurses in the clinic, he told them he had a question he wanted to ask Dr. Taillefer.

Myrna replied that he would have to ask one of them his question. Brent was told Dr. Taillefer was in Alaska and would not return for several weeks.

From the serious expression on Myrna's face and the somber tone of her voice, Brent concluded that Dr. Taillefer must be up in the Far North for something serious. Otherwise, the nurses would have been anxious to share some exciting news about Dr. Taillefer with him and his mother. He recalled hearing reports about Dr. Taillefer's trips to places like Alaska, where he went out to Eskimo villages. He once heard that the doctor had mushed in the snow behind a dog sled. Brent remembered hearing the legend that if a pretty young Eskimo girl sat on your sled, you had to marry her. Brent asked Myrna if Dr. Taillefer owned a dog sled.

Myrna replied that that was a strange question, saying that Dr. Taillefer was not a musher.

Myrna told Gwyn that something serious was happening to Dr. Taillefer. He was in court, on trial, a defendant in a lawsuit.

Brent remembered walking through the swinging doors in the hemophilia treatment center, past the treatment room to the first door on the right, down the long hallway, the door of Dr. Taillefer's office. The door had a glass window in the upper half. Dr. Taillefer's desk was near the far wall. He could sit in his comfortable chair, behind his desk, his back to the wall, facing the door, and detect people through the door window before they opened the door to the room.

What impressed Brent about Dr. Taillefer's office was the mask mounted on the wall above his chair. The mask was a gift from Clyde Hugo and his wife, Ellen, presented to Dr. Taillefer to show their gratitude for his work in their village of Anuktuvuk Pass[99] in the winter of 1971. Dr. Taillefer had explained to him how the Eskimos in the Nunamiut[100] village in the Brooks Range of northern Alaska crafted the masks. Brent always rejoiced while drawing or creating designs that satisfied his artistic creativity. The mask was of great interest to him.

Brent was fascinated to learn that the original Anuktuvuk masks were fashioned when Eskimo fathers returned to the village after hunting wild game. Eskimos are happy people who laugh a lot and share humorous recounts with their children. They revel over surprises. Once, when returning to the village, the men realized that they had no surprises to bring home to their children after their hunting journey. They chopped curved chunks of wood from a willow trunk to create facial masks. They made slits for eyes and the mouth, and they decorated their creations with pieces of fur from the wild animals they had trapped. The Eskimo men donned the masks they had fashioned and moved into the village, their faces covered with the wooden masks, to surprise the children of the village. To the glee of the children and the other adults, the masked men were received with joy and merriment. Brent was profoundly impressed by the human spirit behind the creation of the masks. There is something that characterizes humans no matter where they live. Despite the harshness of their existence, the Eskimos expressed themselves through their art.

---

99 Anuktuvuk, which means "place of caribou droppings," is the only existing Nunamiut settlement in Alaska. Anuktuvuk Pass is one of the few places the caribou can traverse the Brooks Range of mountains in northern Alaska during their annual migration.

100 Nunamiut Eskimos are inland people living in the Brooks Range in northern Alaska, whereas most Eskimos live along the seacoast. Their principle diet is meat from caribou. "Eskimo" is an Indian word meaning "meat eater."

The mask on the wall behind Dr. Taillefer's desk was made with the aid of the ulu. The blade was cut from a steel handsaw. The curved edge was sharpened. A round piece of bone was attached to the upper unsharpened edge for a handle. The sharp ulu blade was used for scraping the fat from the inside of a caribou hide, followed by stretching the hide over a piece of curved wood carved from a willow tree trunk. The skin was moistened with tundra tea made from moss; black tea was not available in the village, for there was no village marketplace in 1971. To complete the mask, wolverine fur was attached for eyebrows, and caribou fur was used for the moustache and beard. Tinting of the brownish animal hide, to highlight the cheekbones with a subtle reddish hue, was accomplished by mixing human blood with the tea, a reminder that human blood has importance in multiple different ways. The fur was attached with sinew from the animals, a substitute for thread, using a needle crafted from bone. Brent was delighted to learn how resourceful humans are.

One of the persons Brent had met at the hemophilia treatment center, while sitting in the waiting room, ten years earlier in 1980, was a shy, soft-spoken young man from Vader, Washington, who had moved to Anchorage with his mother. This young man, Brad Craigdon, like Brent, had hemophilia and was well. He had been infused many times for treatment of bleeds with concentrate before heat treatment or viral depletion had been incorporated in its production. The Oregon hemophilia center outreach personnel continued to direct his care after he moved from Washington to Alaska. The doctor, nurse, physical therapist, and psychologist evaluated him during the annual hemophilia clinic they conducted each year in Alaska. They continued to ship concentrate to Brad's home, which assured him of an uninterrupted supply for his infusions. They arranged for Dr. Aaron Kingston, an Anchorage hematologist, to provide Brad's medical care in Alaska. Frequent telephone conversations with the center assisted Dr. Kingston in providing optimal hemophilia care for Brad, his Alaska patient. In

1986, the Oregon Hemophilia Center, during an outreach evaluation of Brad, recommended completing the blood test for HIV infection, which had recently become available, to determine whether Brad had become HIV infected, although he seemed well. Results of the blood test revealed that Brad Craigdon was infected with HIV, the virus that causes AIDS. In 1986, AIDS was not a frequent topic of discussion in Alaska.

Brad, twenty-seven years of age at the time he found out he was HIV-positive, was understandably sad when he learned of his test result. He became sullen, withdrawn, and felt that life was hopeless. He became unemployed and continued living with his mother in their home, a short distance northeast of Anchorage in Wasilla, west of Palmer, along Highway 3. He seldom left the house after he discovered he was HIV infected. Before his HIV test result was revealed, he'd held an interesting and pleasant job as a filing clerk in an Anchorage law firm. After Brad Craigdon learned that he was HIV-positive, he became depressed.

With the recommendation, advice, and assistance of an Anchorage attorney, Brad agreed to seek damages against the pharmaceutical manufacturer of the concentrate that had produced the medicine that was contaminated with HIV. Rather than suing Cutter, a division of Miles Laboratories, who made the concentrate, the attorneys' strategy included a combined lawsuit listing Brad Craigdon as the plaintiff, with three defendants, including Dr. Taillefer.[101]

During this trip to Alaska in 1991, Dr. Taillefer was spending his days in the federal courthouse in Anchorage. The first information Dr. Taillefer received about the lawsuit filed against him on behalf of the plaintiff, Brad Craigdon, was the notice that he was required to

---

101 The three defendants were Cutter, a division of Miles Laboratories, the pharmaceutical manufacturer of the concentrate Brad had been infused with to treat his hemophilia; Oregon Health Sciences University (OHSU), the location of the Hemophilia Treatment Center; and Dr. Anton Taillefer, the director who gave him the contaminated concentrate.

attend a meeting with an attorney on July 12, 1990. He met attorney Bert Benson, an assistant attorney general for the State of Oregon, and his legal assistant, Margaret May Mills, in room 3153 on the third floor of CDRC at the Oregon Health Sciences University. The plaintiff alleged that Dr. Taillefer had failed to warn him of the risk and dangers of HIV infection from the concentrates Dr. Taillefer prescribed for him. Remembering that he had always enjoyed a close, comfortable relationship with his patient Brad Craigdon, the doctor couldn't imagine that Brad would be suing him. The doctor was astounded, for he regarded Brad as a nice young man. He was shocked to learn of the lawsuit.

The doctor did not subscribe to a medical malpractice insurance plan. He was employed by the State of Oregon; therefore, in court, he would be defended by the attorney general's office. Dr. Taillefer did not have deep pockets, a phrase attributed to trial attorneys' impression of doctors who receive high incomes, a likely source for reaping high settlements. Mr. Benson reviewed the plaintiff's suit for Dr. Taillefer, followed by discussion. Midway through the deposition, before all the facts were revealed and a strategy was proposed, Dr. Taillefer was surprised again, an ominous surprise. Nurse Myrna suddenly rushed into the room and told the attorney and his assistant that Dr. Taillefer must be immediately released. His house was on fire. His mother died in the blaze. The intended court date for the trial of Dr. Taillefer was postponed.

On Monday, September 24, 1990, two months after his home burned, Dr. Taillefer boarded Alaska Airline Flight 154 for San Francisco at 7:30 AM. He was met at the airport by attorney Lance Penser and was driven in Mr. Penser's black sedan to Mr. Penser's law office in the Ice House of San Francisco, a remodeled wooden structure that had served as a depot for blocks of ice before refrigeration was installed in homes and shops of the hilly city on San Francisco Bay. The law office was located in a trendy section of the city, where fashionable offices replaced old traditional structures. Mr. Penser had been solicited by Miles Laboratories for the defense of the Craigdon suit. The tall, well-groomed attorney, with reassuring confidence, reviewed the plaintiff's claims that Dr. Taillefer had prescribed infusions of HIV infected concentrate without warning the plaintiff of the possible hazards from viral contamination. He made notes and assessed Dr. Taillefer's character and appearance as well as his credentials. Mr. Penser was satisfied with Dr. Taillefer's ability to appear in court to stand trial. He weaved through the heavy traffic, returning the doctor to the San Francisco airport for his return to Portland.

The next morning, Tuesday, September 25, a deposition was scheduled in an upstairs room of Baird Hall at OHSU. In addition to Mr. Benson and Margaret May Mills, the principal attorney and his assistant representing the plaintiff, Mr. Craigdon, were present to depose Dr. Taillefer with questions and statements. Marty Bachman, a famous trial lawyer from Philadelphia, had been solicited by Brad Craigdon's Alaska attorneys to spearhead the trial. AIDS was a new topic; new fields were to be opened. Attorneys had no experience in AIDS trials. Mr. Bachman and his assistants grilled Dr. Taillefer for three hours while recording his answers to the questions they asked. Several times they asked him the same question, phrased differently, attempting to detect inconsistencies in his answers.

"Did you prescribe Koate for Mr. Craigdon for infusions to treat his hemophilia?" Mr. Bachman asked Dr. Taillefer.

"Yes, I did, "Dr. Taillefer replied.

"Was the medicine you prescribed contaminated with HIV?"

"Possibly. It might have been," Dr. Taillefer answered.

"You mean, Doctor, that you do not know if the medicine contained HIV or not?" the interrogating attorney replied.

"How could I know? I did not test the medicine," Dr. Taillefer patiently answered.

"Didn't Mr. Craigdon become HIV-positive?"

"I am not allowed to answer your question. A person's HIV status is confidential," Dr. Taillefer answered. "You have access to Mr. Craigdon's medical records. His test results are listed in those records."

"I demand that you answer my question. Is Mr. Craigdon HIV-positive?" Marty Bachman asked.

"I yield to whatever is in his records, which are before you."

Sensing he had not yet successfully reduced the doctor's bearing, Mr. Bachman continued. "Did you give Mr. Craigdon HIV, Dr. Taillefer?"

"I do not know if the medicine I prescribed for Mr. Craigdon had HIV in it or if it did not," Dr. Taillefer replied.

"Dr. Taillefer, when did you inform my client, Mr. Craigdon, that he was infusing with HIV infected concentrate to treat his hemophilia?"

"Oh, I'm not sure. We informed all the hemophilia patients who were infusing with concentrates that there was a suspicion of a possible harmful substance in the blood supply used as the source of their clotting factor," Dr. Taillefer conceded.

"And when was that?" Mr. Bachman, who was seated across the large wooden table from Dr. Taillefer, demanded while pounding on the table.

"As soon as the Medical Advisory Committee recommended notification."

"What year was that, Dr. Taillefer?"

"I think it was in the early nineteen eighties."

"Did you instruct my client to stop infusing the contaminated medicine?" the animated attorney asked while glaring at the doctor.

Dr. Taillefer responded to the question. "No, I did not. We repeated the advice of the Medical Advisory Committee, who published a proclamation stating that the risk of dying from a head bleed if concentrate was not infused when needed was greater than the risk of dying from an HIV infection."

"So, you are saying you knew there was a risk of HIV infection if the concentrate you prescribed was infused?" Mr. Bachman quickly replied.

"I didn't say that."

"Oh, you mean you are saying there was no risk?"

"Mr. Bachman, please, I didn't say that either."

Marty Bachman continued grilling Dr. Taillefer. "Dr. Taillefer, are you a board-certified hematologist? Do you run a clinic that specializes in treating patients who have a bleeding problem?"

"Mr. Benson, must I answer these questions?" Dr. Taillefer asked his attorney.

"Yes, Dr. Taillefer," Bert Benson answered. "You are required, during a deposition, to answer the attorney's questions."

"You have my credentials in the papers before you, Mr. Bachman. If you would have examined them, you would already have the answer to your question," Dr. Taillefer softly replied.

"Answer me, Dr. Taillefer, are you a hematologist? Are you a doctor who has specialized in treating patients with bleeding problems?"

"No, I am just an ordinary doctor," Dr. Taillefer admitted. "I'm not a blood specialist; I'm not a hematologist."

HIV and AIDS was new territory for attorneys as well as for doctors. A great amount of information must be assimilated in preparation for a trial. There was no indication that Craigdon's suit against Dr. Taillefer would be set aside. Attorneys had an opportunity to establish a new area of expertise. They would become knowledgeable by preparing for the trial of AIDS issues relating to the blood supply and concentrates. If one suit was not favorably settled, they would at least gain experience and establish a knowledge base for future settlements and court trials.

During the late winter of 1991, on February 21, Dr. Taillefer received a telephone call from the attorney general's office at Oregon's state capitol in Salem. John McCulloch, special trial counselor to the Oregon attorney general, overseer of Bert Benson, wished to meet with Dr. Taillefer and prepare him for the Craigdon trial, which had been reset for June 1991. Dr. Taillefer mounted his gray Moto Guzzi motorcycle April 23 to visit Mr. McCulloch's office in the Justice Department Building in Salem. Dr. Taillefer usually commuted daily from his home to the hemophilia treatment center on a bicycle, a distance of five miles. When he had an out-of-town appointment, he rode his Moto Guzzi or drove one of his old trucks to the appointment.

In the State Office Building, Mr. McCulloch welcomed Dr. Taillefer into his quarters, a somber subdued suite paneled in dark wood. Dr. Taillefer placed his white Shoei motorcycle helmet in a corner of the room, on the polished wooden floor. He attempted to minimize his appearance as a motorcycle guy. He appeared as a tall, trim, middle-aged man, sporting gold-rimmed spectacles and a gray moustache, with a casual country-folk manner but with confidence and self-assuredness. The attorney questioned the doctor about his recollection of the plaintiff, Brad Craigdon. He wanted to know what type of person he was … what were his personal qualities. Was he excitable, reliable, and dependable? How did he present himself—with confidence or was he withdrawn? Mr. McCulloch began to instruct Dr. Taillefer regarding his personal appearance, reminding him that his appearance and presence before the jury was the most important aspect of the trial. The jury, not the judge nor the attorneys, would decide the fate of Dr. Taillefer in the courtroom.

"You must not wear motorcycle clothes at the trial. There must be no leaking of information to the plaintiff's attorneys that you even ride a motorcycle. They could manipulate motorcycle culture to make you appear disrespectful before the jury."

Mr. McCulloch advised the doctor that he must dress like a doctor is expected to dress. He continued speaking in a serious tone of voice, instructing Dr. Taillefer that he needed to purchase a new jacket and match it with a stylized dress shirt, coordinated necktie, and slacks. And he must wear well-shined black dress shoes.

Mr. McCulloch continued to prepare Dr. Taillefer for his appearance before the court. He coached him, saying that he must always answer questions simply, without long answers. He should never make a statement or volunteer information that he was not asked. He must answer questions promptly, without hesitation, and look directly at the jury when replying to questions. He was to impress the jury that he was interested in their interpretation of what he had to say, relaying to them that he considered their opinions important.

Mr. McCulloch warned the doctor that he would be questioned by several attorneys, including Mr. Bachman of Philadelphia. The plaintiff's attorneys would ask him questions in different ways. Using his deposition before them, they would attempt to demonstrate differences in his answers in court compared to the recorded answers to questions in his deposition in order to discredit him before the jury.

"Regardless of the temperament of the plaintiff's attorneys, no matter how many times they rephrase the same question, do not lose your composure. Remain calm. Always relay to the jury an impression of sincerity, honesty, and confidence," Mr. McCulloch warned Dr. Taillefer.

After he was excused from the coaching session, Dr. Taillefer thought that John McCulloch reminded him of Chester, a long, lanky cowboy on the television program *Gunsmoke*, the sidekick of Matt Dillon, who walked with a limp and spoke with a drawl. He returned to Portland on his gray chrome-trimmed Moto Guzzi, cruising up the I-5 Freeway, savoring the sweet rumble from the twin Bub exhaust pipes. He'd discovered that the attorney's demeanor, his home-spun friendliness, was a skillful ploy that threw adversaries off guard. John McCulloch was not a backwoods attorney working for the government, one who had no interest in defending a public employee. He was a local Oregonian, born in Portland and a graduate from law school at the University of Oregon, whose skills in the courtroom elevated him to become the special trial counselor to the attorney general. He served the Oregon Department of Justice in addition to maintaining a private law practice with his daughter, Sue-Del McCulloch. He had successfully served a broad spectrum of clients in the public and private sectors of Oregon.

Multiple coaching sessions with Dr. Taillefer, directed by John McCulloch, finally culminated in not a perfect witness, but an acceptable defendant for the trial to be held in Alaska. The State of Oregon, where Dr. Taillefer attended to the needs of persons affected by hemophilia at the treatment center, had a cap on liability, limiting the amount a person could request in suit against a doctor to $250,000. There was no cap on liability in Alaska. Therefore, the attorneys for the plaintiff, Brad Craigdon, filed their lawsuit in the Ninth Federal District Court in Anchorage, Alaska. The suit listed Dr. Taillefer as a defendant, suing him as well as the university, where the treatment center was located, and Miles Laboratories, who had manufactured the Koate that Brad Craigdon had infused for treating his hemophilia.

Chris, Dr. Taillefer's oldest son, who had just turned twenty-four, drove his father to the Portland International Airport on Saturday May 11, 1991, where he boarded Alaska Airlines Flight 1406, departing at 8:30 AM for Anchorage. The attorneys, Bert Benson, John McCulloch, and their assistant, Margaret May Mills, had checked their bags and were seated in the airport waiting area to board the same flight. Dr. Taillefer kept his distance from them, as if he was sending them a message implying he was displeased to be there. He regarded the event as an unjust burden, an intrusion into his life.

His daughter Mary came to the airport to see him off, not knowing when her father would return to Portland from Anchorage. As a going-away gift, in hopes of raising her father's spirits, she presented him with Mark Twain's book *The Innocents Abroad* for his reading pleasure during the trial days ahead in Alaska. She recalled letters her father had mailed to her on his trips to Alaska native villages beginning when she was three years of age, in 1967, letters she had saved.

After the flight arrived in Anchorage on Saturday, the four persons from Oregon crowded into a rental car with their bags and drove to the Captain Cook Hotel, where they had room reservations. They had no idea how many nights they would sleep in the Anchorage hotel.

The next morning, Dr. Taillefer walked to the Holy Family Cathedral, where he attended the 10:00 AM mass. Worship services that Sunday morning included unusual guests. The bishop introduced families from Magadan who had traveled from Russia. Their home, across Chukchi, on the Sea of Okhotsk, in eastern Russia, on the sixtieth parallel, was the destination for a group of Alaskan aviators during the past months.

An association of small airplane owners had received permission to fly their airplanes to Magadan in a group. The Berlin Wall had come down in 1989, but the Soviet Union was still ruled by Mikhail Gorbachev, General Secretary and Ruler. The Soviet Union would not be dissolved until a few months later, during Christmas 1991. The airplane pilots, after visiting the Russian town, invited the Russian families to visit Anchorage, as a gesture of friendship toward their emergence from Soviet suppression.

Sunday afternoon, May 12, Dr. Taillefer was confined to Mr. McCulloch's hotel room, reviewing papers and documents as well as listening to coaching instructions regarding his appearance before the jury. Finally, Dr. Taillefer, who had become restless—his thoughts were not about the forthcoming Alaska trial—walked out of the hotel room and followed a wide paved path, walking alone along Cook Inlet, rejuvenating his spirits with the view of the sharp snow-covered mountain peaks visible to the west across the open water. The low position of the sun above the western horizon created a pink glow on the snow-covered mountains across the deep blue water of Cook Inlet and Knik Arm. The prominent Mount Susitna dominated the other peaks, as if that majestic mountain ruled the others. It resembled a father of a large family surrounded by his children.

Monday morning, May 13, included an early breakfast meeting in the hotel café, attended by the attorneys, their assistant, and Dr. Taillefer. They explained that their planned strategy in court required the assistance of local Anchorage attorneys. Boxes and boxes of papers related to the trial demanded organization and efficient access. Via car, they traveled the short distance to the law office in Anchorage, where Darrel Higgins assisted them and provided storage with easy access for rapidly retrieving papers and documents during the trial. After introducing Dr. Taillefer to Mr. Higgins, the three attorneys returned to the federal courthouse for the scheduled 9:00 AM jury selection. The federal courthouse in Anchorage is a large, imposing cement fortress-like structure with courtrooms on the upper level. Entrance includes passing through security, a safeguard against carrying pocketknives or any concealed metallic objects detectable with X-ray machines.

Dr. Taillefer was instructed by Mr. McCulloch that his presence was required during the jury selection. The trial was in the Ninth District courtroom of the U. S. Federal Court, presided over by the Honorable Judge James Fitzgerald. Opening remarks were presented by the plaintiff's attorney and by the attorney for the defendant. The attorney's opening remarks for the plaintiff contended that Dr. Taillefer had failed to warn the plaintiff, Brad Craigdon, of the risk of HIV infection, which leads to AIDS, from the concentrate he was infusing for treating his hemophilia. Dr. Taillefer and Miles Laboratories, the manufacturer, should have known and warned Mr. Craigdon of the risk by December 2, 1982, the attorney stated.

Although three defendants were listed, only Dr. Taillefer would sit in the courtroom during the trial. If the jury found him guilty of failure to warn, the other two defendants, Miles Laboratories and OHSU, would also be assumed guilty. If he were acquitted by the jury, complaints against the other two defendants would be dismissed. The attorneys, John McCulloch and Bert Benson, represented Dr. Taillefer as well as OHSU. Mr. Lance Penser, from San Francisco, represented Miles Laboratories. Mr. Marty Bachman, from Philadelphia, represented Mr. Brad Craigdon. Each of these attorneys was assisted by Anchorage attorneys, comprising a filled courtroom before Judge Fitzgerald. The requested retribution sought by the plaintiff included twenty million dollars[102] from Dr. Taillefer and each of the other two defendants, totaling sixty million dollars, a huge amount of money. Dr. Taillefer, well dressed, sat silently, motionless, listening to the opening statements until the court was adjourned by Judge Fitzgerald until the next day at 9:00 AM. The judge addressed the jurists, instructing them that they must not discuss the case outside the courtroom. He cautioned them to refuse offers to make comments to the newspapers if requested to

---

102 In 1990, $20,000,000 and $60,000,000 would be equivalent to $32,950,000 and
$98,850,000 in 2008, calculated as the gross price index (Measuringworth 2009).

do so. At the end of the day, Dr. Taillefer walked from the federal courthouse back to the Captain Cook Hotel. In the evening, he walked to McDonalds for a Big Mac dinner with french fries, followed by a pleasant evening walk along Cook Inlet.

On the morning of his fourth day in Anchorage, Dr. Taillefer had his breakfast alone in his room, to avoid his attorneys. The *Anchorage Daily News* of Tuesday morning, May 14, printed news of the AIDS trial. Dr. Taillefer clipped the article from the newspaper and mailed it to the hemophilia treatment center in Portland.

The plaintiff's attorneys continued to present their arguments during the remainder of the week in the federal courthouse. Dr. Taillefer, gray-haired, with a trimmed moustache, sat quietly during those days, listening to the attorneys. He was dressed neatly in a brown tweed jacket, with coordinated brown slacks, a pale blue dress shirt with a thin brown stripe, matching necktie, and polished brown shoes. He looked through his metal-rimmed spectacles directly at individual members of the jury, one after another, sitting in the wooden jury seats.

He remarked to John McCulloch during a court intermission that the judge's eyes were closed as if he were asleep, referring to Judge Fitzgerald. The judge, wearing his black robe, had had his eyelids lowered as he leaned backward in his swivel chair behind the elevated court desk where he presided. Mr. McCulloch cautioned the doctor not to be misguided, not to be fooled by the judge's lowered eyelids. He was not sleeping. He knew what was going on.

Saturday and Sunday, the eighth and ninth day in Anchorage for the trial, were days off from court appearances. But John McCulloch forbid Dr. Taillefer to fly home for the weekend to be with his family in Portland. Instead, he was allowed to place telephone calls to three of his children, Mary, Jennifer, and Christopher. Mr. Lance Penser, the San Francisco attorney defending Miles Laboratories, who was staying in the penthouse suite on the top floor of the Captain Cook Hotel, with a panoramic view of Cook Inlet, in contrast with Dr. Taillefer's lower level simple hotel room, flew back to San Francisco Friday evening, to return to Anchorage

Monday morning. Dr. Taillefer returned to Holy Family Cathedral to attend the Sunday morning mass. The attorneys coached and directed him in their hotel room Sunday afternoon in preparation for the defense arguments. In the evening, as the spring daylight hours lasted, he jogged along Cook Inlet, where whales were visible near the shoreline.

Monday morning, May 20, the tenth day in Anchorage, was a beautiful, windless day with clear blue skies, a comfortable temperature. A muffin shop was discovered down the street from the hotel. The shop was busy at breakfast time, for coffee and a raisin muffin were a pleasant beginning to the day. Dr. Taillefer wondered why some little shops were so successful while others failed. Maybe if he lost in this trial, he could open a muffin shop in Portland. His time would be used better, and more income would be earned than he received as a doctor spending his days in court being sued.

In the federal district courtroom, there was continuing testimony by the plaintiff's witnesses. The mother of the plaintiff testified, stating that her son had been devastated by the effect of knowing he was HIV-positive and that he would die of AIDS. He had followed the recommendations of Dr. Taillefer, who prescribed medicine that would allow him to overcome the effects of hemophilia and lead a near-normal life. Instead, Dr. Taillefer gave him medicine that was contaminated with a deadly virus, which sealed his fate. Why didn't Dr. Taillefer warn him of the dangers of the medicine?

The testimony of Brad Craigdon's mother was disturbing. Dr. Taillefer didn't blame Brad or his mother for their reaction to such a terrible sentence. He also would have been devastated if someone informed him that he would become stricken with AIDS. But Dr. Taillefer attempted to maintain his composure without revealing any turmoil from her testimony. He had known Brad's mother for more than fifteen years, during which time he had advised her on methods to care for the problems resulting from her son's recurrent bleeds. She had always been cordial, without any indication of ill feelings toward him, in contrast to the animosity displayed in the courtroom.

At the noon recess, Dr. Taillefer needed a respite from the tension of the court. He walked to a shopping mall in downtown Anchorage for lunch. He was impressed with the modern shops, including a large Nordstrom store. He was becoming very weary of the trial. He considered bolting out of there. Running away. In the evening, after a pleasant walk along Cook Inlet, he retired to his small hotel room and read half of Brad Craigdon's deposition, printed on a stack of sheets of white paper, before falling to sleep.

Tuesday morning, the eleventh day in Anchorage, hay fever bothered Dr. Taillefer, resulting in red eyes, sneezing, and a stuffy nose. His symptoms were allayed some after he ingested a Fred Meyer cold capsule. The plaintiff's side completed their witnesses' testimony. News on television in the hotel room announced that the Portland Trail Blazers defeated the Los Angeles Lakers in basketball.

After sitting motionless all day in the courtroom, the doctor wanted to be out-of-doors in the evening. He left the hotel for a brisk one-hour walk before driving the rental car a short distance South of Anchorage, where a body of water juts inland from Cook Inlet, representing a fjord between the Kenai Peninsula to the south and the Chugach Mountains to the north. The waterway is blind, not a passageway. The magnitude of the tide is one of the greatest of any body of water in the world, five meters. During high tide, it is an inviting body of water several miles wide and more than forty miles in length. After the seawater rushes out at low tide, which requires five hours, a large mud flat remains. In 1778, Captain James Cook led an expedition into the body of water that now bears his name, Cook Inlet. Seeking a Northwest passage, he dispatched William Bligh from *HMS Bounty* to explore this arm of water. Bligh was thwarted, unable to discover an outlet, and forced to reverse passage of his ship for the second time, to turn again, hence the name "Turn Again Arm."

On that Tuesday evening, Dr. Taillefer witnessed a spectacular sight when he drove the rental car eastward along Turn Again Arm. The tide had rushed out, leaving a pod of black-and-white killer whales stranded in the tide pools, including two adult males and two females with two juveniles.[103] After stopping the car and parking along the roadside, when he was out of the car, Dr. Taillefer heard the juveniles making a shrill sound, as if they were crying for their mothers. The juveniles moved about in the tide pools and splashed water with their tails onto the adults to prevent the skin of their parents, who were trapped, unable to move about, from becoming dry. Autos blocked the road as people stopped to view the whales. A man carrying wet blankets waded out in the mud to the adults, covering them for their protection. However, he was arrested by the patrolmen from the Department of Fish and Wildlife for disturbing the whales, a reminder that law enforcement officers tend to demand what is legal, rather than considering what is reasonable for the circumstances. The newspaper the next morning reported that the tide returned and the whales were able to make their way back into the sea.

Wednesday, May 22, the twelfth day in Anchorage, was a beautiful cloudless day. The defense began its presentation with Bert Benson questioning witnesses. When Dr. Taillefer walked back to his hotel room from the courthouse, at the end of another long day in the courtroom, a care package from home, mailed by his daughter, Julie, was waiting for him. It contained photographs, books, and letters, including one from his twenty-one-year-old-son, Nicholas. The package also contained snacks, teas, and a drawing from his three-year-old granddaughter Laura Annie. On the thirteenth day, Dr. Taillefer became discouraged as the trial continued. He sought solace, a time for reflection, during a long evening walk on the coastal trail, proclaiming out loud, out of hearing range of his attorneys, that he didn't want to be with any more lawyers!

On the fourteenth day in Alaska, Friday, May 24, court session did not convene, to allow attorneys time to prepare their procedures.

---

103 Orcinus orca, the killer whale, is the largest of the oceanic dolphin family. The males are six to eight meters in length, and the adult females produce a calf every five years.

Dr. Taillefer rented a mountain bike, a convenient way to explore the coastal trail. In the evening, John McCulloch, Bert Benson, Margaret May Mills, and Dr. Taillefer were invited to dinner at the home of the Anchorage attorney and his wife, Darrel and Maxine Higgins. The Higgins's home was in a lovely residential area with wide streets, where modern single-story residences are set back from the curbs. While enjoying dinner, an unannounced guest arrived in the backyard, visible though the large bay window. Mrs. Higgins had recently planted two new trees in her garden. A tall shaggy brown moose on skinny legs stopped before each of the new trees bearing delicate new green leaves, and munched his way down to the ground, leaving only bare dirt where the trees had briefly stood. The moose, who may have been smiling, trotted away, leaving the dinner guests to consume the barbecued chicken the Higgins had prepared for dinner.

The next morning, Saturday, May 25, no court was in session. The Oregon attorneys, Margaret May Mills, and Dr. Taillefer hired a guide to float them down the Kenai River on an inflatable raft. The river is wide and shallow, where the easily visible salmon are caught when migrating up the shallow gravel streambeds. As they drifted from Cooper's Landing to Lake Skilka, the water was difficult to visualize in places because of smoke from a forest fire on the Kenai Peninsula.

The third day off from court, Sunday, May 26, after again attending mass, Dr. Taillefer set out on the yellow mountain bike for a ride along the seacoast of Cook Inlet. Alaska has fabulous bike paths. But he discovered that others, in addition to bicycle riders, traveled the wide paved bicycle paths. As he was descending a hill on the curved path through the trees, he heard a warning cry behind him. "On your left, coming past you!" Although he was descending the hill at a fast pace on the bicycle, he was soon overtaken and passed by two helmeted persons on roller blades. He wondered how they stopped themselves without crashing to the ground.

Upon returning to the hotel after the bicycle ride, the doctor ate dinner alone in his room. He read the Sunday paper, which recounted the adventures of Beethoven. West of Anchorage, families own summer homes on the shore of Lake Susitna. Along the lakeshore, floating docks had been constructed, where the homeowners moor their float airplanes when they fly to the lake for summer weekends. Some of the homes had been badly damaged when the owners were absent. The damage was caused by falling trees. Inspection revealed that a beaver had gnawed the tree trunks, causing the large trees to fall onto the houses. The irate owners discovered that the gnawsome beaver was living beneath one of the floating docks. The homeowners flew their seaplanes to the lake, moored them to the docks in front of their homes, and set a trap for Mr. Beaver. While the owners were sleeping during the night, the beaver, which they had labeled Beethoven, gnawed the mooring lines, setting the float planes adrift. The homeowners, according to the Sunday paper, were concerned about catching Beethoven to prevent further damage to their lakeshore homes, and they were wondering how they could recover their seaplanes, which were adrift. The last report that Dr. Taillefer read in the newspaper about Beethoven indicated that the homeowners' attempts to catch Beethoven were unsuccessful.

The number of days of residence in Anchorage for the defendants from Oregon continued to increase. The sixteenth day, Monday May 27 was a holiday, Memorial Day, without a scheduled court session. The attorney for Miles Laboratory, Lance Penser, left his penthouse suit for the weekend, flying to San Francisco. Dr. Taillefer and his attorneys remained in Anchorage. From 10:00 AM until 3:00 PM, they assembled in the law offices of Darrel Higgins, reviewing depositions and documents. Dr. Taillefer reflected that he was becoming weary of Anchorage and the court proceedings. The day was overcast with a light rain, which did not prevent him from going on a bike ride along the coast trail. He had his dinner in the hotel room, where he wrote letters to be mailed to his children and grandchildren, a total of ten letters.

The trial resumed on Tuesday, the seventeenth day in Anchorage, a cool, cloudy day. Prior to appearing in court at 9:00 AM, Dr. Taillefer telephoned Mr. T. K. Hammaer, an officer in the Portland Bureau of the

IRS, who had been assigned to handle his delinquent income tax. The previous summer, records for filing income tax were destroyed in the fire that consumed his home. Even though Dr. Taillefer submitted a copy of the *Oregonian* that included a full front page of his burning house, the IRS would not accept his excuse for lack of receipts and records. The telephone call to the IRS was not effective. His delinquent income taxes were just one more conflict demanding his attention.

The trial moved into the defense phase of arguments, with attorneys calling witnesses. Dr. Erik Dunthorp was called by John McCulloch to the witness stand. Dr. Dunthorp, director of the New England Area Comprehensive Hemophilia Center, and member of MASAC[104], testified as an expert witness for the defense of Dr. Taillefer. Dr. Dunthorp, who flew to Anchorage from the University of Massachusetts, in Worcester, told the jury that Dr. Taillefer had responsibly prescribed concentrate for Mr. Craigdon according to the knowledge currently available. He recounted for the jury that by the time the agent that causes AIDS, HIV, was discovered, Mr. Craigdon was already infected. Experience has revealed that HIV infection from infusing concentrate in hemophilia occurred in the late 1970s—1978 or 1979—or early 1980s—1981 or 1982, before any virucidal measures were included in the manufacture of concentrate.

During the afternoon, three persons arrived in Anchorage from the hemophilia center in Portland: Dr. Larry Watson and nurses Sue Underwood and Myrna Campbell. Sue had retired from the hemophilia center. She was called as a witness to attest to the medical nature of the treatment center that provided direction for Mr. Craigdon's hemophilia care when he lived in Vader, Washington, prior to his move to Alaska. Sue, Mr. McCulloch reasoned, with her unsophisticated speech and Southern drawl, would prove to be an effective witness to testify before the jury. On the eighteenth day in Anchorage, Wednesday, May 29, Mr. Viktor Mack from Cutter Biological was called to testify, defending

---

104 Medical and Scientific Advisory Committee of the National Hemophilia
  Foundation

the worthiness of Koate, which Dr. Taillefer had prescribed for Mr. Craigdon. The day was cool and windy, a day for a good bicycle ride. Dr. Taillefer enjoyed riding into the wind, struggling against nature, a struggle that can be physically won, in contrast to a struggle against society, which will be lost, resulting in discontent and frustration. Following the ride in the fresh air, and the purchase of a birthday card for his son, Nick, Dr. Taillefer met with Dr. Elisabeth Jergens, who was scheduled to testify the next day, and the nurses for dinner in the hotel dining room.

The trial resumed on the nineteenth day in Anchorage, a cool, overcast morning, Thursday, May 30, with the testimony of Dr. Jergens from the hemophilia center at Cornell Medical Center in New York City. She attested that Dr. Taillefer had provided directions and recommendations for Mr. Craigdon's hemophilia care in a timely and proper manner, using all the knowledge available in the 1970s and 1980s. During the midday court recess for lunch, Dr. Taillefer visited the Anchorage Museum, which housed a commendable bookstore as well as many Russian artifacts. During the afternoon session in court, Dr. Larry Watson, a hematologist and hemophilia treater from the Oregon Hemophilia Treatment Center, testified for the defense of Dr. Taillefer, reinforcing the impression that Dr. Taillefer's prescribed treatment for Brad Craigdon had been appropriate and timely. Following dinner in his room, Dr. Taillefer reviewed his expected testimony with John McCulloch until 11:30 PM, while observing the late May evening daylight, which persisted until 12:30 AM.

On the twentieth day in Anchorage, Friday, May 31, the clerk of the court announced, "All rise." The Honorable James Fitzpatrick, wearing his long black judge's robe, entered from a side door near the rear of the courtroom. The judge took a seat in his swivel chair behind his wooden desk in the center of the courtroom. From the front entrance of the courtroom, the members of the jury, in single file, entered and assumed their seats in the jury box at the side of the courtroom. Dr. Aaron Kingston, the Anchorage hematologist who provided care for

Brad Craigdon in Anchorage, sat in the witness stand. Before sitting in the dark brown armed wooden witness chair, Dr. Kingston repeated the oath administered to him by the clerk of the court, swearing to God to tell the truth while holding up his right arm. His testimony was followed by Sue Underwood, the retired nurse from Portland, who had served in the hemophilia treatment center from its beginning and had participated in the medical care of Mr. Craigdon before he moved to Alaska. Dr. Kingston and Mrs. Underwood testified that Dr. Taillefer provided excellent care for Mr. Craigdon, and the doctor was always concerned about Brad Craigdon's well-being.

Although hay fever continued to be troublesome, Dr. Taillefer was more comfortable as the trial proceeded, despite sitting so many days before the jury. He received telephone calls when he returned to his hotel room, as well as letters from his family in Portland, including a letter from his fourth daughter, Mary. There would be birthday parties in Portland for his son Nick, June 1, and for his granddaughter Laura, June 5. But he was stranded in court in Anchorage. He would much rather enjoy attending birthday parties in Portland. During lunch recess from court one day, John McCulloch and Bert Benson informed Dr. Taillefer that they would withhold him from testifying until the next Monday. He told them that he was weary of his court appearance and wanted to proceed as quickly as possible and return to his customary life away from the court.

The weekend arrived, Saturday, June 1, and Sunday, June 2, the twenty-first and twenty-second days in Anchorage, where the daylight extended into the evening until 1:00 AM. The testimony of the plaintiff was reread. Dr. Taillefer was coached by John McCulloch, who maintained that Mr. Marty Bachman would attempt to discredit him before the jury. Mr. Bachman, the well-known trial lawyer from Philadelphia, he predicted, would utilize Dr. Taillefer's sworn disposition. He was expected to ask Dr. Taillefer questions based upon statements in the disposition in order to reveal a conflict in his testimony in court before the jury compared to his statement in the deposition. John McCulloch warned Dr. Taillefer to study his deposition and only offer answers that were recorded. "Give direct, brief answers," Mr. McCulloch reminded him. He was not to offer statements beyond the answers to questions Mr. Bachman[105] put before him. On Saturday evening, Dr. Taillefer and Sue Underwood each selected a bowl of soup in the hotel café at 9:00 PM. The bright Alaska springtime daylight continued for several more hours. Outdoors, the drone from the engines of airplanes disrupted the evening silence as pilots capitalized on the long hours of daylight, hauling supplies to villages in the bush.

Sunday morning brought pleasant weather, with intermittent clouds in the sky. Following a breakfast in the hotel restaurant, discussion and coaching for the trial continued between Sue Underwood, Margaret May Mills, Bert Benson, and Dr. Taillefer as they drove north from Anchorage on Highway 1, on their way to the Matanuska Valley. There, they noted dandelion stems growing to a height of two feet while supporting bright yellow blossoms three inches across.[106] For lunch, they sat in the café of the Palmer Hotel, thirty-seven miles northeast of Anchorage. From Palmer, they could view the Chugach Mountains in the east and the Alaska Range to the north and west that includes Mt. McKinley, rising to 20,320 feet.

On the twenty-third day in Anchorage, June 3, a beautiful Monday morning, Dr. Taillefer talked on the phone with his daughter Kathy and her husband, Steve, and to Myrna and Josephine in the hemophilia center in Portland. He received a letter from his daughter Jennifer. Dr. Taillefer was called to the witness stand on this day to begin his defense testimony. He was in the witness chair, before the judge and jury, from 9:00 AM until 5:00 PM, except for lunchtime. He was questioned by John McCulloch. He felt relieved to be testifying after sitting silently for so many days. His spirits improved.

---

105 Marty Bachman, a Philadelphia trial attorney, was labeled as "Smarty Marty" during the trial because of his demeanor.

106 The Matanuska Valley produces cabbages that achieve two feet in diameter, weighing five to ten pounds, an effect of extended hours of daylight in the springtime and early summer.

The twenty-fourth day, June 4, testimony continued, with Dr. Taillefer resuming his position in the witness chair. He was cross-examined by Marty Bachman for the entire morning, until the court's noon recess. Mr. Bachman had miscalculated Dr. Taillefer's courtroom appearance before the jury. In his recollection of Dr. Taillefer's deposition in Portland last September, nine months previously, Mr. Bachman had assumed he could demonstrate to the jury that the doctor was poorly qualified to direct a hemophilia treatment center. He was expected to give vague, confusing, inconsistent answers to questions during cross-examination. The plaintiff's attorney assumed Dr. Taillefer would have the appearance of a slovenly, casual backwoods doctor who was unsure of himself. Mr. Bachman demanded to know, "Dr. Taillefer, are you a hematologist?"

Dr. Taillefer's response to Mr. Bachman's demand: "No, I am not a hematologist."

"But hemophilia is a blood disease. How can you direct a clinic serving persons with a blood disorder if you are not a blood specialist?" the short-statured, intense, well-dressed Philadelphia attorney demanded to know, as he peered with a piercing gaze over the gold metal rims of his spectacles.

"Hemophilia is not a blood disease, "Dr. Taillefer softly replied with assurance.

"Well, then," Mr. Bachman retorted, while parting his thin lips and showing his teeth, attempting to smile, which was more like a sneer, "Dr. Taillefer, if you say hemophilia is not a blood disease, what kind of disease do you say it is?"

"Hemophilia is not a disease."

"What? You say it is not a disease? What is hemophilia, then?" Mr. Bachman impatiently queried, his back turned to Dr. Taillefer while facing the jury.

Dr. Taillefer waited for Mr. Bachman to turn around so that he could face him directly before replying to his question. He answered the attorney by characterizing hemophilia as the result of a disturbance in blood clotting, not a blood disease. The disorder affects the entire person. In the treatment center, there are hematologists as well as other medical specialists. His role was to assure that modern, excellent medical management was identified and provided to persons who had hemophilia. Dr. Taillefer said he was a specialist, an experienced and qualified hemophilia treater although he was not a hematologist.

Despite several maneuvers, Mr. Bachman failed to discredit Dr. Taillefer. He was unable to demonstrate inconsistencies between his deposition and his testimony. John McCulloch may have impressed Mr. Bachman as a superficial attorney just doing a routine job of defending a case assigned to him by the attorney general's office when he attended the deposition in Portland. He was taken aback when he discovered that Mr. McCulloch favorably impressed the jury. Dr. Taillefer was a creditable defendant and Mr. McCulloch was a strong attorney. Mr. Bachman discovered that Dr. Taillefer had been well coached. He was well prepared for his defense by his attorneys, Mr. McCulloch and Mr. Benson.

Dr. Taillefer was aware that the plaintiff, Brad Craigdon, was not always present when court was in session. He was also sensitive to Craigdon's avoidance of looking directly at him whenever he was present in the courtroom. He had always liked his former patient. He assumed Brad was following the advice of his attorneys by avoiding his former doctor's gaze. He felt sorry for his patient. He was bothered that Brad's mother wouldn't look at him or speak to him after all the years of association. Dr. Taillefer reasoned that perhaps that's the way it has to be in court. He was a doctor and didn't understand everything about lawyers.

Lunch was at the Captain Cook Hotel café where two Anchorage newspapers revealed that Dr. Taillefer had testified as a defendant the previous day in Judge Fitzgerald's federal district court. Dr. Taillefer followed the judge's orders and refused to be interviewed by reporters from the newspapers. The articles that appeared were composed by journalists who attended the courtroom hearings without interviewing the doctor or the attorneys.

Following lunch, court resumed. Dr. Taillefer's testimony had been completed during the morning session. The defense rested. Rebuttal witnesses were summoned to the witness stand by the plaintiff's attorney, not Mr. Bachman, but by Mr. Craigdon's Anchorage attorney. A nurse from Providence Hospital in Anchorage was called to rebut Nurse Sue Underwood's testimony; however, the argument was weak and anticlimactic. At 4:00 PM, Dr. Taillefer was released and the court adjourned to allow attorneys time to prepare their closing arguments. Dr. Taillefer shopped for gifts for his children. He discovered a red rubber stamp pad for a birthday gift for his granddaughter, Laura, who would be three years old the next day, June 5. He was pleased to receive a telephone call in the evening from his daughter Jennifer.

On Wednesday June 5, the twenty-fifth day in Alaska, the hemophilia center in Portland reported by telephone to Dr. Taillefer that activities within the clinic were proceeding well despite his absence. They missed his presence and requested that he hurry home, which he certainly desired. When he realized the clinic could function without him, he questioned whether that was good or bad. Perhaps he was not as indispensable as he'd thought he was. Court reconvened during the morning, after Dr. Taillefer discussed details with John McCulloch at breakfast. Closing arguments were presented for the plaintiff, by Marty Bachman, and for Dr. Taillefer, by John McCulloch. Judge Fitzgerald instructed the jury until 5:00 PM, when they were released after being reminded again that discussion of the case was forbidden.

The evening was cloudy and cool as Dr. Taillefer and his attorneys visited an Anchorage tavern. The walls of the interior of the tavern were elegantly paneled with dark wood. Many of the customers, all men, wore jackets with shirts and neckties. They stood leaning against brass rails that surrounded small, round, tall tables and the edge of a long bar. They drank mugs of foaming beers, some smoking cigarettes or cigars, while nibbling tidbits from small plates of food. The view of Cook Inlet from the wall-length windows on the west side was magnificent. Dr. Taillefer was not very sociable; he was surly. He was thinking that the tavern was profane. The white man chased all the Eskimos and Indians away from there, their land, and replaced them with this outlandish tavern, where they did not feel welcome. He realized that the Alaska native people would be absorbed by the aggressive white man. They would not survive many more generations. Anchorage has become a hub for world business, affording access between Asia and North America, but the natives do not benefit. They are too gentle.

Thursday morning, the twenty-sixth day in Alaska, June 6, court resumed at 9:00 AM, with the jury out for deliberation. Dr. Taillefer could only wait. And wait. He returned to the hotel room to patiently sit with his attorneys and Margaret May Mills. They were silent and restless, but they could only continue waiting. The hours passed slowly.

Friday, the twenty-seventh day in Alaska, June 7, a telephone call was received in the hotel room at 3:00 PM. The jury had reached a verdict. The attorneys and Dr. Taillefer scurried from the hotel to the courthouse. They entered the courtroom and were seated. After the judge entered and was seated, the jury was summoned. At 4:30 PM, Judge Fitzgerald asked the foreman if the jury had reached a verdict.

"We have reached a verdict, Your Honor," the foreman responded.

"And what is your verdict? How do you find the defendant, Dr. Taillefer?" the judge asked.

"Your Honor," the foreman replied, "we the jury find the defendant, Dr. Taillefer, not guilty." He stated this clearly.

Acquitted!

The jury had concluded that thirty-two-year-old Brad Craigdon had become infected from infusions of concentrate for treating his hemophilia before December 1, 1982. That was a date agreed upon by the attorneys and the plaintiff—that Miles Laboratories and Dr. Anton Taillefer should have known of the risk of infection and should have warned Brad Craigdon. He was already infected before that date; therefore, the manufacturer of the medicine and the doctor were neither negligent nor liable for not informing him of his risk of HIV infection until 1982.

The contentious and often bitter four-week trial ended. Several jurors began crying after the verdict was read. Judge James Fitzgerald directed courthouse security guards to keep the lawyers, reporters, and spectators in the courtroom until the jury had left the building. The *Anchorage Daily News* immediately requested an interview from Dr. Taillefer as he left the courtroom.

Dr. Taillefer, a sixty-one-year-old pediatrician who had treated individuals with hemophilia for a long part of his career, sobbed and hugged his lawyers after the verdict was read by the jury. Outside the courtroom, he said he felt sorry for all the persons who have hemophilia, those who, like Brad Craigdon, contracted the fatal disease through the clotting medicine that was intended to save their lives. He emphasized that they were innocent victims who got a "raw deal." He had instructed his trusting patients who suffered from hemophilia to take the medicine and their suffering would disappear. They would have a near-normal life and live to become old men. He was wrong.

Dr. Taillefer told the newspaper reporter that he regarded the contamination of concentrate as a great tragedy. He confessed that he was sorry the doctors didn't have access to more information to help Brad and all the other patients before it was too late. The doctors had tried with all of their energy to help their patients, but they were not well enough informed. They were wrong.

At the moment the jury returned to the courtroom with their verdict, Brad Craigdon was not present. He did not hear the verdict read in the courtroom. One of his attorneys stated that he was ill and was unable to drive to Anchorage from his home in Wasilla. Although he did not yet have AIDS, most experts agreed that people infected with the virus will begin to show symptoms eight to ten years after becoming infected. Since the virus, HIV, was not identified until 1985, no one knows for certain when Brad Craigdon became infected. He was tested for the virus in 1986. By 1985, pharmaceutical companies had developed safe concentrates. After that, persons with hemophilia no longer became infected by HIV.

Brad Craigdon's expert witnesses testified that he probably contracted HIV in 1984 because in the early 1980s, he used less concentrate than most severe persons who have hemophilia, and therefore had less chance of becoming infected.

However, experts for Miles Laboratories and Dr. Taillefer cited studies showing that most persons with severe hemophilia who became infected with HIV were infected by the end of 1982 (Del Amo et al. 2006, Darby et al. 1995). They maintained that it was likely Brad Craigdon was infected with the virus before 1983. Dr. Taillefer had saved blood samples from many persons who came to his clinic, including those with hemophilia. The blood samples had been frozen and stored for research investigations. Whenever blood samples from persons who had hemophilia were collected and stored serially over different years and then retrieved and tested for the presence of HIV, the year of HIV infection could often be ascertained. He knew HIV infection occurred in some persons with hemophilia before 1983, as early as 1979 in some instances, before HIV was recognized.

The end of December 1982 became a benchmark in the Craigdon trial because that was when an attorney who was working for Miles Laboratories, the parent company of Cutter, the manufacturer of Brad Craigdon's medicine, wrote a memo advising corporate officers of the company to include an AIDS warning in the concentrate package insert. Brad Craigdon's attorneys considered the memo the central issue of the case. They assumed that the memo would convince the jury that Cutter was aware that the medicine was polluted with the deadly virus. Cutter did not warn users of the risk of the medicine, Craigdon's attorneys assert, for fear that profits from the sale of concentrate would suffer.

By deciding that Brad Craigdon became infected with HIV prior to December 1982, the jury assigned his date of infection beyond the range of anyone's responsibility to warn.

The key to the case was that Brad Craigdon, and all the other persons with severe hemophilia, became infected with the virus before anyone knew anything about the virus. John McCulloch said he was proud of the jury for not finding in favor of the plaintiff during the difficult and emotional trial.

Dr. Taillefer's bag was packed. He quickly returned to the hotel, rushed to the airport, and was on a homeward flight by 5:45 PM. He arrived in Portland at 11:30 PM on June 7, where he was joyously greeted by three of his daughters, Mary, Jennifer, and Kathy, and by his son, Jesse. They held up WELCOME HOME signs they had prepared for their father's return from a month's absence in Alaska.

A Girl with Hemophilia

Wednesday, June 12, 1991, after returning to Portland from Alaska, Dr. Taillefer evaluated Brent in the clinic, which included an assessment of his painful ankles.[107]

"Hey, Ma, there's a girl in the clinic," Brent rushed to tell his mother after she entered the building from the parking lot.

"What do you mean?" Gwyn replied to her son. "Only guys have hemophilia."

"That's what I'd been told," Brent nervously replied. "I thought this was a no-girls clinic. But look, Ma, sitting over there in that wheelchair, that's a girl."

"You're right," Gwyn replied quietly, avoiding attention as she agreed with her son. "We'll ask Dr. Watson or Dr. Taillefer why a girl is waiting in the hemophilia clinic. She appears to be waiting as if she is a patient to be seen by the doctors."

Sally Phillips was thirty-four years of age. She had hemophilia. She was at the hemophilia clinic to visit the orthopedic doctors with her parents and her brother.

When Gwyn sat down, Sally's mother introduced herself. "I am Mrs. Phillips, this is my husband, and this is my daughter and my son. My son and my daughter have hemophilia. When the doctors and nurses came to Pocatello from Portland during a hemophilia outreach clinic, they checked my son and daughter. My daughter has devastating orthopedic problems. She cannot walk any farther

---

107 Note from the daily journal of Dr. Taillefer, June 12, 1991

than from that chair to the drinking fountain. She spends her days in the house on the sofa or in the wheelchair. We thought we would come over here to Portland to see if anything can be done to help Sally walk. She needs a checkup by the orthopedic doctors. We hope they have suggestions that will help her. She cannot get around very well, which makes her feel bad."

"I notice that you appear to be puzzled," Mrs. Phillips continued. "Yes, my husband and I have two children with hemophilia, a boy and a girl, who are now a man and a woman. Hemophilia runs in my family. My son and daughter have cousins with hemophilia in Idaho. The explanation for hemophilia in my daughter is related to another medical condition that affects her. She has Turner syndrome. Rather than having two X chromosomes, Sally has only one X. She has forty-five chromosomes in the cells of her body instead of forty-six, which are present in most women. I passed my X chromosome, which has the hemophilia gene on it, to both my son and my daughter. I do not have hemophilia because I have forty-six chromosomes. That includes an X chromosome bearing a normal gene to cover up the chromosome that has the hemophilia gene on it, "Mrs. Phillips explained to Gwyn. "I am a carrier of hemophilia, but I don't have it."

"I understand. I'm a carrier of hemophilia too," Gwyn responded. "I've met other boys and men with hemophilia before today, but I'd never heard of hemophilia in a girl. The presence of hemophilia in your daughter must be rare; she must be very special."

Turner syndrome occurs when a female has only one X chromosome. Normally females have two X chromosomes, XX. If a gene is located on an X chromosome, an X-linked recessive gene such as hemophilia (h) may be expressed if the normal dominant gene (H) is absent because of a missing X chromosome:

- Normal female $X^H X^H$
- Female hemophilia carrier $X^H X^h$
- Female Turner X^H
- Female Turner hemophilia carrier X^h

Hemophilia can appear in females for different reasons :

- Turner syndrome: X^h

- Female hemophilia carrier marries male hemophilia husband, $X^h X^H$: $X^h Y$, to produce a female with hemophilia: $X^h X^h$

- As a result of lyonization, only one X chromosome in a female is active. If the normal hemophilia gene X^H in a female hemophilia carrier $X^H X^h$ is lyonized (turned off), the hemophilia gene X^h will be actively expressed, resulting in a female with hemophilia.

"Yes, my daughter, Sally, and my son, Steve, are both very special. Both of them have had many bleeds into their joints, which were not treatable until concentrates came along in the 1970s."

Mrs. Phillips's son and daughter were listening to the two mothers talk, comparing notes of bleeds in their children. Steve, Mrs. Phillips's thirty-two-year-old son, said, "Oh, Ma, it's not so bad. I'm attending college and I drive a car." Addressing Gwyn, Steve said, "Now that we have concentrate for treatment of bleeds, I can give myself a shot and prevent pain."

"What do you do, Sally?" Gwyn asked. "How do you spend your days?"

"I like to crochet," Sally cheerfully responded.

"You must have many stories you can recall about hemophilia. Do you have insurance that pays for concentrate?" Gwyn asked Mr. Phillips.

"Oh, yes," he replied with a courteous smile. "We have wonderful insurance that pays for all the costs of my son as long as he is in college, and it pays for Sally since she is disabled."

"You must have a great employer if they pay for the medical costs of your grown children. Hemophilia care is expensive. May I ask who you work for?" Gwyn shyly asked Mr. Phillips. "Some insurance companies will not pay for hemophilia care. They say hemophilia is an inherited disorder; therefore, it is a preexisting medical condition that their benefits will not cover. Other insurance companies have a cap on the benefits of their policies. With two affected beneficiaries on the same policy, the maximum benefit can be quickly reached."

"I'm no longer working. I am retired. I worked for the railroad for forty years, the Burlington Northern in Pocatello. They have been very good to us. They never question our need for help to pay for the medical costs of Steve and Sally. The railroad is a great place to work if you want to raise a family."

When Sally was evaluated by the orthopedist, X-rays of her bones revealed severe joint damage, with almost no knee joint space remaining. The normal joint space was replaced with bone on bone, an absence of the normal cartilage cushion. Arnold Deaton, the physical therapist accompanying Dr. North, reported that Sally's range of motion in her knees was almost nonexistent. Dr. North discussed some possible maneuvers that might benefit Sally. He suggested a diet to help her prevent gaining more weight. Women who have Turner syndrome tend to be short and heavy. If she could avoid weight gain and lose weight, her knees might benefit because she wouldn't be carrying around so much weight. She would also be rewarded physically if she was guided by an exercise program. Arnold Deaton offered to locate a swimming pool for Sally in Pocatello. Non-weight-bearing exercise in a swimming pool twice each week would bring improvement to her daily life. Finally, Dr. North discussed the possibility of knee joint replacement. He said the primary indication for knee joint replacement is to relieve pain. With Sally's mother and father beside her during the orthopedic evaluation, Dr. North explained the process of joint replacement.

Sally preferred to maintain her status quo. Her knees were not painful; there just wasn't any motion. She declined knee joint replacement. When the Phillips family returned to Pocatello, Sally did not enroll in a swimming pool exercise program.

Testing completed in the clinic revealed that Steve and Sally were both HIV-positive. Some persons preferred to complete their HIV tests away from their hometown because of fear that someone they know might discover the test results. Stigma confronted individuals who were HIV infected as a result of the association of AIDS with homosexuality. Sally and Steve began treatment with AZT. However, their health deteriorated and they developed AIDS despite AZT treatment. Mr. and Mrs. Phillips patiently provided the best care they could during the years when their children suffered from recurrent joint bleeds. They finally discovered relief from pain when concentrates became available for infusions at home. They were ultimately confronted with the devastating discovery that the medicine, which had offered so much hope, was contaminated with HIV. After many years of devotion to their son and daughter, instead of a bright future for the rest of their adulthoods, Mr. and Mrs. Phillips buried their son and daughter after they died of AIDS.

The concentrate improved the level of living for Sally and Steve, but ultimately it brought death to both of them because it was contaminated with HIV. Was the improvement in the quality of Sally's life overshadowed by her eventual death from AIDS? Should the doctors have continued to prescribe concentrate after it was recalled because of contamination? Could the pharmaceutical manufacturers of concentrate have eliminated the hepatitis virus, which would also have eliminated HIV? Were the deaths of Sally and Steve preventable?

Part V

Origin of Hepatitis and HIV

Infectious Diseases in Humans Originated in Animals

There had been a lot of discussion about HIV infection and where it came from by 1990, when Brent was fifteen. He questioned why he had never heard of it before. Where did it begin? Who was the first person to get AIDS? He wondered why, if he had hemophilia, he also got AIDS. He had heard that AIDS was one of the "4H diseases," and he wondered what that meant.

Gwyn told her son that some people have said that President Ronald Reagan regarded AIDS as a disease that affects queers. She said what he meant was homosexual men; one of the four Hs stands for homosexual. She pointed out to Brent that a significant source of President Reagan's support came from the religious right and "Moral Majority," a political action group founded by Reverend Jerry Falwell. He said that AIDS is the wrath of God upon homosexuals. Pat Buchanan, President Reagan's director of communications, stated that AIDS is "nature's revenge on gay men" (White 2004).

Despite the increasing deaths from AIDS with the passing of each month, President Reagan's response during his presidency from 1981 to 1989 was indifference. National attention increased in 1985, when the American Hospital of Paris announced on July 25 that film star Rock Hudson had AIDS. Soon after the announcement, in late 1985, U.S. Representative Henry Waxman, Democrat from Los Angeles, proclaimed, "It is surprising that the president could remain silent as six thousand Americans died ... that he failed to acknowledge the epidemic's existence. Perhaps his staff felt he had to, since many of his new right supporters had raised money by campaigning against homosexuals."

Dr. C. Everett Koop, President Reagan's surgeon general, famous for mobilizing the nation in a movement to stop smoking, stated that he was cut out of all AIDS discussion for the first five years of President Reagan's administration by "interdepartmental politics." The reason, he explained: "Transmission of AIDS was understood to be primarily in the homosexual population and in those who abused drugs. The president's advisers," Dr. Koop recounted, "took the stand that 'They are only getting what they deserve.'" At the groundbreaking ceremony of the AIDS health-care organization in Washington, D.C., in 2003, Michael Cover, former associate executive director for public affairs at the Whitman-Walker Clinic, solemnly stated, "In the history of the AIDS epidemic, President Reagan's legacy is one of silence. It is the silence of tens of thousands who died alone and unacknowledged, stigmatized by our government under his administration." Allen White wrote, "How profoundly different might have been the outcome if his leadership had generated compassion rather than hostility."

From 1981 until the end of 2007, 25 million persons died of AIDS, leaving 12 million African orphans (Worldwide AIDS 2007). Gwyn told her son that President Reagan maintained that AIDS was God's justification for punishing people for their sins, the sin of being homosexual. They got what they deserved.

Brent wondered what it meant to be homosexual. He asked his mother if two men who had sex together were homosexual. She replied by confirming that two men, or two women, who had sex together were usually homosexual. The subject of sex was too delicate for him to ask about details from his mother.

Brent quietly asked his mother what the other three *H*s were. Gwyn told her son that the four notorious *H*s stand for homosexuals, hemophiliacs, heroin addicts, and Haitians. Brent wanted to know if he was one of the *H*s. Gwyn answered him by saying that no one likes to be pigeonholed. Who wants to be regarded as some catchy word category? We are all people, individuals, not a label on a filing cabinet drawer. Haitians do not want to be relegated to an AIDS classification, as if they are to blame for the spread of HIV. She told him she didn't think of him as one of the *H*s. She reminded him that she detested the word hemophiliac. She never wanted anyone to call him a hemophiliac. He was not a "thing." He was Brent, not an *H*. He was her son. Her only dear son. And she loved him.

Brent anxiously confessed that there were a lot of things about AIDS and HIV he did not understand. Gwyn reminded her son that if he wanted to know something about HIV or AIDS, he could ask Dr. Strong, who was an expert, or Dr. Watson or Dr. Taillefer. One of those three doctors at the hemophilia treatment center could probably answer his questions, if there was an answer. Some things about AIDS might not be known. AIDS had not been around a long time; it became known only recently. It was a new disease.

Brent demanded to know where AIDS came from. He could not have been aware of a remarkable book, *The River,* written by Edward Hooper, which addressed his query (Hooper 1999). Brent died in 1993; the book was published six years later. One year before Brent's death, scientists concluded that HIV, human immunodeficiency virus, is the direct descendant of SIV, simian immunodeficiency virus, which is present in African Chimpanzees.

Viruses are specific for their hosts. Cows and dogs don't get polio. Polio is a disease of humans. Viruses cannot survive independently by themselves. They require the machinery from the inside of a cell of a host for survival. For polio to infect a human cell, it must attach to the cell before it can invade it. Humans possess a polio receptor site determined by a gene on human chromosome five. Without the receptor site, the polio virus cannot infect the cell and produce disease. Cows and dogs do not possess the polio receptor site. Similarly, the malaria parasite cannot infect human red blood cells unless a receptor site is present on the cell. The malarial receptor site on human red blood cells is the Duffy blood group. Most people are blood group Duffy a, or Duffy b, or Duffy ab. Some people are Duffy silent—they have no Duffy blood group. People who are Duffy silent do not become infected with malaria. The most well-known population of people who are Duffy silent are black people living in Central Africa. They are able to live in Africa without succumbing to malaria. Malaria originally came from birds. The parasite was able to jump a species and infect humans with the evolution of the Duffy blood group. Most infectious diseases of humans came from animals. The origin of infectious diseases of humans that originated in animals is well discussed in the Pulitzer Prize–winning book by Jared Diamond: *Guns, Germs, and Steel* (Diamond 1999). Human measles originated in cattle that harbor the disease of cows: rinderpest. Cattle were also the origin of tuberculosis. Whooping cough (pertussis) originated in pigs and dogs.

The dynamics of change that facilitate the infection of humans from an animal disease, jumping a species, a zoonosis, involves evolution in the agent causing the disease, a virus, bacteria, or parasite, as well as a change in the habits of the recipient human host. Throughout the history of modern man, the greatest killers have not been wars but infectious diseases. Human infectious diseases—smallpox, influenza, tuberculosis, malaria, the plague, measles, and cholera—all evolved from animals. A striking example of jumping a species was the Spanish flu, which was responsible for the influenza epidemic of 1918, which killed twenty to forty million people and infected 28 percent of all Americans, resulting in 675,000 deaths (Billings 2008). More Americans died from influenza than from military combat in the "Great War" of 1917–1918. The influenza of World War I was the result of a virus of birds jumping to humans. Modern molecular research has delineated the genetic mutation that allowed an infectious virus of birds to inhabit a new host—humans (Brown 2005). The phylogenetic and sequence analysis of the 1918 bird flu viral genome illustrates the importance of understanding the adaption of the bird influenza virus to humans (Taubenberger et al. 2005).

1918 was a momentous year, a year of peace, the end of one of the cruelest wars in the history of mankind, an unbearable trench war. Yet a fatal disease emerged at the end of the war that claimed the lives of hundreds of thousands of humans, erasing the aura of peace. Medical science turned its whole might toward combating the greatest enemy of all—infectious disease. Likewise, the end of death and suffering from hemophilia was in sight in the 1980s, bringing peace to those who had previously been assigned a dismal fate as the result of their medical condition. Suddenly, unexpectedly, those innocent persons who had infused with concentrates to relieve their suffering and to extend their life expectancy were stricken when a previously unknown infectious disease emerged within their midst, claiming at least half their lives. The scenario of the influenza of 1918 and HIV/AIDS in the 1980s is similar in that the anticipated peace and enlightenment for hemophilia was shockingly smitten by an infectious disease, as was the anticipated peace for the world at the end of the war in 1918, when it was snuffed out by influenza. However, a difference is apparent between the two scenes. The threat of an infectious disease prompted a vigorous response by the government and medical science in 1918. Within the hemophilia scene, between the scientific/medical and government response and those inflicted with the infectious disease, an element existed not present in the Spanish influenza scenario. The element of interference to be contended with was the profit motive of the pharmaceutical industry who manufactured the vector responsible for the infection of HIV in hemophilia—the concentrates.

HIV is not alone as an infectious disease that came from animals to infect persons, those with hemophilia who infused with concentrates. First there was hepatitis, and then AIDS. Although the source of several infectious diseases of humans is known, the origin of the viruses that cause human hepatitis infection has not been established for all of the different recognized hepatitis viruses. Multiple types of human hepatitis exist, including type A (HAV), type B (HBV), type C (HCV), and others. These viruses have distinct subtypes.

Hepatitis B virus infects 5 percent of the people in the world, one of every twenty persons, 350 million worldwide (Miller and Robinson 1986). HBV is homologous with murine (mouse) leukemia virus and evolved from a retrovirus progenitor, a common ancestor 2,300–3,100 years ago (Simmonds 2000). HBV genotypes A and D are distributed globally, genotypes B and C in East and Southeast Asia, genotype E in West Africa and genotype F in Central and South America. Molecular biological investigations indicate there is intermixing and approximate equal sequence divergence between human genotypes A–E with the sequences recovered from primates (chimpanzees, gibbons, orangutans, and woolly monkeys). No undisputed conclusions on the origin of HBV (hepatitis B virus) exist.

Hepatitis C virus infects 170 million people, with a worldwide global distribution in humans and primates (Simmonds 2000). In the United States, ten thousand deaths occur each year from HCV (Verbeek et al. 2000). There are six different subtypes believed to have diverged from a common ancestor five hundred to two thousand years ago (Smith et al. 1997). The investigation into origins of HCV is tedious because the virus is difficult to culture and infects only humans and close primates.

- Geologists complete research on the origin of mountains and land masses by studying rocks.

- Anthropologists and paleontologists study the origin of animals, humans, and plants by examining bones, teeth, and fossils.

- There are no direct records of viruses from their past; only their effects detectable by damage they may have caused are available for research. Viruses are invisible in the geological and historical world (Simmonds 2000).

HEV (hepatitis E virus) is present in pigs but causes no illness (Smith 2008). Of the two-month-old pigs tested in the Midwestern United States, 79 percent tested seropositive for HEV. Pig HEV is similar to but not identical to human HEV. Infection of pigs with HEV from various parts of the world indicates that pigs are probably the reservoir of HEV.

The origin of HIV, which causes AIDS, is clearer than the origin of hepatitis viruses. AIDS is a human disease caused by infection with HIV, which originated from SIV following the jumping of the virus from one species to another, from chimpanzees to humans. At the time of Brent's death, in 1993, this information had not been confirmed. When a virus jumps a species, a zoonosis, often it is much more virulent in the receptive host compared to the originating host. Some chimpanzees have harbored SIV without adverse effects. SIV infection in chimpanzees doesn't produce a recognizable illness. SIV virus has been present in chimpanzees for many years, perhaps thousands of years. Humans and chimpanzees were unaware of its existence until SIV was discovered during the search for the origin of AIDS. The most similar primate virus compared to the human virus that causes AIDS (HIV) has been discovered in chimpanzees. The infection of humans with HIV occurred when the virus jumped from one species to another: SIV_{CPZ}/HIV-1 (simian immunodeficiency virus from chimpanzees to human immunodeficiency virus type 1).

The transfer of the virus that causes AIDS in humans from chimpanzees has been recognized. But different opinions exist explaining how the virus was transferred from chimpanzees to humans. If explanations attributing SIV transfer to HIV by deliberate design, such as promoted by the CIA, are discarded as being too radical for consideration, three different theories have been proposed, each defended by research.

Three proposed theories for transfer of SIV in chimpanzees to HIV in humans:

- natural events
- oral polio vaccine
- hepatitis B vaccine

Some doctors and scientists believe the transfer of SIV from chimpanzees to humans, which became HIV, occurred by natural processes. The transfer of diseases from cows to humans occurred when humans lived in close contact with animals, when cattle were domesticated, sometimes sleeping in the same quarters with humans. Humans kept chimpanzees for pets. They hunted them. They ate the meat from their bones, and even up to the present time, similar to eating raw fish, sushi, raw chimpanzee brains are eaten as a delicacy in some parts of Africa. Social changes with migration, wars, and truck routes have disturbed the societies that had existed for many years, undisturbed, in Africa.

Edward Hooper and others believed the transfer of SIV to HIV was the effect of medical intervention in Central Africa after World War II, in the 1950s. Because of the rampant polio epidemics in Africa in the 1950s, great pressure was exerted by the World Health Organization (WHO) and others on researchers and scientists to develop a polio vaccine. To manufacture a vaccine, it was necessary to culture the virus outside the body, in the laboratory, in tissue culture. Polio virus will not grow in mouse tissue culture but it will grow in cultures of kidney cells derived from primates. When the polio virus was grown in the cells of primate kidney, followed by attenuation of the polio virus, and then inoculated into humans to provoke an immune response against polio, the response was less than optimal. Subsequent research led to the development of a live polio vaccine given orally. It is suspected that the live polio vaccine included unknown SIV virus—present in the primate kidney cell cultures. At the time of development of the oral polio vaccine, researchers were not aware of the existence of SIV in primate kidney cells. They assumed simian (primate) kidneys were free of harmful viruses.

The presence of HIV in Africa before AIDS was recognized has been established by several examples. In 1976, a survivor of an airplane crash in Africa was given a blood transfusion. The unit of blood was obtained from a local donor. The recipient of the blood transfusion died of AIDS in 1980. After HIV tests were developed in 1984, a stored blood sample collected from a Bantu person in the Belgian Congo in 1959 was reported to have tested HIV-positive. The test results completed on this sample, thirty years after it was collected, attracted great interest, implying that HIV was present in Africa before 1959. However, subsequent research methods have failed to demonstrate the presence of the HIV genetic material in the sample. Attempts to document the presence of the intact HIV in the stored blood sample have been unsuccessful. Blood samples collected in the 1960s from primates in the primate centers in the USA have been shown to contain SIVs. Hooper believes HIV arrived to infect humans in Central Africa in the 1950s, at the time the oral polio vaccine was introduced in Africa.

A British meeting of The Royal Society of London assembled scientists from all over the world to discuss and debate the oral polio vaccine (OPV) theory of the origin of HIV/AIDS. According to this theory, proposed by Tom Curtis in his 1992 article in *Rolling Stone* magazine (Curtis 1992), further supported by the research of Edward Hooper, the AIDS pandemic was triggered by contaminated oral polio vaccine. The scientists who published their presentations from the British meeting in 2001 concluded that AIDS, which is the result of HIV infection, is man-made. The participants at the conference also concluded that the transfer of SIV to humans was connected with medical activities in Africa in the 1970s. The two most prominent suggestions proposing the origin of AIDS before the conference had been the "cut hunter" and oral polio vaccine (OPV) theories. The first theory postulated that an African hunter handled chimpanzees that harbored SIV. Through an accident, such as a knife cut, a hunter was contaminated with SIV when the chimpanzee's blood entered his wound. The SIV jumped a species (a zoonosis) from SIV to become HIV in the hunter recipient. The second hypothesis for the origin of HIV from SIV resulting in AIDS suggested that the manufacture of OPV included the culture of the polio virus in tissue culture of chimpanzee kidney cells that contained SIV.

The British conference of leading nonmedical and nonpharmaceutical investigators of molecular biology, evolution, and epidemiology discussed the important question: When was the first discovery of HIV in humans (Origin of AIDS 2008)? Multiple references had been previously made to the blood sample that had been stored since it was collected in Zaire in 1959, retrieved, and tested positive for HIV as evidence that HIV was present in Africa prior to the distribution of OPV in the 1950s. Some persons have maintained that HIV infected humans in Africa in the 1940s or 1950s. At the British AIDS Conference, the Los Alamos research group, led by Gerald Myers (Burr et al. 2001), reported that at least ten simultaneous but different events have resulted in synchronous epidemics, which they describe as a "big bang theory" for the origin of AIDS in the 1970s, which was the result of a "punctuated origin event." Reviews suggest that the origin of HIV/AIDS from OPV no longer has scientific consensus (Horowitz 2008). Instead, some other man-made event, not natural evolution such as proposed by the "cut hunter theory," must explain the remarkable array of genetic recombinant variants, which the Myers group has described as arising simultaneously in the 1970s. Rather than the OPV theory of the origin of AIDS, another iatrogenic innovation has been proposed: the hepatitis B vaccine.

African chimpanzees were used for the manufacture of HB vaccines in the 1970s. However, rather than culturing HB in tissue culture of cells from chimpanzee kidneys, an in vitro culture, live human hepatitis B virus (HBV) was directly inoculated into chimpanzees, an in vivo culture (figure 5). The donors who contributed the HB virus (homosexual volunteer men from New York City) had been previously immunized with polio vaccine that had been manufactured by growth in simian kidney cell cultures that had been contaminated with SIV. The human HBV that had been cultured in chimpanzees was returned to humans for further growth and an immune response. Blood was collected from the infected humans. The infected serum from multiple donors was pooled to produce four different strains of HB vaccines. A pilot study was conducted with the four HB vaccine strains in hundreds of homosexual volunteer men in New York City and in Central African volunteers in 1970 and 1975. The HB vaccine theory proposes that progenitor SIV viruses were activated when transferred from humans to chimpanzees and then back to humans (Marriott et al. 1996). Pooling the sera and the time interval from the polio vaccination of the donors until harvesting the HB created an environment conducive for viral genetic recombination. The earliest HB vaccines may have activated an HIV-related retroviral gene from one or more primates. The series of events is cited as describing the mid-1970s "punctuated origin event," which is the origin of the HIV/AIDS pandemic. This event, discovered by the Myers group, explains the nearly simultaneous emergence of the ten separate but related AIDS epidemics in Africa in the 1970s. HIV/AIDS emerged suddenly in Africa and North America simultaneously.

The big bang theory for the origin of AIDS explains the simultaneous emergence of AIDS in Africa and in homosexual men. The discussants at the British AIDS conference set aside Hooper's OPV theory, citing that kidney cell tissue cultures from African chimpanzees were not utilized in the manufacture of OPV and this vaccine was not given to homosexual men in New York City (Plotkin 2001). However, Edward Hooper's indefatigable energy and ten years of research, which led to the publication of *The River*, was the spark that ignited other researchers to review existing available knowledge describing the origin of AIDS, culminating in the British conference that was convened to debate and discuss the hypothesis of OPV and the emergence of HIV/AIDS.

Figure 5. Path of SIV to HIV

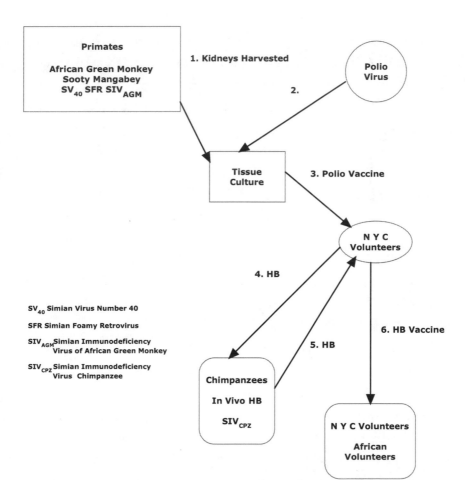

SIV_{CPZ} (simian immunodeficiency virus from chimpanzees) is a close viral relative of the human AIDS virus, HIV-1. There is no evidence HIV existed prior to the 1970s; therefore, the origin of HIV from SIV_{CPZ} prior to that time has been dismissed.

The pathway for the origin of HIV, the virus that causes AIDS in humans, from primates via hepatitis B vaccine, is portrayed in figure 5. Hepatitis B virus (HBV) was obtained by collecting blood samples containing the virus from volunteers in New York City. The live virus was injected directly into chimpanzees (4). The cultured human HBV was returned from chimpanzees to humans (5). The human volunteers mounted an immune response to produce sera for the first HB vaccine. Sera from many volunteers were pooled to form four different vaccine strains (6). The early hepatitis B vaccine was utilized in a pilot study in which hundreds of New York City volunteers and African volunteers were immunized. The return of HBV from the chimpanzees to humans was accompanied by the transfer of the simian immunodeficiency virus, SIV_{CPZ}, to humans. Furthermore, the human volunteers had previously been immunized with polio vaccine (3) manufactured in tissue cultures of primates (1) that had been infected with polio virus (2). The kidney cells utilized for culturing the polio virus contained the simian viruses from the sooty mangabey and from the African green monkey (figure 5).

The distribution of the HB vaccine in Africa coincides with the geographical dissemination of AIDS in Africa after HIV was introduced, followed by its spread by social practices. Cancer of the liver, which is associated with hepatitis B virus, in Africa also coincides with the geographical distribution of the HB vaccine in the 1970s. Debating the origin of HIV/AIDS, the British Conference concluded that it was an iatrogenic outcome of specific vaccine experiments. HIV/AIDS originated from one or more man-made, not naturally occurring, events dating back to the mid-1970s. Implicated, according to the scientists and scholars, is the hepatitis B vaccine.

The zoonosis, the jumping of the virus that causes AIDS in humans, from primates to humans, is explainable by the hepatitis B vaccine. The spread throughout human populations is explainable by natural events, by human behavior. The New York City volunteers were homosexual men, unaware they had been infected with HIV, whose actions unconsciously promoted rapid spread from one person to another, explaining to Brent the reason one of the four *H*s represents homosexual men.

Gwyn explained to her son that those men, like Brent, were victims of a threat that they did not create. They had volunteered to be used to help develop a polio vaccine in the 1950s or 1960s. Later, in the 1970s, they volunteered to offer their bodies to help develop a hepatitis B vaccine. The doctors and scientists unintentionally created the threat when they introduced the viruses of primates into the human volunteers, unaware of the danger that would ensue from their attempts to create vaccines. The men's lifestyle—they were homosexuals—is not acceptable to everyone. Yet some of the same people who refute them did not refuse the vaccines produced as the result of their volunteering to help humanity.

Brent said he comprehended how the primate viruses got into the New York City volunteers, which accounts for the *H* of homosexuals. He wanted to know the origin of the other three *H*s.

At the same time the homosexual men of New York became infected with HIV, black men of Africa became infected with HIV for the same reason. They volunteered to help develop a hepatitis vaccine. They were used by the scientists in a pilot study for a vaccine trial. When the first cases of AIDS were discovered, scientists did not know the illness was easily spread from a man to a woman, not only spread from one man to another man. When a person becomes infected with HIV, he or she is not sick. Other viral diseases cause symptoms. When people are infected with the virus that causes the common cold, they "catch cold." Children who are not immune and who become infected with the virus that causes one of the diseases of childhood, chicken pox, get sick and break out in blisters on their bodies. In contrast, there are no symptoms when a person becomes infected with HIV. The black men of Africa, unaware they were infected with HIV, transmitted the virus to their wives when having sex, without either having signs of illness. Many of their babies became infected with HIV when they were born to HIV infected mothers.

Black men who lived in Haiti returned to their ancestral African lands for a visit. While visiting in Africa, unaware, they became infected with HIV when they had sex with HIV infected African women. They returned to Haiti with the virus incubating in their bodies, which was transferred to Haitian women and spread to other Haitian men. Living conditions in Haiti are impoverished. The spread of AIDS in some parts of the world overlaps the areas of poverty. Haiti is an area of poverty that accounts for another of the four *H*s.

The *Rolling Stone* article, first proposing the oral polio vaccine theory for the transfer of SIV from primates to HIV of humans, appeared before Brent died of AIDS in 1993. Eight years later, the British meeting to discuss the OPV theory arrived at a consensus, endorsing the proposal that the manufacture of hepatitis B vaccine was the event that resulted in the emergence of HIV in the 1970s. And even fourteen years after Brent died, another proposal has been offered, advancing the natural events theory: the cut hunter idea that SIV mutated to become HIV in an African, which spread to a Haitian who was visiting Africa. According to this theory, proposed by Worobey and his associates (Gilbert et al. 2007), an infected Haitian individual, one person, unaware, brought HIV back to Haiti, as early as 1960, followed by infection of homosexual men, or drug users, who spread HIV when they returned to New York City after visiting Haiti. The Worobey group does not refer to the British conference and the hepatitis B theory for the emergence of HIV, which was proposed six years earlier.

Another concept regarding the origin of HIV/AIDS in Africa suggests that HIV, the human virus, was inoculated into chimpanzees. However, research refutes this suggestion. When SIV_{CPZ}, the immunodeficiency virus of chimpanzees, becomes HIV-1, the human immunodeficiency virus that results in AIDS in humans, and is returned from humans back to chimpanzees, the chimpanzees do not become ill. They develop antibodies to HIV, followed by disappearance of the human virus; it is cleared. This is in contrast to the history of HIV-1 in humans. Humans also develop antibodies to HIV-1, but the virus does not disappear. Instead, over several years, the viral infection slowly progresses to AIDS. The suggestion that the CIA inoculated chimpanzees with HIV so that the virus would spread to humans must be tossed into the wastebasket of radical suggestions.

The debate about the origin and arrival of HIV, the zoonosis, SIVcpz/HIV-1, by different paths, continues, each defended by sound and reputable research scientist proponents. Is there only one origin of HIV? Or are there multiple origins? If only one correct explanation exists for the origin of HIV/AIDS, the others must be wrong. Which is the correct explanation for the emergence of AIDS? Will we ever know?

Brent acknowledged that two of the *H*s, homosexuals and Haitians, were accounted for. What about the other two *H*s, especially the one that claimed him—hemophilia?

Some of the people of the first two *H*s shared needles with drug users. People addicted to drugs such as heroin became infected by needles used by HIV infected homosexual persons or Haitians. They are the third label of the *H*s: heroin addicts. To purchase drugs, some of the heroin addicts sold their blood for money.

The pharmaceutical companies that manufactured concentrates from plasma obtained from blood often set up blood collection centers in neighborhoods where the IV drug users could easily drop in to give blood in exchange for dollars, Gwyn advised Brent. In Portland, Oregon, the walk-in plasma donation center operated by Alpha Therapeutics on Southeast Ankeny collected blood from anyone who wanted to sell his blood or plasma in exchange for dollars. The heroin users, unaware of HIV, which had not previously been described, were the source of HIV contamination of plasma used to manufacture concentrates.

Infection with HIV, the final *H* of the four *H*s, hemophilia, although easily explainable, wasn't explained before it was too late. The pharmaceutical companies paid donors for plasma that was not treated to remove harmful viruses such as hepatitis B and hepatitis C. Prior to 1990, a test to detect hepatitis C virus in donor plasma was not available (Sobesky et al. 2008). There was worldwide demand for clotting factors, resulting in efforts to increase production without research to improve safety.

Brent asked whose fault it was that he became infected with HIV—that he had AIDS. Who was guilty?

Gwyn sadly replied that she was not sure who was guilty. Maybe no one was guilty, but many people were wrong.

Brent wanted to know why the drug companies continued producing medicine. If the medicine, the concentrate, was polluted, why didn't they stop making it? He reminded his mother that he had heard of other products that had to be recalled or discontinued. If the grocery store sold lettuce that caused outbreaks of E. coli, the lettuce was taken off the shelves and tossed into the garbage or fed to pigs. When Ford made the Bronco II, it was discovered that it rolled over easily, and Ford quit making that car.

Gwyn said she could think of two reasons why the drug companies kept making concentrate, even after many people suspected the medicine was contaminated with something that could make people sick, instead of discontinuing production. In the first place, the drug companies—such as Bayer, Cutter, Hyland, Armour, and Alpha—thought they were very humane. They didn't want to abandon persons like Brent, leaving them to face the fear of suffering and even death from bleeding, without the medicine they manufactured for him. Even if there was a threat of getting a disease from infusions of concentrate, that threat was less than the risk if no medicine was available. There was a great demand for concentrate from the hemophilia users of the medicine.

Brent cheerfully remarked that he was pleased to know the drug companies cared about him. He was eager to know what the other reason was that the drug companies kept making the medicine, even if it wasn't clean.

The other reason, Gwyn informed her son, was called profit. Money. There was a lot of competition between companies who manufacture concentrate. Lots of dollars were at stake.[108] If a drug company couldn't deliver concentrate, but another company could, the first company might lose business, with loss of their customers to another company. If one drug company could make a purified concentrate, a medicine that had no risk of causing disease, customers of the company still selling dirty medicine would patronize the safer company. To prevent loss of customers while companies scrambled to make a clean medicine, the drug companies that made the older medicine minimized the risk and recommended that it was better to keep using the old medicine; it was proven and had demonstrated its usefulness. Finally, when new purified medicine was successfully manufactured, some people insist that the drug companies shipped all the dirty medicine overseas and saved the new medicine for the USA or Europe. They had a warehouse with shelves full of polluted concentrate, worth thousands and thousands of dollars. Rather than dumping the polluted medicine in the incinerator, they dumped it in Japan, Hong Kong, South America, and other faraway places in the Orient (Bogdanich and Koli 2003).

The action by the drug companies of dumping concentrate overseas to poor people demonstrates that the motive for continuing to sell concentrate, even though it was known to be polluted, was not for a compassionate reason, Gwyn confided to Brent. She told him the motive was to make a profit, a money motive. In November 1984, a Cutter internal memo noted an excess inventory of unheated product filling the shelves of their warehouse. They proposed to "review international markets" to see if more unheated product could be sold. Cutter instructed its Hong Kong distributor that "we must use up

---

108 Sales in concentrates produced in the USA in 1995 amounted to 2.4 billion dollars.

stocks" of unheated medicine before switching to a "safer, better" heat-treated product (Bogdanich and Koli 2003).

The plasma fractionating industry, which includes the pharmaceutical manufacture of concentrates for treatment of hemophilia, became a multibillion dollar enterprise. Great amounts of investments had been made in time, personnel, facilities, and equipment. Competition between manufacturers was intense. Rather than risk loss of production, sales, and market share, to competitors, by pausing to improve safety, the producers of concentrates increased production. Their goal was to capture as much of the market as possible rather than produce a safer product.

Prevention of HIV and Hepatitis

Questions remain unanswered. Why wasn't research completed to purify the concentrate so that it would be safe and not cause infections of hepatitis and HIV in people with hemophilia? If the drug companies could charge thousands of dollars for concentrate, why couldn't they spend a few dollars on safety? Why did the drug companies buy blood from people who were likely to be infected with hepatitis? Didn't the government require any regulations?

A person was required to possess a driver's license to drive a car. To drive a car, insurance was mandatory. To catch a fish, a fishing license was necessary. Many regulations exist in our society. Why weren't there regulations to protect the blood supply? Why were the drug companies paying people who lived on the street for their blood, or paying people who were so poor they had to sell their blood? Some of the people who sold their blood surely used the money to buy drugs.

The FDA and the American Red Cross were in charge of the nation's blood supply. What were the requirements to be eligible to sell your blood? Were there any?

The drug companies have defended their action, saying they did not know how to purify the donor plasma, to remove the hepatitis virus from plasma without destroying the AHF clotting activity.

Donna Shaw, an unbiased nonmedical journalist, who was not part of the pharmaceutical industry, reviewed the safety of the manufacture of concentrates: "On the Trail of Tainted Blood—Hemophiliacs Say U.S. Could Have Prevented Their Contracting AIDS," published in the *Philadelphia Inquirer* April 16, 1995. If Donna Shaw's article had appeared fifteen years earlier and hepatitis had been depleted from the plasma to make concentrates, even though doctors and scientists may have been unaware of HIV, the destruction of HBV would have also destroyed HIV even if that virus had not been discovered.

During World War II, Captain Emanuel Rappaport of the U.S. Army Medical Corps observed that many of the wounded soldiers returning from overseas to the Schick General Hospital in Clinton, Iowa, developed hepatitis (Shaw 1995). All the men had one thing in common: they had received battlefield transfusions of plasma. The plasma transfusions were from sources that included pools of dozens of donors. It was apparent that if only one donor harbored the hepatitis virus, the entire lot of plasma would be infected. In 1945, Rappaport published, in the July *Journal of the American Medical Association*, his conclusions that pooling of plasma greatly increases the risk of hepatitis among recipients. In 1946, Rappaport proposed screening of donors and research to develop methods for killing viruses in blood products. He predicted that it was likely that this condition would be encountered more frequently in the future.

Heat treating plasma for killing hepatitis virus was developed by army medical researchers in the 1940s. Why wasn't this method applied to concentrates made from pooled human plasma for treatment in hemophilia until 1983? By 1983, most of the persons with hemophilia had already become infected with the hepatitis viruses and HIV. Ten thousand individuals who had hemophilia in the United States were infected with HIV by the late 1970s and early 1980s. Other countries purchased supplies of American-made concentrates, which resulted in thousands of persons with hemophilia throughout the world becoming infected with hepatitis and HIV leading to AIDS. Pharmaceutical manufacturers of concentrate, the fractionators, responded by declaring that they did not know until the early 1980s how to kill the viruses without destroying the clotting activity in the plasma.

In 1941 and 1942, doctors recognized that whole blood was too fragile to survive transportation and transfusions in the battlefields.

Seven commercial pharmaceutical manufacturers were contracted by the army to prepare freeze-died plasma for the battlefields, including Hyland, a subsidiary of Baxter Healthcare Corporation, and Cutter, part of Miles Laboratories. WWII was the first war to use blood transfusions. Prior to that war, there were few blood banks. Captain Rappaport knew that in Europe and the United States, other doctors were also observing outbreaks of homologous serum jaundice, presently known as hepatitis B. He reported that the incidence of hepatitis after infusions of pooled plasma was fourteen times more frequent compared to transfusions with whole blood.

In 1962, seventeen years after Rappaport's published study, the surgeon general's office of the U. S. Army supported his conclusions and declared that pooled plasma was the vehicle that caused homologous serum jaundice. The report confirmed that the larger the plasma donor pool, the greater the risk for hepatitis. During WWII, plasma was pooled from fifty blood donors, which increased in size as the war progressed. The army concluded that the likelihood of jaundice appearing in a recipient after a blood transfusion was small. However, when blood is pooled during processing of the plasma, the incidence of jaundice increases.

Although the military attempted to kill hepatitis in plasma in the 1940s while retaining its health benefits, the attempts were not successful because the etiology of the ailment causing serum homologous jaundice had not been discovered. No laboratory animal studies had been completed to demonstrate susceptibility to the human viruses. Volunteers from prisons, from the military, and from state hospitals were used in experiments until the high risk of illness and even death was recognized. Doctors knew in the 1940s that albumin, fractionated from plasma, could be heated to sixty degrees Celsius (140 degrees Fahrenheit) for ten hours to destroy viruses without altering albumin's usefulness. By the end of the war, heat-treated albumin became an alternative for plasma. By 1950, an army-led research team, headed by J. G. Allen, demonstrated that plasma heated to 33 degrees Celsius (90 degrees Fahrenheit) for three to six months destroyed the hepatitis virus, but the Allen method also inactivated clotting factors. Later modification of the heating process preserved the clotting factors. In 1952, during the Korean War, army doctors infused pooled plasma that had been irradiated with ultraviolet light to destroy hepatitis. Ultraviolet irradiation was unsuccessful; more than 20 percent of the recipients developed hepatitis.

In 1964, Dr. Judith Pool at Stanford University Medical Center successfully developed a new procedure for replacing the clotting factor missing in hemophilia. The dramatic improvement resulted in an entirely new forecast for hemophilia. She discovered that freezing a unit of plasma, followed by slowly thawing just up to the melting point, resulted in some sludge in the bottom of the unit, hence it was called cryoprecipitate (cryo), which contained the clotting proteins. The plasma from single donors was not pooled. A volume of ten cc, two teaspoons, of cryoprecipitate had little risk of hepatitis if the donors were carefully screened. A person affected with hemophilia could receive one or even ten units of cryoprecipitate, to elevate their clotting factor. A person whose clotting factor in his blood was less than 1 percent of normal because of hemophilia could be infused with cryo to elevate his clotting factor level to 50 or even 100 percent of normal. A person with hemophilia could treat his bleeds at home if he could properly store the frozen bags of cryo. In 1966, Hyland, a division of Baxter, further freeze-dried cryo to produce a desiccated powder stored under vacuum in a small bottle; it was called factor VIII concentrate. By injecting a small volume of water into the vial of concentrate, the reconstituted clotting factor could be easily infused into a hemophilia recipient.

A. G. Redeker, in 1968, at the University of Southern California, asserted that Allen's heat treatment of plasma was not completely without danger of transmission of hepatitis. Allen had moved to Stanford University by then, and he countered that Redeker had not been thorough in his research. He asserted that Redeker's studies were based on plasma obtained from two commercial fractionators, Hyland and Courtland Laboratories in Los Angeles, who collected plasma from paid donors from skid row. Large numbers of plasmas, from thousands of donors, were pooled together to form one huge lot for fractionating into plasma components, including factor VIII. The donors sold their blood for money and were at high risk for carrying disease such as hepatitis. Therefore, the plasma required heating for longer periods of time than utilized by Redeker. Allen said that neither the National Research Council nor any other government regulators had inspected Hyland's or Courtland's records. He stated that the fractionating laboratories had not adhered to his standards described in an army-financed report in 1969. By the time of Allen's report, the National Institute of Health had already approved the commercial sale of the first freeze-dried concentrates. These concentrates had not been heat-treated. They were manufactured from the plasma pooled from thousands of paid donors.

Researchers at the National Institute of Health , in an article published in the *Journal of The American Medical Association* in 1970, warned that just one unit of plasma contaminated with hepatitis virus could render an entire pool infectious, even if it was diluted ten million times.

By 1976, most hemophilia treaters were prescribing the new easy-to-use concentrates for treatment of bleeding in hemophilia in the United States. The government, through the Maternal and Child Health Division of the National Institute of Health, began funding comprehensive hemophilia care centers to assure that care for hemophilia was provided, and to assist in training for the infusions of concentrates at home rather than in emergency rooms or in hospitals. The quality of life for persons who had hemophilia improved, as observed by less pain and suffering with an increase in life expectancy. Life-threatening incidents such as head injuries could be managed. Surgery such as appendectomies and even joint replacements could be performed, correcting immobilization from joint deformity.

By the late 1970s and 1980, hepatitis contracted from infusions of concentrates became a leading cause of death in hemophilia. The U.S. government, the pharmaceutical fractionators, and even some hemophilia treater physicians, maintained that hepatitis was an acceptable risk considering the significant benefits from the concentrates. Federal regulations permitted the sale of the medicine with a WARNING OF HEPATITIS label affixed to the bottles of concentrate. The fractionators declared that the large demand for concentrates could not be met with only volunteer plasma donors. The American Red Cross blood banks, which are responsible for the nation's blood supply, when questioned regarding the logistics of producing enough AHF concentrate from their volunteer donors to fulfill the demand for concentrates to supply all the persons who have hemophilia, replied that it wasn't possible to do so.

Hepatitis was considered by the fractionating industry as an unfortunate but unavoidable downside to the industry. The government and the industry reasoned that most persons who infused concentrate for treatment of hemophilia would live longer with the medicine than without it, justifying the risks. The government did not demand procedures to destroy hepatitis viruses in blood. The pharmaceutical fractionators were directed to utilize the available screening tests for their paid donors; however, the antibody tests were not sensitive enough to detect the hepatitis virus in every instance, and no test for hepatitis C became available until 1990. If a person was infected with hepatitis only a few days before donating plasma, antibodies would not have been present, and the infective virus would not be detected. Some scientists claimed the concentrates were dangerous because of their viral threats.

Dr. Judith Pool, at Stanford, where Dr. Allen was also conducting research, sent a letter in 1974 to federal health officials, warning against a national blood donor policy that allowed paid donors to continue donating plasma as the source of hemophilia concentrates. Investigations had established that a strong association existed between paid blood donors and development of hepatitis in recipients. Many paid donors lived in suboptimal conditions, where breeding grounds for viruses and diseases existed. The World Health Organization accused the commercial fractionators of exploiting poor donors in their plasma collection centers in South America, Central America, Asia, and Africa, which were established in the 1960s and 1970s. Dr. Pool objected that the proposed government policy did not encourage the use of volunteer donors; instead, it assumed continuation of the dangerous, wasteful, expensive, and unethical purchase of plasma by the pharmaceutical houses.

In 1975, the World Health Organization advocated an all-volunteer system for plasma donation. However, federal regulators sided with the commercial industry, agreeing that the benefits of using paid donors outweighed the risks to the recipients of plasma products. The Food and Drug Administration replied to objections of a paid donor system by proclaiming that for biological products, safety meant relative freedom from harmful effects to persons affected by a product when prudently administered considering the character of the product in relation to the recipient at the time of utilization.

In 1977, the World Health Organization requested that pharmaceutical manufacturers of concentrates kill viruses in their commercial products for the sake of future generations who would infuse to treat hemophilia. The request was repeated in 1979, urging increased efforts; however, the federal regulators stood by their policy of favoring commercial fractionators.

On July 16, 1982, the Centers for Disease Control in Atlanta confirmed the first AIDS cases in hemophilia in the United States. Three cases were reported. Epidemiologists began to suspect that AIDS was spreading through blood and its derivatives, which raised serious concerns for persons with hemophilia who were recipients of concentrates derived from plasma. No test was available to determine which batches of pooled plasma were infected. No heat-treated concentrates were sold in the United States, despite their use in treating hemophilia in Germany.

The manager of Cutter's plasma procurement division acknowledged in 1983 that there was strong evidence suggesting that AIDS is spread through plasma products. American fractionators knew of Germany's advanced production of heat-treated concentrate. An internal Cutter memo in January 1983 cited a loss of concentrate sales if competitors produced a heat-treated concentrate before Cutter was able to do so, suggesting urgency in development of the new product. In March 1983, CDC warned that blood products appear to be responsible for the appearance of AIDS in hemophilia. Improved methods in the heating process protected the activity of the AHF clotting factors when the medicine was heated at 140 degrees Fahrenheit for seventy-two hours, as had been done for albumin since the 1940s, leading to the FDA approval of Baxter's heat-treated product in March 1983. Cutter responded, noting that in May 1983, when Baxter's Hyland Pharmaceutical Division's heat-treated factor VIII concentrate came onto the market, they had been beaten to the marketplace and needed a temporary solution that would preserve their market position. In May of 1983, France decided to withhold importing concentrates from the United States until they developed a better solution. Cutter sent a letter to France and to twenty other countries, proclaiming that AIDS had become the center of an irrational response because of unsubstantiated speculation that AIDS may be transmitted by blood products. Cutter gave the impression that they were improving their products, without announcing that they expected to soon release a heat-treated concentrate.

On February 29, 1984, Cutter was the last of the four companies that produced concentrates to receive approval in the United States for its heat-treated product. After their new heat-treated concentrate was marketed, Cutter continued producing the old non-heat-treated concentrate until August 1984. They defended their action by stating that they had several fixed-price contracts, and the old product was less expensive to produce. Some customers, Cutter maintained, doubted the new medicine's effectiveness. They cited a shortage of plasma for producing the newer heat-treated concentrate. There was concern by some hemophilia treaters that heat treatment might alter the properties of the proteins in concentrate, which could increase the incidence of inhibitors in recipients. Cutter cited that a delay in offering the newer medicine was the result of requirements by the government. Although Cutter discontinued selling non-heat-treated concentrate within the United States in 1984, they continued sales overseas under the trademark of their parent company, Bayer Corporation. In November 1984, they noted that an excess inventory of non-heat-treated concentrate existed.

In response, they reviewed international markets to determine if the older product could be sold. They sold the older medicine to Asia and Latin America to avoid being burdened with large inventories of unmarketable older non-heat-treated concentrate, while the newer heat-treated concentrate was sold in the United States. By the end of 1984 and the beginning of 1985, Hong Kong asked Cutter for the new medicine. Cutter replied that they must use up the old supply first. When persons with hemophilia in Hong Kong began testing HIV-positive, doctors in China who cared for persons with hemophilia became concerned that Cutter might be dumping HIV contaminated concentrate into lesser developed countries. In May 1985, a medical emergency was recognized in Hong Kong that resulted in a request for the newer heat-treated concentrate. Cutter responded by declaring that the newer medicine was being supplied for treatment of hemophilia in the United States and in Europe, with only a small amount available for the most vocal individuals with hemophilia in Hong Kong.

The United States Food and Drug Administration's regulator of blood products, Dr. Harry Meyer Jr., contended that the companies that produced concentrate had broken an agreement to voluntarily withdraw non-heat-treated concentrate from the market. The FDA, in May 1985, called together officials from the companies and ordered them to comply and immediately cease selling the old medicine. The FDA wanted to keep the news away from the public and quietly resolve the issue without alerting Congress and the medical community. Cutter stopped shipping non-heat-treated concentrate overseas in July 1985, stating that there no longer appeared to be any markets where they could sell substantial quantities of non-heat-treated concentrate.

Doctors and patients in the United States and overseas were not informed of the concerns of officials within the companies that manufactured concentrate. Many of the concerns were recorded on internal memos. Companies existed under different names—such as Cutter, also known as Miles Laboratories, Bayer Corporation, and Rhône-Polenc ... all the same company.

In 1985, the FDA approved a solvent-detergent method for deviralizing plasma, a method developed at the New York Blood Center by Alfred Price and Bernard Horowitz. Later, Horowitz stated that theoretically, researches could have attempted to kill viruses sooner in concentrates, but they did not know that HIV was on the horizon. In 1980, Dr. Horowitz said that killing the viruses without destroying the clotting activity was considered a difficult problem. One of the spokesmen for the American Blood Resources Association, a group from the blood products industry, maintained that the problem was complicated. David Bell pointed out that in addition to selection of the proper temperature and time, stabilizing compounds must be identified. There was concern that the body's immune system might reject a clotting protein that had been altered by heat treatment, treating it as a foreign protein, which could result in an allergic reaction or production by the body of an inhibitor to the clotting factor in the concentrate. The effort to meet required government approval, first using animals before humans, was time consuming amounting to years of effort.

When AIDS appeared on the scene in hemophilia, there was an acceleration to overcome the fear that had existed in the 1970s: that heat treatment would inactivate the clotting activity of plasma. The problems were overcome and heat treatment was shown to destroy HIV without harming clotting activity. If efforts to similarly destroy hepatitis viruses had been employed in the 1970s, perhaps AIDS could have been avoided in hemophilia.

Allen, who retired from Stanford in February 1987, referred to his own work with heat treating plasma, and said, as part of a Kentucky lawsuit, that no medical, economic, or social reason could justify ever using unheated pooled plasma or its clotting products. He referred to large plasma pools as "highly profitable but medically bankrupt." Back in 1940, he had written to the army about heat treating plasma. In 1971, he made recommendations that commercial fractionators heat treat their concentrates.

Charles M. Heldebrant, director of research and development for Alpha Pharmaceuticals in 1993, testified that his company did not begin a procedure for destroying viruses until 1982. The directive to conduct research on heat treatment of plasma originated in the marketing department in order to keep pace with competitors; the motive was not intended to produce a safer concentrate. The process of heating plasma at 140 degrees Fahrenheit for twenty hours, which was developed within four months, included further purification of concentrates before heat treatment. Nothing in the process was so innovative that it could not have been completed earlier. The same heat treatment destroys both hepatitis viruses as well as HIV.

A class-action suit was filed in Chicago in 1993, representing all the persons in the United States with hemophilia who were infected with HIV as a result of infusions of concentrates. The pharmaceutical companies that produced the concentrates sold HIV contaminated products even though they were aware that methods existed to purify the medicine, the suit contended. Five defendants were listed, including four U.S. pharmaceutical manufacturers who produced concentrates in the 1970s and 1980s: Cutter, Hyland, Alpha, and Armour. The fifth defendant was the National Hemophilia Foundation, who, the suit contended, was too financially dependent upon the pharmaceutical manufacturers to be an effective advocate for those who have hemophilia. In 1995, the federal appeals panel dismissed the suit, saying such a lawsuit would bankrupt the U.S. plasma industry, which had worldwide annual sales amounting to $2.4 billion (Shaw 1995).[109] The defendants denied wrongdoing, saying they acted as rapidly as possible once the risk was known.

---

109 With the introduction of recombinant and monoclonal AHF, the cost of antihemopilia concentrate has increased from ten to twenty cents per AHF unit in 1995 to seventy cents to one dollar per AHF unit in 2009. The annual sale of U.S. produced AHF concentrate has probably increased from $2.4 billion in 1995 to $10 to $20 billion in 2009, although the exact amount has not been revealed. Bayer announced Kogenate was its third best-selling product in 2009, generating sales of 888 million Euros (1.26 billion dollars). (Bayer 2009).

Manufacturers of concentrates have been named as defendants in several hundred lawsuits. When verdicts have been returned after a trial, they have favored the pharmaceutical companies in eleven of thirteen cases. For different reasons, the plaintiffs have not received a favorable verdict. The time allowed was a factor in some cases. In the suit filed in federal circuit court in Alaska, Craigdon vs. Miles Laboratories in 1991, the jury decided that the doctor involved, Dr. Taillefer, and the manufacturer of the concentrate, Koate, had not failed to warn the hemophilic plaintiff of the risk of HIV by 1982, a year agreed upon when knowledge of a risk of infection from infusion was established. In many parts of the world, contamination of concentrate with HIV has resulted in many infections with the virus that causes AIDS in hemophilia. Many lawsuits have been filed in a variety of countries. Thousands of persons who had hemophilia died from AIDS after receiving the polluted concentrates. Governments have punished a variety of officials for failure to impose regulations that would have detected the risk of infection sooner. A test for detecting who had been infected was not available until 1985, too late to determine when most people were infected with HIV (table 4).

Part VI

Onset of AIDS

Signs and Symptoms of AIDS in Brent

B rent tested positive for HIV in 1987. He remained well until the end of 1991, when he began to exhibit signs of infection.

From tests completed on stored blood samples collected from people with hemophilia, it was discovered that most persons who had been infused with concentrate became infected with HIV in the early 1980s (Devean and Bucquet 1993). By the time Brent showed signs of AIDS, he had most likely been infected with HIV for ten or twelve years.

Breathing became difficult. He was tired. He had no appetite. He lost weight. He had pneumonia. Brent had never been hospitalized for hemophilia. He had not needed surgery nor had a life-threatening bleed from hemophilia. With the onset of AIDS he became a very ill young person and required hospitalization. His lungs had become overwhelmed with pneumocystis, one of the hallmarks of AIDS.

One of the doctors in the hemophilia center, a specialist in diseases of the blood and cancer, Dr. Ned Strong, had experience treating AIDS illness and was familiar with pneumocystis infections. He began guiding Brent's AIDS care. To treat pneumocystis pneumonia, Dr. Strong prescribed intravenous pentamidine, a powerful drug that had to be slowly dripped into Brent's vein while he was carefully watched over by the nurses in the hospital on January 6, 1992. He recovered from his near-fatal pneumonia. He rallied and improved enough to return to his home from the hospital. Dr. Strong recommended continuing monthly pentamidine treatments, one of the medicines Brent had received before he became ill. These treatment sessions were by inhalation rather than the intravenous treatment he received after he became ill. Without pentamidine, Brent would have died.

Brent cried out that the inhalation treatments with pentamidine were awful. Sucking that stuff deep into his lungs made him sick. For the inhalation of nebulized pentamidine, he was required to exhale, hold his breath, and then suck in the vapor from the mouthpiece by taking a big deep breath. He hated it.

Dr. Strong solemnly told Brent that pneumocystis pneumonia is an infection that is labeled a reportable disease. It is not a contagious disease. But as a doctor, he was required to report Brent to the public health department. They kept track of all such cases. They wanted to know what happens to people who have pneumocystis infection.

Brent asked Dr. Strong if that meant that he was going to die. He wanted to be told how much longer he would live. Dr. Strong quietly told Brent with dignity that at the most, he would live one year.

The public health department required that all HIV-positive students must be reported to the principals of the schools they attend. If Brent was reported as HIV-positive to the school, he knew he would be expelled. Only kids who were drug users or having sex would become HIV infected, most everyone thought. Whenever AIDS or HIV came up for discussion, nearly everybody associated those topics with homosexuality. Brent was not a homosexual person. The school and the public health department had not considered that there is another way a young person can become HIV infected besides drugs and sex. The other way is by having hemophilia. Hemophilia cases are not spreading HIV by using drugs or having sex. The school was aware that Brent had hemophilia, but they were unaware that he was HIV infected.

The school board is obligated to assure that each enrolled student has access to an education. That applies to all the students as well as to an individual student who has a health problem. HIV is an infectious disease. HIV is not a contagious disease that is transmissible through normal contact in a school. Brent did not pose any health risk to other students. But AIDS was a red flag that could quickly alarm students and teachers and would most likely result in cessation of Brent's attendance at school.

His mother requested a school conference. It was scheduled for January 25, 1992, after he had recovered from his pneumonia and returned to school. The high school principal and Brent's teachers intended to meet with Brent, his mother, and the hemophilia center staff, including Myrna Campbell, the clinic nurse; Hanna Whitman, the social worker; and Dr. Taillefer, the clinic director, behind a closed door in a quiet, private room at the high school. The purpose of the conference was to notify the school that one of their students, Brent, was HIV-positive. Brent, his mother, and the persons from the hemophilia center sat solemnly and respectfully in the shiny, hard school chairs, without conversing with one another in the school room, waiting for the arrival of the school principal and Brent's teachers.

Suddenly, before the principal and the teachers arrived in the room, Brent unexpectedly stood up and exclaimed loudly, "I quit." Brent firmly said this with confidence, looking at those astounded persons in the room. "I will choose my own destiny." He was responsible for his own existence. Brent ended his high school education in the middle of the eleventh grade, his junior year at Oswego High School. He walked out of the room and the school building with determination, never to return to school. His unpredictable action was a sign that he did not simply exist; instead, he decided what his existence would be. After he returned home, he told his mother he would not allow the school the opportunity, as if it were a pleasure, to expel him from high school because he was HIV infected.[110]

No longer attending high school, Brent became very ill. He was treated again by Dr. Ned Strong with intravenous pentamidine. He had been receiving six hundred milligrams of AZT daily while enrolled in an AZT study group. AZT was declared ineffective for Brent when his T-4 helper cells dropped to $20/mm^3$. Brent developed pneumocystis pneumonia and was bronchoscoped in the hospital on April 29, 1992. He rallied, improved with treatment, and returned to his home in Lake Oswego.

---

110 Conversation with Gwyn McCann on August 31, 2007

Making Big Bucks

Living at Home: Out of School

Brent's parents had separated; his father no longer lived in their home. Brent was close to his father. He missed him. His mom was reasonable— she tolerated Brent's father's visits to the house to see Brent, but he couldn't live there anymore.

Brent kept busy at home, filling the hours by drawing, reading, and playing video games. Gwyn continued teaching English classes at Riverside Community College.

Brent had two best friends from high school. One, Hutch, was his special drawing friend, who would spend hours with Brent. He was often at Brent's home. One of Brent's favorite activities was looking through Marvel Comics. He and his friend practiced drawing illustrations that resembled the figures in the comic books.

Hutch said to Brent that maybe when he finished high school, he would go off to college and study to become a scientist. Brent agreed that science was cool. But he had always thought Hutch would become an artist. He drew so well. He pointed to the muscles on the caricature Hutch had just finished sketching. Brent and Hutch laughed as they thumbed through the papers covered with colorful sketches of cartoon characters they had completed. Muscled men were depicted dynamically rescuing terrified women with long blond hair curling over their pointed breasts. Bolts of lightning struck in the background, reflecting from the curved, sharp sabers grasped in the tightly clenched fists of their drooling saviors.

Hutch agreed that he would always keep drawing and sketching. But he wanted to do something big, something important. He confided to his drawing buddy that someday he wanted to have a wife. He wanted to earn lots of money to buy her a nice house and all the nice things women want. Hutch, whose real name was Hutchinson Kimberly Johnson, said that his mother had told him she would like to live in a nice house, a home where she would proudly receive her friends and family for tea. Hutch's mother worked as an assistant for a naturopathic doctor. Since the divorce from her alcoholic husband, when Hutch was a small child, she had to struggle. Her income was barely adequate for herself and her teenage son. If he became a scientist, he could make new medicines, do research, and maybe find a cure for Brent's hemophilia. He could work in a laboratory of one of the drug companies that made Brent's medicine. Performing research in a drug company's laboratory would be great. It meant earning good money and making discoveries. His mother's dreams of nice clothes, a new car, and a pretty house would come true.

Brent advised his friend that he was right and wrong at the same time.

Hutch quickly responded, sounding puzzled as to how he could be both right and wrong.

Brent told his friend that he was correct about one thing: he would make good money working for a drug company.

Hutch cheerfully agreed. He had heard that working for a drug company paid well. But he questioned where he was wrong.

Brent told Hutch that his father had informed him that most research and scientific discoveries were no longer made in drug companies' laboratories. In the old days, his father said, one of the main purposes of drug companies was to discover new medicines that could be useful in treating people's illnesses. But for the past ten or twenty years, the main purpose of the drug companies is marketing. The discoveries of new medicines are made in research laboratories of universities and scientific companies, such as Genentech. The drug companies sometimes provide money to scientists in the universities for their research. But the main goal of the drug companies is not to make new discoveries. No, the main effort of the drug companies is to make money to assure stockholders that their company has a good cash flow, a good return on their investments. The drug companies follow the methods the scientists successfully develop at the universities or scientific companies. After they adopt the method to produce a new medicine and the medicine is approved by the government, the FDA, the drug companies launch an intense marketing strategy. Universities can't do marketing, but drug companies can, and they are good at it.

Brent said his father told him that in the United States, there are no government cost controls on medicines. Many countries have cost controls that regulate the price a drug company can charge for its new medicines, but not in the States. The drug companies can charge any price they want for products they sell since there is no regulation (Chen 2007). If someday Hutch worked for a drug company in the USA, he would be working for a company that makes a lot of money through marketing, but he would not be making any scientific discoveries. While he would be able to buy nice things for his mother and his wife, if he was lucky enough to find one, Brent told Hutch that he wouldn't discover a new medicine for hemophilia.

"I know what you mean, Brent. If you hadn't quit school, you could have been in one of our discussion groups in government class. Our class at Oswego High divided into small groups that were assigned subjects to discuss and present to the rest of the class," Hutch updated his friend about school.

"Okay, Mr. Smart Guy, what did your group talk about?" Brent demanded. "Bring me up to date. What did I miss by quitting school?"

"Just calm down for a second, okay? And I will give you the benefit of my advanced wisdom," Hutch chided, clearly sensing that he had struck a note of advantage in the discussion with his friend.

Impatiently, Brent burst out at Hutch, "Tell me now what you talked about. Right now!"

Slowly, as if he were savoring his advantage, watching the reaction on his friend's face, Hutch began recounting the activities of his high school group and the discussion that he and four other students had exchanged in their class. "Our assignment was to discuss capitalism and a free market." Hutch told Brent that a mother of one the girls in the discussion group had diabetes and gave herself insulin shots. "The question we posed to ourselves," Hutch related to Brent, "was how much should a person with diabetes have to pay for insulin? Should a person who needs insulin to live receive the medicine as a basic right, or should a drug company be permitted to charge for the insulin? Should they make a profit from selling insulin? Is it ethical to make money because someone is suffering?"

"What you're telling me is nothing new," Brent guffawed. "People make money from other people's suffering all the time. That's the nature of the way things are."

"Shut up and listen for a few minutes," Hutch demanded. "Do you want to hear about our discussion or not?"

"Okay, go ahead and speak your piece. I'm interested," Brent reassured Hutch.

"We decided there is a conflict between capitalism, representing free marketing, and what is best for society," Hutch soberly stated. "In the case of insulin and diabetes, researchers discovered that insulin could be made from pig pancreases. After the discovery of insulin, drug companies began producing insulin to sell. Their motive was not new scientific discovery. They intended to sell insulin to the thousands of people all over the world who have diabetes. They sold it to make a profit for their shareholders in their companies."

"Is making a profit bad or good?" Brent asked.

"Aha!" Hutch quickly responded. "You're catching on. It's both good and bad."

Brent wanted further explanation of what his friend said—how something could be good and bad at the same time. Hutch began to explain what he meant.

Scientists in the universities where insulin was discovered couldn't make insulin for all the diabetics in the world. Their responsibility does not rest with making insulin for everybody who needs it. Their efforts are directed toward discovery. To make insulin for all the diabetics in the world, a drug company begins production using the method of discovery perfected by the scientists. In a free society, the government does not begin production of a new medicine. The government must assure that the benefits of a new discovery become available to the people without actually producing the products. In a free society, the products are produced by a commercial drug manufacturing company whose purpose is to make a profit. Successful production by the drug companies depends upon marketing. Without a profit, drug companies will not produce and market the product. Thus, making a profit is possible only because people suffer; they have a need to treat their suffering, which the drug companies can fulfill by providing their medicine. They make a profit by the suffering of other persons.

"I heard about insulin and genetic engineering, stuff they call recombinant technology," Brent remarked.

"That's right" Hutch quickly acknowledged. "Insulin is now manufactured by recombinant technology, no longer from killing those squealing pigs to cut out their pancreases."

"Was the way to make insulin using recombinant techniques discovered by the drug companies?" Brent asked.

"No way, Jose!" Hutch quickly responded. He explained that methods of insulin production by genetic recombinant techniques were discovered by scientists at universities. After they were trained and graduated from the universities, they joined a company called Genentech—whose purpose is to make biological medicines using genetic techniques that will be useful to people with different kinds of disorders without harming the bodies of those who need the medicine to live. After Genentech successfully makes the medicine with new genetic techniques, the drug companies get the methods from Genentech and begin manufacturing the medicine in large quantities to sell all over the world, which is capitalism. Companies make medicines to sell because they can earn lots of money. In countries where there is no capitalism, no free market, few drugs are developed. Making insulin with recombinant genetic techniques instead of squeezing the juice from dead hogs' pancreases came about in America rather than China because the companies who make insulin get to keep the money, instead of the government.

Brent reminded his friend that the production of insulin was similar to the marketing of concentrates by the drug companies. He had heard from his father that what has driven new discoveries in America has been the spirit of capitalism and free marketing. But his father also said that the spirit of capitalism may have been polluted, just as the concentrate was polluted with a virus.

"Oh, come on now," Hutch replied. "How can a virus spread into an economic concept like capitalism? It's not a human, living thing."

"No, you're right; capitalism isn't a living body like a human being. A virus can't infect it. But it was infected by something else just as harmful as a virus," Brent confirmed. "Rather than an infection by a virus, capitalism has been infected by greed!"

"Wow! You mean the spirit of capitalism has been eroded by greed so that capitalism is no longer a positive force in our society?" Hutch asked. "How did that happen?"

Brent and Hutch continued discussing the fact that capitalism is less effective as a resource for innovation because of its pollution with greed, which is explainable by deregulation. Because of human nature, society needs governance, regulation. It's an economic principle that people forget in the United States. According to economists, the obligation of a capitalist is to be responsible to stockholders by generating a profit for their investments. It is not to guarantee the quality of the products they are selling (Magnuson 2008).

Despite the economic downturn in the United States and around the world in 2009, without cost controls, pharmaceutical companies continued to reap a profit. While many companies downsized or ceased to exist, pharmaceutical companies expanded regardless of an increased unemployment rate, mortgage foreclosures, and rising poverty. Their action, demonstrated by the purchase of Wyeth Drug Company by Pfizer for $65 billion in January 2009, attests to their capitalistic goal, to make a profit for their stockholders, irrespective of the bleak times for most citizens (Pollack 2009). The purchase allows Pfizer, already number one in the pharmaceutical industry, to solidify its rank and to become diversified in the health-care industry, the effect of lack of regulation in the United States.

Hutch remarked, "Because you suffer from hemophilia, a lot of people are making big bucks. I guess the motto of the companies who manufacture drugs is 'When people bleed, there is a need.'"[111]

"Yeah, pretty cool, Hutch," Brent cheerfully replied to his drawing buddy. "How about this for the drug companies: 'When people have pain, our bankroll will gain.'" Brent and Hutch laughed as they contested with each other to come up with the cleverest slogan reflecting the profit motive of the drug companies. Brent quipped, "Okay, Hutch, how about this rhyme? 'When I bleed, there is a need, answered by greed!'" Brent and Hutch, delighted by their cleverness, doubled over with laughter.

Ride in a Black Mercedes-Benz

"I have to tell you," Brent confided to his friend Hutch. "You know what Dr. Taillefer told me?"

"No, I don't know Dr. Taillefer. Is he your doctor?"

"Yes, he's one of my doctors who help treat my hemophilia."

"Well, what did the good doctor say?" Hutch asked.

"He said he always wanted to ride in a Mercedes Benz."

"What does riding in a Mercedes have to do with the cost of medicine?" Hutch skeptically demanded to know.

---

111 Total compensation to the CEO of Wyeth, Bob Essner, for the year 2007 was $24.1 million. Wyeth produces Xyntha, an antihemopilia concentrate for treatment of bleeds in hemophilia. (RE: http://www.fiercepharma.com).

"Now who's the smart guy?" Brent had quickly sensed his advantage over his friend. "This is what Dr. Taillefer told me." He related the tale he'd heard from his doctor. "One of those fat drug companies that sell concentrate—I think it was Cutter … or maybe it was Armour—invited him to come to a meeting at a fancy Southern California resort. All expenses paid. The drug company invited a bunch of doctors, twenty or thirty of them, to their meeting—paying all their expenses."

Hutch had heard of doctors going to meetings in nice places, paid for by drug companies trying to woo their business. The drug companies can write off the cost of the meeting as a huge tax break. They could easily spread the same amount of information with a telephone conference and spend a lot less money. Sometimes doctors are just as guilty as drug companies when it comes to luxury. The doctors take care of sick and suffering people who pay for their services. With some of the money the doctors earn, they go on cruises. Travel agencies offer cruises for doctors that they label as educational so that doctors can write them off as a tax deduction—the cost of a pleasant cruise up the Nile River in Egypt, enjoying the luxury of fine dining and beautiful scenery in exchange for a one-hour lecture each day aboard a luxury liner. The doctors and the travel companies are living a high life as the result of the profit they make by other people's suffering.

"But what about your Mercedes story?" Hutch reminded Brent.

Dr. Taillefer had told him that the drug company flew him to Palm Springs in California. It was necessary to fly to Pasadena, the closest airport to Palm Springs. When he arrived at the airport, a limousine was waiting for him. Not just for him, Brent learned later from his mother. When she asked Dr. Taillefer if he went alone on the trip, he said no. Although divorced, he didn't go alone. He took a pretty blond woman with him. Dr. Taillefer and his girlfriend were impressed when they climbed into the limousine after their arrival at the Pasadena airport. It was a stretch black Mercedes with soft leather seats. A chauffer drove them to Palm Springs, where there was a room reserved for them at the Stouffer Renaissance Esmeralda Resort in Indian Wells. The hotel room had a queen sized bed.

For three days, Dr. Taillefer and his girlfriend relaxed in the hotel room or at the poolside, enjoying the clear sunshine and cloudless blue sky. The doctor went to meetings in the conference room for two or three hours each day and listened to talks by other doctors. At the end of each afternoon, the drug company hosted a happy hour, where the doctors and their wives, or girlfriends, were served fine liquors and fancy hors d'oeuvres. Afterward, in the balmy dessert evenings, the group of doctors, their guests, and the drug company executives attended an elegant dinner in the hotel dining room. During the day, when the doctors were at the meetings, Dr. Taillefer's girlfriend sat by the pool in her bikini, soaking up the sunshine. If she wanted to, she could have played golf. Directly across the road from the hotel, a beautiful golf course rolls over the hills, replacing the native desert mesquite and paloverde with watered green grass. Golf courses extend for twenty miles in Palm Desert, sucking the water for the fairways from the Colorado River. The girlfriend wanted to try golf for the exercise. But she was advised that walking on the golf course was not allowed. Golfers were required to drive electric golf cars. The cost for one round of golf was $250 per person, which the drug company would pay. The only expense Dr. Taillefer had to pay from his own pocket was for the girlfriend's suntan lotion.

"Wow!" Hutch exclaimed. "That lucky doctor is living well because of you. Your pain is his gain. Because you are a bleeder, all those doctors and the drug salesmen got to stay in a fancy resort—wined, dined, and tanned—and sleep in a big bed between fancy sheets with their wives or girlfriends."

"Yup, and Dr. Taillefer got to ride in a fancy Mercedes with his girlfriend." Brent quipped. "I guess it's all part of capitalism. I thought to myself, 'I pay, you play, and the drug companies get rich' when Doctor Taillefer told me his story."

Empowerment

Sketches at the Zoo with a Friend

For several years, Brent had created drawings and sketches. Drawing was an important outlet for him, helping satisfy his search for the meaning of his life. Brent first met Milan Bennett on Thanksgiving of 1990. Brent's mother had invited Milan and his wife, Barbara, to the Perry's home for the holiday. They had just moved to Portland from Massachusetts. Barbara was a new faculty member at the Riverside Community College where Gwyn held a faculty appointment..

Milan was an artist. He struggled to find a gallery that would sell his work. Eventually, Milan joined the faculty at the community college. Brent showed some of his drawings of comic book characters to Milan. Brent's drawings included human figures as well as guns. The drawings of the guns were highly rendered with many details, including numbers inscribed into shiny polished surfaces. The human figures were of muscled men who were often portrayed in anatomical fisted positions. Every muscle was accentuated, bulging, as if working, which created a body image reminding Milan of a sack full of walnuts. The drawings were poignant, representing images of masculine power, as if Brent was identifying power through an image.

Responding to Brent's mother's suggestion, Milan began tutoring Brent in July 1992. Brent was interested in becoming an artist, in drawing, even though he knew he was dying and that his body was withering. Milan admired and respected his spirit; he understood Brent. The two of them together were a physical contrast. Milan was a solid, tall, robust man, standing more than six feet, with long black wavy hair, a curly beard with some graying, and a neat moustache. He gazed meaningfully and directly at a person through his rimmed spectacles. Brent was short for his age; he had become frail in appearance as he became ill. Milan believed Brent was transforming images of power of the muscled men to his own power. Drawing was important to Brent because he was consciously selecting a central motif, power, which reflected his behavior and gave him a sensation of efficacy and satisfied his search for meaning in his life. Milan knew that what a person draws shapes how he behaves. Drawing allows an individual to experience ableness, which facilitates a situation that could happen to any of us.

Milan sensed that Brent needed to loosen up; he was too rigid. Milan recognized that a good place to unravel would be the zoo, a great place to study art. The first site in the zoo Brent and Milan visited was the monkey house, a happy place to draw the spirit in your life, to draw what's in your mind. Brent and Milan sketched with black marker pens on large, thick white pages while sitting side by side but independent of one another. Brent did not copy Milan's drawings. He didn't even glance at his mentor's sheet. Brent hated it. He detested drawing monkeys.

"Those dumb animals won't sit still," Brent complained with exasperation, his face turning pink. He was correct; the monkeys would not sit still and pose for an artist. When drawing a monkey, the artist cannot look down at his paper, then look back up at the monkey, and then look back to his paper. The monkey would not be there; it would be gone.

"You have to be fast, really fast, to draw a monkey," Milan patiently emphasized, understanding Brent's frustration. The zoo visit seemed to be a disaster.

Then, suddenly, Brent's drawings changed. He had let go. He'd made a leap. His caricatures, which had illustrated anatomical muscled men, turned to something completely different. He was not drawing landscapes or body parts; instead, he was drawing what was in his mind when at the zoo. The zoo loosened him up. Brent transformed his mind-set from muscle men to monkeys. Brent knew anatomy thoroughly. He could precisely illustrate the masseter muscle of the jaw of a chewing giraffe. Suddenly, while at the zoo, he no longer drew an arm or a leg—he drew an animal. He began owning it all. His drawings became fluid, beautiful, and adept. Although Brent was young, he was wise. He was aware of his limited time left to live. He understood that he could not control his living or dying. However, as long as he was alive, he could control his actions, his life. Although Brent could not control the conditions of his life, the potentials within himself could be activated by his decisions (Frankl 1984). He was pleased with himself.

"Look what I did," Brent exclaimed to Milan, proudly displaying his drawings, which he'd completed rapidly, sketching a baboon, a giraffe, or an elephant in a minute or a minute and a half. Brent was honest and did not subdue his boastfulness when he was completed with an animal drawing. Milan recognized that because he was dying Brent had surrendered himself, which required supreme courage, an observation that was heartbreaking for Milan. Rapidly, Brent completed black-and-white drawings of different animals. Glancing at each animal sketched by Brent, a viewer could readily see Brent in each animal character he sketched. His chimpanzee was contemplative. The most profound was the elephant, which reflected Brent's wisdom. Brent's baboon displayed another of his qualities—churlishness.

Brent could see the artist he wanted to become if only he could live and not die. He was confronted with death because his body was a finite thing. But he was capable of defying and braving even hopelessness. He had to make a choice at the moment—he could be bitter or he could be not bitter. He needed to choose how to live. He must choose between frustration and engaging the monkey. He chose the latter, which made his thoughts come alive on the page, an action that gave him power, a power different from the muscle-bound figures he had caricaturized in his previous drawings. Awareness of the transformation for Brent that day at the zoo was a striking call to teaching for Milan. He reflected, recognizing to stay alive as an artist, he must grow with his work and become fulfilled by teaching, learning from his students. Brent provided that opportunity.

"Can you imagine what difference there would have been if Brent had photographed the zoo animals, rather than drawing them, and mounted their photographs in a nice photo album?" Milan pondered. "None of the power of the animals would have been transferred to Brent."[112]

The first visit to the zoo for Brent with Milan was the most profound, although there were others. There was no regression on subsequent visits. Brent continued to quickly produce animal sketches, more than forty. Because he knew that monkeys do not pose for a sketch—they do not sit still—rather than copy the appearance of an arm or a leg, Brent created his impression of a monkey from his mind. People attending the zoo stopped to look at his animal sketches. Some were heard to say to one another, "Just look at him. He is so young to be a professional artist." Such a comment brought a smile of satisfaction to Brent's face.

Brent was pleased with his sketch of the chimpanzee he completed in the zoo in 1992. He was unaware that the animal he admired was the reservoir of HIV, the virus that was killing him ... However, the animal was not at fault for Brent's infection with HIV. It was man's intervention in Africa that assembled the conditions for the transfer of the animal virus, SIV, to humans to become HIV. This is an example that humans are not always conscious of the impact their actions have on innocent animals and other humans.

Milan and Brent were together for activities at other times in addition to drawing at the zoo. At first, Milan was uncomfortable discussing HIV with Brent. But he encouraged Brent to express his feelings through his drawings. "Brent could draw anything," Milan said. He acknowledged Brent's feelings. Brent was aware of Milan's insight into his thoughts. When Brent turned sixteen, he had begun

---

112 Comment during an interview with Milan Bennett November 12, 2007

to practice driving his father's car. Sometimes Milan would ride in the passenger seat beside him. Sarcastically, Brent smugly told Milan, "You don't need to worry about me," implying that if they crashed, what difference would there be? Brent was going to die anyway.

Brent began to show signs of illness, even though he was attending weekly sessions of pentamidine inhalation to ward off pneumonia, and swallowing with difficulty four AZT tablets four times daily to slow the progression of HIV infection to AIDS. Milan and Barbara continued to encourage him. In June 1992, they enlivened his spirits with a drive over the mountain and through the forest to the seashore so that he could enjoy running in the sand on the beach and splashing in the waves lapping the shore. They had left the car parked in the sunshine with the windows rolled up while they walked along the beach. When they returned to the car from the cool ocean breeze and wet sand, they discovered that the interior of the parked car was intensely hot. Milan was worried. Brent was too frail to withstand the heat. He ran the car's air conditioner, opened all the windows, and fanned the air to drop the stifling heat. They returned to the beach cabin where they were staying and were surprised when Brent sarcastically reminded them that fate had not yet claimed him. Then he celebrated by quaffing down three bowls of Cap'n Crunch with cold milk. He required an infusion of concentrate to control bleeding in his ankles after the run on the beach. They'd brought the medicine with them, along with a supply of needles, alcohol swabs, syringes, and Band-Aids, to complete an infusion, a new experience for Milan and Barbara. They telephoned Lee, Brent's dad, who instructed them how to assist Brent, who knew how to mix the medicine and insert the needle for infusion into his arm vein.

On July 18, 1992, a birthday party was scheduled for Brent's mother, her forty-seventh. She was out of the house, busy gathering supplies for making crazy hats for the party. No one else was at home except Brent and Milan, who happened to be visiting, when the telephone rang.

Brent answered to discover that the hospital was calling. Brent was told, with a warning, that his white blood cell count, his T4-helper cells were very low. The caller had assumed that he was talking with a parent. He did not ask who was answering the telephone. Brent became agitated, as if another blow had confirmed his fate. Previously, he had attended a movie with his father and Milan. The movie, featuring Arnold Schwarzenegger in *Terminator II*, encompassed the central theme that history is predestined. Later, Brent scrawled *No fate!* on the wall, as if his fate was also sealed, predestined.

After Brent died, his zoo drawings were framed and displayed on the walls of the art gallery at Riverside Community College in Portland, Oregon. The display of Brent's drawings was open to the public, hosted by Milan Bennett, Monday evening, March 27, 2000, through Friday, April 28. The art showing was well attended. On the opening evening, refreshments were served to the gathering of the people who acclaimed Brent's zoo animal drawings. Although the monkeys were not swinging before the viewers and Brent was gone, the power of the monkeys that was transferred to Brent remained in his drawings. Milan has become the art department chairman. He has successfully displayed his own completed works in different galleries and has sold numerous paintings. He continues to teach and paint, empowered by the lessons he learned from a dying youth, a youthful artist who refused to accept fate but was relentlessly overtaken by fate, a fate that disregarded his beliefs and decided his outcome.

During their days together, which artist developed the most, Brent or Milan? An unimportant question. More importantly, Milan recognized through art that power was transferred from monkeys to Brent—and from Brent to Milan.

Why Me?

A recurrence of pneumocystis pneumonia dragged Brent down again in the spring of 1992. Instead of enjoying the cheerful pink, red, and blue colors of the rhododendrons and camellias poking out of the bright green ferns surrounding the home beneath the tall trees, he suffered malaise and weakness from his illness and nausea from the pentamidine treatments. He rallied again. But in the autumn, another recurrence of pneumonia weighed him down again. Brent became discouraged after recurrent treatments and recovery. He did not recover to the full vigor of his pre-AIDS days. The toll on Brent's body was evident. He knew he would not have had AIDS if he did not have hemophilia.

"Just how did hemophilia get into our family?" Brent demanded to know. "Explain it to me, Mom. How did it land here?"

"Well, you see, this is how it is," Gwyn replied to her son. "My mother—your grandmother—had four daughters, including me. Each of us, independently, inherited the hemophilia trait from our mother, although we show no signs of hemophilia. Our mother, who also has no signs of hemophilia, carries the mutant hemophilia gene."

"Yeah, but how did Grandma get it? Where did all this hemophilia gene stuff come from?"

"Her mother, my grandmother, your great-grandmother, was tested, and she did not have the mutant hemophilia gene," Gwyn answered.. "She didn't carry the trait." (Table 1, figure 1)

"And your grandpa didn't have hemophilia, did he?" Brent stated.

"You are absolutely correct. Grandpa did not have hemophilia," Gwyn confirmed. "Yet my mother had not one but four daughters who carried hemophilia. That indicates that passing the gene to a daughter was not a one-time thing, as if she had a mutation in one of her eggs. No, all four of her eggs that developed into her four daughters possessed the mutant hemophilia gene, indicating that all the cells in her body contained the mutant gene. And if the mutant gene did not come from her mother, where did it come from?" Gwyn asked Brent, making sure he was following her logic.

"I don't know," Brent admitted. "It couldn't have come from your grandpa; he wasn't affected with hemophilia."

"You're right—and at the same time, you are mistaken," Gwyn anxiously replied, gratified that Brent was following her conversation. "You are correct that Grandpa didn't have hemophilia. And yet the mutant gene probably came from him."

"I don't get you, Mom." Brent uneasily squirmed in his seat, admitting he couldn't understand his mother's logic. "If my great-grandpa didn't have hemophilia, how could he pass it on to his daughter?"

"Well, this is what I have been told," Gwyn replied seriously. "Most likely, the mutation was in one of Grandpa's sperms, the one that fertilized Grandma's egg to make a new baby, the egg which became my mother. The hemophilia gene was not in all of Grandpa's cells of his whole body, but a mutation could have occurred when one of his sperm was made."

Appearance of hemophilia in the McCann family was similar to the first presence of hemophilia in Queen Victoria's royal family. The mutation of the antihemophilia factor (AHF) gene was present for the first time in Brent's maternal grandmother (Individual 2000, figure 1), and in Queen Victoria (Individual 0001, figure 3, Appendix II).

The genetics counselor at the hemophilia clinic had explained to Gwyn that mutations occur all the time. She continued to reassure Brent that although the word "mutation" sounds bad, its effect is not always harmful. Mutations are the source of change that allows animals, plants, and people to adapt to new needs of nature and their surroundings. Mutation is the source for evolution and also sometimes the cause of genetic disease such as hemophilia (Nachman and Crowell 2000).

"Yeah, Ma," Brent blurted out, implying that his mother was lecturing to him. "First, I have to deal with hemophilia. Next, HIV ... then AIDS whacks me. And now you're telling me I have to add another threat to my troubled life—mutation. How can so much happen to a nice guy like me?" (table 3).

Gwyn gave her son an affectionate embrace while reassuring him that he was special.

One of the miracles of nature is the capacity for organisms, including plants, animals, germs, and humans to reproduce like offspring from generation to generation. Living things breed true; that is, they beget their own kind. Maple trees reproduce to make new maple trees. Zebras bring forth newborn zebras, not lizards or other kinds of animals. Gwyn reminded her son that some people explain the order in life by the creationist theory, which is, according to the book of Genesis, where everything is made by God. She had been raised that way in a family headed by a Protestant minister.

She continued by saying that in contrast with creationism, there are theories of evolution. All living things on Earth have a common origin. For the evolution of life to produce different forms, alteration in genetic material must occur. Genetic information is carried in parcels of DNA called genes. Genes must have the capacity for occasional alterations to create the opportunity for evolution to proceed, which allows the development of new types of living creatures. Such alterations in genetic material are called mutations. It is likely that most new mutations are lost—they disappear—and the organism doesn't complete development or perishes. Sometimes a process, called selection, allows a mutation to survive, which begins a new chain, establishing the mutant gene in future populations and resulting in a change in a trait or establishment of a new species.

Persons affected with hemophilia have reduced biological fitness; that is, their life expectancy is shortened, and they have reduced reproductive fitness. They have fewer children than men who do not have hemophilia. The reason men who have hemophilia have fewer children compared to men who are not affected with hemophilia is not biological. There is no decreased fertility in hemophilia. It is because they are less likely to marry, and when they do marry, fewer children are conceived, by choice. If hemophilia is biologically deleterious, why doesn't it disappear from the earth? What keeps the hemophilia trait going? If all males who have hemophilia in the entire world were destroyed, would hemophilia disappear from the face of the earth, never to be seen again? Or would it appear in the next generation? The answer is that hemophilia would reappear. The explanation comes from studying mutations.

The mutation rate is the rate at which a mutation takes place in a germ cell for each generation. In their excellent comprehensive discussion of mutation rates, Vogel and Motulsky (1986) cite the mutation rate for hemophilia type A as $2.2 - 5.7 \times 10^{-5}$. This means that once in the 45,454 times the hemophilia gene is reproduced, a mutation occurs. For hemophilia type B, the mutation rate is thought to be about one-tenth as frequent, $2 - 3 \times 10^{-6}$. Since a female has two X chromosomes, the likelihood of a mutation of the hemophilia gene occurring in females is twice as great compared to males who have one X chromosome. However, males make many more sperm, spermatogenesis, compared to the number of eggs made by females during their lifetimes. Different kinds of sperm are produced in fertile males, but the kind of sperm that can fertilize a female's egg to create a new life, the "egg-getter" sperm during the years a man can reproduce, numbers about sixteen billion (Hooge 2008). Each time a sperm is made, the hemophilia gene is copied. Considering the mutation rate, a man's sperm would produce thirty-five thousand hemophilia mutants during his lifetime. Theoretically, one or two out of every fifty thousand fertilized human zygotes (eggs) would contain a new mutation for hemophilia. During a lifetime, extending over thirty or more reproductive years, a woman ovulates approximately four hundred times (Human Ovulation Process 2005). Considering the mutation rate, only 1 of every 110 woman would produce an egg bearing the hemophilia mutation.

Brent wanted to know why a mutation hit his family right in the middle of their clotting-factor gene. Why not the Benson family, who lived in the yellow house across the street, or the Halversons, who lived at the bottom of the hill? In his biology class and in a *Time* magazine, he had learned of mutations causing other diseases besides hemophilia. There was a girl in his English class, Cindy Johnson, who had eyes of a different color. She had one blue eye and one brown eye (heterochromia). The girl's different eye colors were caused by a mutation. Her mutation was not inherited. The mutation occurred after fertilization in the developing embryo, affecting only the cells in one of her eyes. Her mutation was not in the sperm her father gave to her mother, nor in her mother's egg, which came together to begin forming her life. It wasn't passed on to her from one of her parents, and she would not pass it on to her children, as the mutation is not present within the egg cells of her ovaries. Brent told his mother that Cindy had a schematic mutation.

Gwyn laughed and corrected her son, telling him the word is a *somatic* mutation rather than a schematic mutation. Brent wanted to know why it was called a somatic mutation. The term somatic is derived from the Greek word *soma*, which means body. A somatic mutation is a mutation in the cells of the body. An inherited mutation is called a germinal mutation, referring to the reproductive cells

Brent returned to his question—why factor VIII? Why did his family get hit with a mutation in the clotting factor gene that affected him? He'd learned in his biology class that mutations happen all the time. He wanted to know why he didn't get a mutation in a gene that causes webbed fingers or red hair. Why the hemophilia mutation? If he had a choice, he would have preferred a mutant gene that didn't do so much damage to his body. He asked his mother if some genes mutate more often than other genes. Gwyn didn't know the answer to his question; however, research has suggested that there may be instability in the hemophilia A gene. The DNA region of the hemophilia A gene may have increased susceptibility to mutations (Lozier et al. 2002).

Brent shifted his questioning by reminding his mother that her father, his grandfather, was a minister, a man who was supposed to be close to God. After hemophilia was discovered in him, did she or his grandfather pray for him, pray that the hemophilia would go away? If God is good, and in charge of everything that happens in the universe, why does he allow mutations? Why didn't he stop Brent from having hemophilia?

Gwyn replied by saying that she believed God is good and all the events in our lives are controlled by God. But they are controlled in ways we do not always understand. All mutations are not bad; some are good. God's intent when he made Brent was to create a special person, which he did. She didn't know in God's scheme of things whether mutations are more common in some genes than in others. Perhaps scientists knew the answer.

Answering Brent's question about why, if God was good, he would allow the creation of something harmful to his body, like hemophilia, Gwyn suggested that God also made the ocean and the land. But components of things God has made interact. A fierce storm occurs when cold air over the ocean moves toward warm land, producing a hurricane. He made the land and the mountains, but sometimes they interact and a terrible earthquake happens, destroying the people God has created. Similarly, the particles in genes can interact. Although God made all the nucleotides that are the components of the genes, sometimes the nucleotides interact or are mistaken when they are copied, causing a mutation in the gene. Genes do not operate in a vacuum. At the basic level, there is no conflict between creationist theory and evolutionist theory of life. She told her son that according to creationism, God made the elements and the atoms, which are the building stones for the molecules. The molecules interact to form substances that are affected by mutations, allowing evolution to act through selection, according to evolutionist theory.

Brent became discouraged and said that maybe his life was not intended to have any meaning. "What is the meaning of my life?" he asked his mother.

She told Brent that his life does have great meaning. It is precious. An example of the meaning of his life is the great happiness he brought to her. She recalled what Viktor Frankl wrote after he was freed from Auschwitz at the end of World War II: "What keeps people going when confronted with hopelessness is their recognition of the meaning of their lives" (Frankl 1984). But often people do not discover the meaning of their lives; instead, they surrender and succumb to their distress. Rather than discovering the meaning of their lives, they give up and die without it unfolding before their eyes. She told Brent that HIV infection and AIDS was just as much a hopeless confrontation to him and the other persons with hemophilia as a concentration camp was to the prisoners during the war. The meaning of Brent's life was more than making him happy; it was about making her and their family happy. She continued, telling her son that persons with hemophilia, like him, had contributed more to the understanding of human diseases than any other medical disorder, a testament to the meaning of their lives. Progress leading to the discovery of the cause of HIV and AIDS came from studying hemophilia men who were infected with HIV, which demonstrated how HIV is transmitted. Thousands of persons infected with HIV around the world have benefited from the research and clinical trials of medication in HIV infected guys who have hemophilia.

Research in genetic engineering has resulted in the successful manufacture of recombinant FVIII for the treatment of hemophilia to produce clotting factor without utilizing pooled blood collected from thousands of donors, a model for the manufacture of deficient components in other genetic disorders.

Understanding human mutations in other genetic disorders has advanced by studying mutations in hemophilia. Gwyn continued telling Brent that although men and boys have hemophilia, they may have it for different reasons. The inherited mutations causing hemophilia are not all the same, even though the affected persons all have the same disorder (Hill et al. 2005). She pointed out that Brent had the most common mutation in hemophilia, the intron 22 inversion in the F8 gene, which causes nearly half of all cases of hemophilia (Oldenberg and El-Maarri 2006). Some other persons had the same kind of hemophilia that he had, but they had it for a different reason. In some persons, rather than an inversion, a different mutation occurred, such as a deletion, a splice-site mutation, a frameshift mutation, a missense or a nonsense mutation. Gwyn may not have been aware that some persons with hemophilia have a compound mutation: two mutations in one gene on the X chromosome (Theophilus et al. 2001).

Brent was uncomfortable with his mother's discussion. He winced, looked down at the floor, and sarcastically muttered that not only mutations but all of hemophilia is nonsense.

She replied by saying that it was not nonsense. The knowledge gained by studying hemophilia in persons like him helped discover the cause of other genetic disorders. No one wants to be different, but sometimes people are different. It is important to understand the differences and what to do about them.

A Cure for Hemophilia through Genetic Engineering

Hemophilia will most likely be the genetic disease that will be cured—not just treated but *cured*—with new genetic technology, which will benefit many people who are affected not only with hemophilia but with other genetic disorders as well.

New research in hemophilia and AIDS will make it possible to transfer the hemophilia gene from the cells of a person who does not have the hemophilia mutation into persons like him who have the mutant hemophilia gene. This is called gene transfer.

In gene transfer, a person with hemophilia, like Brent, would have a normal gene inserted into his muscle cells so that his biceps and quadriceps produced clotting factor. He would no longer have to take shots.

There would be no need to replace all the mutant hemophilia genes in his body. The cells containing the inserted gene would gradually take over and make factor VIII, ignoring the cells that don't know how to make the clotting factor.

Researchers are learning methods of gene transfer and gene replacement therapy through experiments in hemophilia (Mannucci 2002). Scientists have reasoned that if a virus can invade a person's cells, similar to what happens during an infection with an adenovirus, and maybe even HIV, perhaps the normal hemophilia gene can be attached onto the virus and get a free ride into his cells, where it will replace the activity missing in the mutant gene and do some good (Kay 2001).

Gene transfer therapy can be thought of as hitchhiking. However, there are still technical problems that must be overcome before a young person like Brent, who had a mutant hemophilia gene, would be able to get a shot, like an immunization, that would cure his hemophilia (Gene Therapy 2008). His life, and the lives of all the other persons who had hemophilia and HIV, made a difference, improving the future for many other people all over the world.

Of all the genetic diseases, hemophilia is the most attractive model for developing gene treatment. After the threat of hepatitis and HIV have taken their toll in hemophilia, life expectancy is expected to reach nearly normal, the result of infusions with safe, virus-free concentrates. Hemophilia is a genetic condition with organized medical care, where monitoring recipients of gene therapy for long periods is possible and efficient in the treatment centers where a hemophilia community exists (Resnik 2009). The recent past experience treating hemophilia with infusions of safe medicine for recurrent bleeding episodes in persons who did not become infected with HIV has witnessed an increased longevity to sixty-three years in severe hemophilia and to seventy-five years of age in milder hemophilia (Darby et al. 2007). The aspects of gene therapy can be closely monitored through organized clinical trials. The drive for financial gains by the pharmaceutical manufacturers to perfect treatments for genetic diseases through gene therapy will not only benefit the stockholders, but also the persons affected by a variety of disorders in addition to hemophilia (Graw et al. 2005). Hopefully, with gene therapy, rather than receiving lifelong repeated numerous infusions, a single treatment or perhaps more than one, but not numerous treatments, would cure a person's hemophilia and extend his life to normalcy in quality and longevity.

A Birthday Party for Brent

During the month preceding Brent's seventeenth birthday, October 4, 1992, Gwyn became concerned about his well-being. Brent seemed dejected. His health was failing. He looked like he had lost hope. On September 2, she cornered her son. "Wouldn't it be fun to celebrate your birthday with a big bash this year?" she asked. Her cheerful exclamation suddenly rekindled the dormant spark within him. He became enthused for living. Brent became excited as he reflected upon whom he wanted to invite to be with him on his seventeenth birthday. Instead of just another day going by, he had control of his special day. He would invite his family, his friends, and all the people he cared about to come to his birthday party for a celebration. Although he might be ill, he could still do something that would be festive for others, exciting, almost notorious.

Brent knew it would be his last birthday, Gwyn later reflected.

The birthday party was at the Stalking Tiger Restaurant in North Portland on October 4, 1992. Everybody was there. Brent's eighty-one-year-old grandfather, Reverend Eric McCann, and his wife, Prudence, flew up to Portland from Santa Cruz in California. Brent's three aunts came from Atlanta, Georgia, Yakima, Washington, and Grants Pass, Oregon, with their families, including Brent's cousins. Even Brent's doctor came to the party, wearing his thick black leather jacket, black leather pants and boots, soft black leather gloves with cuffs to the mid forearm, and his white helmet, riding his Moto Guzzi. Brent's family and friends gathered together in a large room set aside for them at the restaurant. Old folks, young folks, babies, children, and adults all celebrated together the joy of Brent's life; he was the center of the festivity. From the long tables where the birthday guests were seated in chairs close to one another, balloons of different colors drifted upward toward the high ceiling, tethered on colorful ribbons. The tables were dusted with sparkling glitter. Small cups held a lit candle in front of each place setting. Although the concept of a "Last Supper" is solemn, sobering, especially when the individual is only seventeen years of age, the ambiance in the celebration room was not of dejection. The guests were somber within themselves while outwardly appearing as birthday party guest are expected to appear. They wanted Brent to remember the birthday party as a happy day.

Gwyn knew Brent wanted it that way. He wanted the people he loved to remember him as a happy guy, not as a suffering, bitter person. The guests were conscious of the significance of the day. While lifting champagne glasses and feasting on birthday cake, no one discussed hemophilia or AIDS. With Brent, they talked about sports, fast cars, and his drawings. The guests knew they would never attend another of Brent's birthdays, but there was no referral to that hopeless thought. Instead, Gwyn raised a glass of champagne in a toast to her son for his courage and idealism. His aunts—Louise, Larissa, and Lea—all agreed that the wonderful birthday party, which brought the family and friends together from afar, was testimony to Brent's special personality. His grandfather proclaimed that Brent had demonstrated steadfastness and courage despite adversary. Although there were many times when Brent could have deviated from pleasant and acceptable behavior, he continued to move forward in a positive manner, his cousin offered. Amid the birthday cake, festive balloons, decorations, and champagne, Brent's radiance was a sparkling lesson in the value of living for the moment, a tribute to the beauty of life. His mother reflected that many positive events in Brent's life created beautiful images to be retained in contrast to memories of the hardships, which she would let go.

Brent was hospitalized again for treatment of pneumocystis pneumonia from December 25, 1992, Christmas Day, until January 1, 1993, New Year's Day. After he returned home, he was weak and tired, without an appetite. He continued to be nauseated from the pentamidine treatment he received in the hospital. He didn't leave the house.

Part VII

HIV in the School

Two Brothers with Hemophilia and HIV

O n Monday, December 28, 1992, Brent lay in a hospital bed. The joy of his birthday party slowly faded as his illness progressed and he deteriorated. On that same day, in southwest Oregon, twenty miles east of Roseburg on Mountain Highway 138, in the small town of Glide, carved out of the forest, where the Little River and the Umpqua River collide, the entire town's people filled the community hall three days after Christmas. They were there to say good-bye to David and Peter Witbeck. The two brothers—David, age seventeen, and Peter, age fourteen—died a day apart from AIDS. David and Peter both had hemophilia and became infected with HIV after treatment with infected concentrate. Peter died at 2:00 AM on Saturday morning, December 26, 1992, the day after Christmas. David, his older brother, died the next day in the same hospital. They lay resting beside each other, the two young brothers buried on the same day in the Roseburg cemetery. David and Brent were the same age; both were born in 1975.

Siblings in other families attending the hemophilia treatment center also succumbed to AIDS after receiving HIV contaminated concentrates, including Sean and Chris Cairns, Steve and Sally Phillips, and Joe and Tim Singler.

Carmelita, the mother of David and Peter, an attractive, vivacious, resourceful Hispanic woman, and her husband, Dale Witbeck, a soft-spoken logger, raised their dark-eyed handsome sons and their sister,

Maria, in a small wooden house with only a rutted dirt driveway, in the rural Oregon logging community.

David Witbeck was born June 28, 1975, in Corona, California. A week after Carmelita brought her newborn son home from the hospital, he was circumcised in the doctor's office. Following the circumcision, Carmelita returned to their home, where the young mother put her infant son into his crib for a nap. She was alarmed when she checked her baby and discovered bright red blood splattered all over his crib and blankets. She wrapped him in a blanket and rushed him to the hospital. The doctor sutured the bleeding site and gave the infant a vitamin K shot, followed by a saline intravenous infusion.

While the doctor was busy attending to her son, Carmelita telephoned her family and discovered unsuspected, surprising information. Carmelita was born in 1954 in Salinas, California, to parents of Mexican descent, who had eight children. Carmelita, the youngest of the eight children, was not raised with the family. Her father, born in 1899, three hundred miles south of Mexico City in the region of Oaxaca, died in 1995 at ninety-six years of age. Her mother, from a small family, was born of a father who lived in Mexico and had hemophilia. Carmelita does not know how old her grandfather was when he died, but he had a brother who died from a bleed at age thirty. One of her sisters has had five sons with hemophilia; another had two sons who were affected with hemophilia. For the first time, she discovered there had been males in the family who were affected with hemophilia. Before her son bled after circumcision, Carmelita was unaware of hemophilia in her family. After receiving the family information, the hospital was able to obtain cryoprecipitate from the Red Cross blood bank, which was infused into the infant, resulting in cessation of bleeding from the circumcision site.

Carmelita, her husband, and their first child moved to Roseburg, Oregon, where Dale, found work as a logger. In 1976, they moved to Glide, twenty miles from Roseburg. The hemophilia treatment center in Portland supplied Carmelita with concentrate to keep in her home in

Glide. Arrangements were made with a doctor in Roseburg to provide infusions for treatment of bleeds in the Mercy Medical Center, using the concentrate Carmelita brought with her to the hospital. Carmelita telephoned the hemophilia treatment center doctor on call when her son had a bleed. The on-call doctor notified the Roseburg hospital, explaining that Carmelita was bringing her son to the emergency room for an infusion of concentrate, which satisfied the hospital's requirement for a doctor's order for the procedure and the medicine.

Acquiring the technique for infusing her son was a goal for Carmelita. She learned the steps leading to infusions, including storing the medicine, mixing the water and the medicine, sterile technique, disposal of used needles ... all the components of infusion except actual insertion of the needle into her son's small arm vein. Carmelita brought David to the clinic in Portland on the Greyhound bus and stayed for several days. Sue Underwood, the clinic nurse, instructed her in the technique of intravenous infusion and reviewed all the steps in the procedure to avoid infection at the venipuncture site. Carmelita practiced inserting the butterfly into a ripe orange to simulate a venipuncture. From oranges, she moved to nurses and doctors, practicing inserting the butterfly needle into the arm of Sue and Dr. Taillefer to experience "hitting the vein." She learned to put pressure at the venipuncture site after the tourniquet was removed and the needle was withdrawn from the vein, with her thumb on a cotton ball. Following her return to her home in Glide, she continued bringing the medicine to the emergency room of the Roseburg hospital until the nurses were convinced that she could infuse her son at home when he had a bleed. She was eager, proficient, and motivated. She soon demonstrated to the nurses that she could infuse her son.

The ability to infuse her son was an important advancement in his medical care. Although the Roseburg hospital was only twenty-five miles from her home, much closer than the two hundred miles to Portland, when transportation was dependent on an old, unreliable Oldsmobile running on worn tires during the wintertime over a snow-covered mountain road, it was not always possible to treat every bleed.

A second son, Peter, was born September 26, 1978, weighing nine pounds, four ounces. He was not circumcised after birth because his brother had hemophilia. When Peter was three months of age, Carmelita carried her new son, who had no signs of bleeding, on the Greyhound bus to Portland, accompanied by her first son, David, for tests to determine if he was affected with hemophilia. The completed tests revealed that Carmelita's second son also had hemophilia. A third child was born in 1979 to Carmelita and Dale Witbeck, a healthy baby girl, Maria.

Carmelita traveled four hundred miles round trip to have her sons treated at the hemophilia treatment center. If their old Oldsmobile wasn't running, Carmelita packed her three children on the Greyhound bus to make the trip. The family usually stayed over one or two nights. They found accommodations in the Ronald McDonald House, in the downstairs apartments at CDRC, or at the Caravan Motel.

At six years of age, in 1981, David became a student in the Glide public school. His brother, Peter, began attending school in Glide in 1984, followed by their healthy little sister, Maria, in 1985.

David's recurrent knee bleeds, despite infusions with concentrate, resulted in a contracture that prevented him from straightening his knee. He was hospitalized in the Portland Shriners Hospital in March 1982 and fitted with a Hessing brace to promote knee extension. The bent deformity of David's knee was accompanied by a synovitis, which was treated with infusions of concentrates three times each week. David's synovitis did not improve. He was rehospitalized in Portland in 1983, where an open surgical synovectomy was completed on his knee after he was infused with concentrate to restore his factor VIII to normal.[113] A few days after surgery and infusions with concentrate, David was allowed to go home, where his mother continued to infuse him daily for two weeks while the surgical wound of his knee healed. Carmelita had acquired the necessary skills to infuse both her sons at home.

---

113 Closed synovectomy through arthroscopy has often replaced open synovectomy.

While David was recovering from knee surgery with daily infusions of concentrate, five-year-old Peter developed a swelling on top of his head in May 1983. Beneath his long black hair, Peter's scalp was raised up three inches from his skull. His mother infused him with concentrate at home, which checked further bleeding, but the absorption of the blood beneath his scalp was slow. The top of his head became mushy, with his ears opening downward toward his shoulders, an appearance suggesting a giant mushroom. With a head wrap to apply gentle pressure, and infusions of concentrate, Peter's head slowly regained a normal appearance after two months and several trips to Portland.

Carmelita had been a passionate pianist. In the family's small home, she played for her children on an old well-polished upright piano. She sold her precious piano to help pay for the costs of caring for her sons, sacrificing the principle source of her joy outside of her children. Neighbors and friends worried about Carmelita making trips to Portland in her old car. The automobile dealers in the small town and around the countryside respected Carmelita's efforts to provide for her sons while subsisting on the meager income from her husband's forest jobs. They surprised her with an unexpected gift, a dependable car.

In 1984, Carmelita was told to return the concentrate she stored in her refrigerator in her home to the hemophilia treatment center. The medicine was being recalled following the illness of another young boy who had been infused with medicine from the same batch, the same lot number. Of the twenty-four vials of medicine Carmelita had possessed in her home, she had already infused twelve vials before the recall was announced.

In 1985, the HIV antibody screening test became available at the public health department in Roseburg. Results of the blood test revealed that David, age ten, and Peter, age seven, were HIV antibody positive. Their HIV infection was evaluated with the Western Blot test, confirming the presence of HIV. The boys were well, without symptoms of HIV, although they had been infected for several years prior to their testing.

When David was twelve years of age, in 1987, one of his school friends became ill with chicken pox. David developed a severe case of shingles, the first indication that his immune system was damaged, a sign of AIDS. Instead of pea-sized pox lesions, half-dollar-sized blisters appeared on his body, completely covering his genitals, producing excruciating misery. He was hospitalized and isolated in Doernbecher Children's Hospital in Portland as a very ill child. David was treated with intravenous acyclovir, a new antiviral medicine.[114]

Peter's first sign of HIV-associated illness also appeared when he was twelve, in 1989, as an asthmatic-like attack. Carmelita had to learn another medical procedure— operating a nebulizer to administer inhaled medicine for Peter.

After the boys recovered from their first illnesses associated with HIV infection, they began to show signs of weight loss. David became thin, wasted in appearance. He was enrolled in the AZT trial study. Later it was discovered that he was included in the study arm of patients receiving the real medicine, AZT, rather than the placebo arm. However his general health continued to fail, although his spirits remained cheerful.

At the local school in the family's small town of Glide, David could not play football. However, he was appointed as the football manager, a position that allowed him to participate in the football games without being on the playing field. During one of the autumn Friday evening football games, the game play resulted in the opposing high school team overrunning the bench on the sidelines. The padded uniformed players swooped up David and carried him across the goal line. He was pleased and shouted, "Do it again!"

Although David and Peter were three years apart in their ages, AIDS began to affect their general health at nearly the same time, with weakness, weight loss, and infections. One of the troublesome symptoms was the development of thrush. They developed sore mouths

---

114 Gertrude Elion received the Noble Prize in Medicine in 1988 for the development of acyclovir.

with patches of white plaque, requiring mouth rinses with chlorhexidine and ketoconazole troches, medicines they didn't like. They would exclaim that they wanted no more of that mouth medicine, that awful stuff. Their mother replied to them that it was up to them to make the choice. Begrudgingly, they accepted the antifungal medicine to help relieve their sore mouths, which had prevented them from receiving adequate nutrition.

Brothers at Hemophilia Summer Camp

Despite their illness, which restrained their activities, Peter and David were never angry, never bitter.[115] They were good at coming out of a medical crisis. They had many friends and were sociable with other youths, although they were almost constantly together. A highlight each summer for David and Peter was hemophilia camp. Peter was outstanding at camp, the only camper who could hit a grasshopper on the fly with a BB gun (plate 14). David was famous among fellow campers for his driving skill. Campers had climbed into the back of the camp doctor's rusty old GMC pickup, a truck with a wooden bed, except for David and his friend, who were riding up front in the passenger seat of the truck cab with the doctor. Doctor Taillefer drove the old truck across a meadow where the horses grazed, with the campers joyfully bouncing in the back. To entertain the happy group, the doctor shifted the truck into grandma gear, engine running, opened the driver's door, jumped out of the slowly moving truck, and intended to run completely around the truck and back to the driver's door while the truck was slowly moving forward. He had successfully completed that maneuver previously while entertaining truckloads of campers a day or two earlier. However, something went wrong during this outing. David, who had been sitting next to the doctor, slid over beneath the steering wheel as soon as the doctor jumped out the door. He stepped

115 Conversation with Carmelita Witbeck on Monday, January 23, 2008, in her home in Roseburg

on the gas, and the truck took off bouncing across the meadow, the campers laughing with glee as the frustrated doctor ran behind, trying to catch the truck. Eventually, when the doctor became worn out and couldn't run anymore, he sat down in the grassy meadow to catch his breath. The truck came up beside him and stopped. David, peering out the driver's window, remarked, "Hey, Doc, can we give you a lift?" David was a hero after that day.

Each morning at sunup, the camp director, Wilbur Campbell, walked through the cabins of the camp and loudly shouted, "Polar bear!" That was a signal for the most adventurous campers to rise from their warm sleeping bags, before breakfast in the mess hall, and bolt out the door to the riverbank. At Wilbur's signal, a shrill whistle, they jumped from the bank into the frigid stream, demonstrating their courage and earning a bead for polar bearing. Many of the campers preferred to remain as long as they could in their warm sleeping bags rather than suffer the shock of a numbing dawn immersion. David and Peter earned polar bear bead awards every day for their chilly morning cannonball plunges. A camp activity planned by Wilbur included Brent, David, Peter, and seven other campers assembling at midmorning to scramble into the forest with Dr. Taillefer for a nature hike. As part of a lesson on how to survive if lost in the forest, the doctor discussed edible plants with the young campers. After the review of plants, each camper was instructed to collect as many of the ten plants as he could find. They ate daisies, which Brent thought tasted like carrots. Peter and David were hesitant to follow Dr. Taillefer's example when he ate stinging horse nettles. They discovered that a green nettle leaf could be rolled up with the irritating side inward, chewed, and swallowed without burning their mouths.

At the end of the day, when the doctor sat down for dinner at the mess hall table, he discovered a plateful of plants that the young campers had gathered and heaped onto his dinner plate. All eyes turned toward the doctor as the campers demanded he eat the stuff on his plate. "How do you like your dinner, Doc?" David chuckled along with all the other campers as Doc quaffed down a bitter frond from a sword-leaf fern, finishing off the meal with sour sorrel leaves.

While David and Peter were off at hemophilia camp, Carmelita, who was divorced from the kids' father, and her daughter, Maria, enjoyed a girls' week at home.

AIDS in School

Small-Town School Confronted by HIV and AIDS

In March 1987, word spread that a student infected with HIV was attending public school in Glide, Oregon. Carmelita had informed the school that her son David was HIV infected. The Witbeck family's identity was kept from the public until the school board could learn about AIDS and develop a plan to assure the safety of the staff and the students. Letters were mailed to the parents of students, confirming that an HIV infected student was attending the school. A meeting was convened to explain the nature of HIV infection. David continued to attend school. He finished the school year without incident. Later, the school learned that David's brother, Peter, three years younger, was also infected with HIV. In 1987, information obtained from the public health department indicated that HIV infection leads to AIDS, which was assumed to always be fatal. The Douglas County health officer, Sharon Thrall, informed the school that there was no risk of spreading HIV to other students in the school setting.

From August 1987 until January 1993, twenty articles appeared in the Roseburg newspaper, the *News-Review*, discussing issues of AIDS and HIV in response to the presence of David and Peter Witbeck in the public school.

The Witbeck family moved August 25, 1987, from Glide to Roseburg, a larger town with a hospital, where medical care for the boys was more accessible. David was twelve, and Peter was nine. Carmelita notified the Roseburg school that her sons were infected with HIV as a consequence of receiving tainted medicine to treat their hemophilia. They were expected to enroll in Winchester Elementary School within the Roseburg School District in September. Richard Eisenhauer, the Roseburg superintendent of schools, scheduled a press conference for August 24, 1987, in response to the boys' proposed enrollment, that was attended by Bob Allen, chairman of the AIDS Council for Douglas County (Martin August 25, 1987). Superintendent Eisenhauer announced at the press conference that an Individual Education Plan (IEP) would be developed in preparation for the two brothers' admission to Winchester school. The plan was intended as a precaution to protect the health and well-being of the brothers as well as the school staff and all the other students attending the school.

School Board Response to HIV

A group of strongly united parents urged the Roseburg School Board to refuse enrollment of David and Peter in the Winchester Elementary School when they learned the brothers were HIV infected (Martin, September 10, 1987). At the Wednesday night meeting, September 9, 1987, an overflow crowd of more than eighty parents of children enrolled in Winchester listened to Sharon Thrall tell them that the chances against transmission of HIV in a school setting was about 9,999 to one. She quoted one study of forty thousand AIDS cases. None of the reported cases were transmitted from one schoolchild to another. She explained that HIV is transmitted from person to person by having sex, sharing needles by drug users, or infusion of blood from a donor who is infected with HIV. Dr. Thrall attempted to relieve the anxiety of the parents by stating that transmission of HIV from saliva is nearly impossible. To become HIV infected, it would be necessary to pour two quarts of saliva into an open wound.

The parents of Winchester schoolchildren were filled with fear and reacted with comments and actions. Dr. Thrall was interrupted at times during her discussion. One man shouted, "Don't give us statistics!"

Another suggested keeping the brothers at home rather than having them attend classes.

Twelve audience members spoke one by one, delivering a unanimous message—they didn't want to take the chance cited by Dr. Thrall, even though it was a tiny chance of infection. HIV infection and AIDS was a frightening threat for them.

One parent, heading a group called "Concerned Parents" delivered a petition to the school board, signed by two hundred adults. The petition requested a separate space to be created for classroom instruction of the HIV infected students if they were admitted to the school. They demanded that the boys must be physically isolated, with barriers separating them from the other students. The petition read, "We, the undersigned residents of School District Number Four, are petitioning the school board, the school administration, and the parents of the two students who have tested positive for the AIDS-related virus to find an alternative to teaching these two students in the public school."

A mother of a student posed a question to the board: "What are you going to do when a child has blood-to-blood contact?"

"What will you do to protect yourself from my pending lawsuit?" one parent asked the board.

"Listen to us," some parents proclaimed. "We have spoken to several doctors, and they have announced that they would not let their children attend a school with an HIV infected child."

The prospect of transmission of HIV from one child to another resulting in HIV infection worried several parents. "You can't be there every minute," a mother of a student emphasized. "There is no such thing as a school recess without body contact."

"It's not what we know; it's what we don't know that scares the heck out of me!" a father of a student exclaimed.

"What options do we have as parents to send our kids to other schools?" a parent stood up and asked.

"Is there a possibility you could design and create a sterile classroom at Winchester Elementary School?" one man questioned.

"We are scared about this disease. The board's decision could mess up the lives of children," the parents with two children at Winchester directed toward the school board. "We have no doubts about the school board's good intentions. But what in your conscience gives you the right to say yes to this policy?"

"I don't care about those kids, those two brothers, who are HIV infected. I have to care about my kids," a mother of a student offered.

Another parent whose children attended a different school within the school district injected, "We must talk about quarantine. Those kids ought to be at home. It's too bad they have HIV. We are not discriminating against them; they should be quarantined."

Most of the parents attending the school board's meeting were not interested in or concerned with the policy formulated by the school board. They were alarmed by the pending arrival of two HIV infected students and the possibility of the spread of the deadly virus. They regarded the school board's policy as "political."

As pointed out by Mary Martin in the Roseburg newspaper (Martin September 20, 1987), there is no escape from the AIDS virus. Before the Witbecks moved from Glide to Roseburg, AIDS was a faraway threat to the people who lived in those two small towns. Some had read in the newspapers about movie star Rock Hudson, who died of AIDS in 1985. Hudson was a handsome, popular Hollywood movie actor. From 1984 until 1985, he played the role of Daniel Reese in the ABC television soap opera *Dynasty*, where his speech began to deteriorate. He had been diagnosed as HIV infected June 4, 1984. While ill in Paris, he issued a press release July 25, 1985, announcing that he was dying of AIDS. He chartered a Boeing 747 airplane and was flown back to Los Angeles with his medical team. He was transferred by helicopter to Cedars of Lebanon Hospital. The doctors declared there was no hope for his life. He returned to his Beverly Hills home and died at sixty years of age on October 2, 1985 (Rock Hudson 2008). On the television program *Dynasty*, he had kissed Linda Evans, promoting concerns by viewers, wondering if she would also become ill with AIDS. But infectious disease specialists claimed AIDS is not spread by kissing or casual contact.

David's and Peter's identities and grade levels had been kept confidential before they were scheduled to begin attending classes the following Monday. The Concerned Parents group was aware that the source of the boys' HIV infection was through contaminated medicine used to treat their bleeding cause by hemophilia. The two handsome, innocent boys were not drug users, nor were they homosexual. At the meeting, the school board presented their policy on handling AIDS and other infectious diseases in school. The board voted in favor of the communicable disease policy by a vote of four to two, approving it subject to reviews at the next board meeting one month later. Included on the board voting in favor of the policy was the boys' Roseburg pediatrician, Dr. Larry Hall, who was familiar with hemophilia.

HIV infection and AIDS was a new medical condition for all practicing doctors. Doctors had not been taught about AIDS in medical school. AIDS didn't exist when they were student doctors. Dr. Hall stated that although the doctors of the medical community had significant concerns about the threat of HIV, they would be willing to support this policy.

School superintendent Eisenhauer stated that federal and state regulations exist, and they dictate the type of education each student must be offered. "We are obligated to follow the laws." He explained to the parents' group, that each student has a right to a free and appropriate education within the least restrictive environment. He patiently and understandingly explained that a student must attend school unless health risks preclude normal procedures—and then other ways must be found to teach the student. He defended the board against charges of being "political." "Every aspect of the law—the rules, regulations, and medical concerns—had to be addressed. That is one of the functions of a school board."

One person asked Dr. Thrall if she and the Douglas County Health Department approved and recommended the school board's HIV and infectious disease policy. Dr. Thrall responded by saying that it was not the health department's job to approve or disapprove of school policies. She said they had reviewed the policy to assure that public health and medical concerns were basically correct. She said that she had children who were six and seven, and she would not hesitate to send them to Winchester school.

School board chairman Stenbeck, after listening to testimony from parents for more than an hour, told them that the school board had their interests at heart. They had done their research. In any decision the school board made, they were at risk for a lawsuit. But they must protect the rights of all students.

School board member King said he had heard valid questions from the audience and would like to hear answers before making up his mind. Another board member, Wagner, asked for a postponement of the decision on the AIDS policy until the next board meeting in one month. She wanted to wait until she attended the parents' meeting that night and had an opportunity to listen to the parents' comments. Dr. Hall of the school board labeled the parents' testimony before the school board as "responsible concerns" and reminded parents that although "zero risk does not exist in infectious diseases," HIV has never been discovered to be spread by casual contact. Board member Kimmel asked for a thirty-day delay on approval of the AIDS policy, noting that admission of the two brothers to Winchester school was a separate issue from policy approval.

Board president Stenbeck concluded the board meeting by saying, "Try to remember—this is not us against them. I hope we are all friends, united with each other to help our children." He recommended approval of the AIDS policy, followed by subsequent amendments. "The brothers are going to be in school whether we have an AIDS policy or if we don't have a policy. Without a policy, we are simply falling backward, ignoring the rights of the boys to be in school."

The next morning, Thursday, September 10, 1987, Superintendent Eisenhauer announced that the boys would be admitted and begin attending classes the next Monday, September 14, 1987. "The plan proposed by the school board is to ensure that students have access to their right for continuing public education," he stated. "For each child attending school, the IEP must be formulated by a multidisciplinary team including parents, school officials and teachers, health department personnel, and the child's physician."

Community Discussion of HIV in the School

Thursday evening, September 10, 1987, a public meeting was held in the Winchester Elementary School gymnasium (Martin September 11, 1987). More than three hundred people attended the meeting, which lasted five hours. Superintendent Eisenhauer presided. A videotape produced by the Oregon State Health Division was shown to the crowd at the beginning of the meeting. After viewing the video, Eisenhauer introduced a panel of speakers, including Dr. Robert McAlister, the AIDS program coordinator for the Oregon Health Division; Dr. Larry Hall, Roseburg pediatrician and school board member; Dr. Sharon Thrall, Douglas County health officer; and Kathy Crenshaw, Winchester school principal. The intention of the meeting was for medical and school personnel to inform the parents of schoolchildren of real and overblown fears of spreading HIV. Each panelist spoke one at a time, followed by questions submitted from the audience. These were written on cards that were handed to the speaker.

Dr. McAlister identified two types of epidemics: AIDS, he said, "spreads because people at risk, such as promiscuous homosexual persons or intravenous drug users, continue to endanger themselves. AFRAIDS," he continued, "is the pathological fear of contracting AIDS. In the first high-risk group, there is too little fear of AIDS in persons who exchange blood, semen, or vaginal secretions with other high-risk persons. At low risk are persons who have casual contact with saliva, tears, blood, urine, and feces of other persons." He maintained that no instances of AIDS have been contracted through casual contact, including use of water fountains and toilets, or when shaking hands or sneezing.

Dr. Thrall echoed Dr. McAlister's message and reminded parents that HIV infected persons may be around them at any time in many places, such as at work or in schools. She emphasized that all persons in all situations should refrain from risky behavior and take precautions in handling body fluids. An example against HIV transmission from one person to another was apparent in the Witbeck household, if the parents of schoolchildren would stop and reflect for a moment. The two HIV infected brothers shared the same house as their sister, mother, and father. In close living conditions, the same toilet, bath towels, dishes, bathtub, and bed sheets were all shared without spreading HIV to others in the family. No one in the family became infected. None of the parents who objected to the enrollment of the HIV infected brothers in Winchester school appeared to recognize the evidence before them— that HIV is not contagious even when there is close contact. They only needed to acknowledge that the mother of the boys, Carmelita, and their little sister, Maria, did not become HIV infected, despite the intimacy of sharing the same household.

- Hysteria associated with HIV infection masked critical thinking.
- HIV is an infectious disease with limited risk of infection

Superintendent Eisenhauer restated during the meeting that all children have legal rights to a free education in America, in the least restrictive environment. He explained the rules and regulations that govern contagious illnesses and school attendance in Oregon. Although the parents' concerns for the health of their children are important, the school district is obligated to follow state and federal guidelines in making plans for students. He reminded the parents attending the meeting that the mother of the two boys with hemophilia came forward voluntarily because she was concerned for the health of all the children, including her sons. She could have avoided informing the school that her sons were infected with HIV. Although the two brothers were intending to begin classes the next Monday, September 14, the school board would not meet until Tuesday afternoon to review the final IEP. Therefore, the boys would not begin classes until Wednesday, September 15.

The superintendent reviewed the precautionary measures listed in the school board policy. He displayed an emergency kit, the type that would be placed in several locations throughout the school. He held up a yellow nylon bag and revealed the contents, which included paper towels, gauze, plastic gloves, Lysol and Band-Aids. He warned of the danger of emotionalism and driving people underground from fear of reporting infection or illness to authorities.

The audience listened closely to the speakers; many took notes. Toward the end of the meeting, some parents began to speak of their concerns and fears. At times, the discussion became emotional. The parents who spoke and asked questions did not want their children to attend a school with HIV infected students. The panelists answered the questions that they read from the cards handed to them by the parents. Some parents were frustrated with the format of written questions, saying they preferred dialogue and spoken questions. A group of thirty walked out. By 11:00 PM, sixty persons remained. Some said they had to go home to attend to their children.

By 12:30 AM, the audience had decreased to about fifty persons, and everyone was weary. A parent called for a show of hands at the end of the meeting, asking whether parents favored admission or rejection of the HIV infected brothers. Ten parents were in favor of admitting the brothers, and thirty-five supported excluding them from enrolling in school.

The superintendent told the parents their concerns would be carefully considered when composing the IEPs. They included caution when using the toilet, the water fountains, riding the school buses, and the extent of physical activities permitted.

By the end of the long meeting, four issues that concerned parents were identified:

- The possibility of contracting HIV infection through blood. Most parents said they were not willing to accept the risk. Winchester principal Kathy Crenshaw responded by saying, "I am a parent of children attending Winchester Elementary School. I assure you that we are taking every conceivable precaution."

- The rights of a few compared to the safety of many. "Why would those boys want to attend school if they knew the virus could be passed on?" a man asked. Another man asked, "Why is the minority more important than the majority?" Dr. Hall responded, "I am sure, as a parent, you would want your child to have a normal life too."

- What are the options for parents who do not want their child to attend Winchester if HIV infected children are enrolled? Superintendent Eisenhauer replied, "Options include homeschooling or private schools. Transfers of students between public schools are generally not allowed unless there is a hardship. But it is the right of parents to request a transfer."

- Confidentiality of HIV infected children. A mother asked, "Won't everyone know who the boys are anyway?" A second mother questioned the wisdom of confidentiality: "If these kids have hemophilia, shouldn't the other kids know so they can help protect themselves from injury?" Superintendent Eisenhauer said the IEP team would work with parents to seek their wishes regarding confidentiality.

The next morning, Friday, September 11, 1987, the *News-Review* of Roseburg published the school board's communicable/infectious disease policy:

- Sharp objects, including needles, will be disposed of in safe containers.
- Needles used by health personnel will not be resheathed.
- Persons with cuts or open lesions will wear bandages or gloves.
- Rubber or plastic gloves will be worn whenever possible when performing first aid.
- Contact of the skin with blood or body fluids from other persons will be avoided. If exposure occurs, the affected skin will be washed with soap and water.
- Contact of the mouth, eyes, or other mucous membrane areas with blood or other body fluids should be avoided.
- Surfaces on which blood has been spilled will be cleaned promptly with soap and water and a disinfectant.
- Blood-contaminated items such as gloves, bandages, and paper towels will be placed in a sealed plastic bag with disposal in a garbage receptacle.
- Hard containers will be used when disposing of sharp blood-contaminated materials.
- Any incident in which blood from one person contacts mucous membranes or broken skin of another will be promptly reported to the supervisor.
- Disposal of all menstrual materials from restrooms will be through sealed containers daily.
- Particular precautions will be applied in such situations where blood contact is more likely, such as contact sports.
- A record will be kept by all persons treating blood-related accidents.

- First-aid kits will be provided at various locations in all schools of the Roseburg School District, along with a source of water, soap, and disinfectant.
- Written summaries of infectious control procedures will be posted in locations in all schools.

Sharon Thrall, Douglas County health officer, offered a list of health measures to teach children and adults to protect themselves against contact with the HIV:

- Wash hands with soap and water periodically throughout the day and after restroom use.
- Don't share implements that can pierce the skin or transmit blood. These include razors, ear piercing devices, and toothbrushes. "Peoples' gums sometimes bleed when they brush their teeth," Thrall says.
- Don't use drugs. Needles used by more than one person can spread the AIDS virus. Other drugs, including alcohol, cloud judgment.
- For parents, set an example for children. Clean up blood spills safely and promptly, using soap and water and a disinfectant. Usually soap and water kills the AIDS virus on the skin, in a dishwasher, or within a clothes washer. Disinfectants can be used to make sure.

On the front page of the Sunday *News-Review,* September 13, 1987, the article written by Mary Martin discussed the past week's AIDS dilemma at Winchester Elementary School (Martin, September 13, 1987). Martin reported that the parents of students who would attend Winchester when it opened on Monday had undergone a week of soul-searching, debate, and intense study. What was keeping them awake at night was fear of a tiny virus, HIV, one sixteen-thousandth the size of a pinhead. The infinitesimally small virus was causing a large commotion.

Some parents did not want the brothers to attend school. Other parents welcomed their enrollment.

A parent of a Winchester schoolchild spoke before the school board, which met the week before the opening of school, and said, "My reaction is to pull my child out of the school. Their admission to the school infringes upon my rights and infringes upon the rights of my child."

Another parent said, "It's too bad they have it. We are not discriminating against them ... but I believe these kids should stay home from school." Many parents vowed that they would take their children out of the school if HIV infected children were allowed in the classroom. The only parents who spoke publicly at the school board meeting were those who believed HIV infected children should not be allowed to attend the public school. Some of those parents had formed an organized group. On Monday, before the school board meeting, they began circulating a petition opposing attendance. By Wednesday, they had collected three hundred signatures of adults who supported exclusion of the HIV infected boys from school. The petition was submitted to Superintendent Eisenhauer at the board meeting Wednesday evening.

Parents telephoned school board members and asked such questions as "Is the possibility of getting AIDS greater than the possibility of surviving AIDS? If so, are you willing to risk the lives of our children?" By Saturday morning, one board member, Keith Cubic, had received five telephone calls opposing attendance and one call favoring enrollment. One mother of a Winchester student, who opposed entry of the boys into the school, said she had been telephoning other parents over the weekend to gauge their feelings. "So far," she reported, "I have talked to fourteen parents who intend to take their kids out of the school." Other mothers, she said, are also telephoning, but there is no final count yet. Because they are vocal, the group was well known to newspapers and to television stations.

Enlightenment of Some Parents

There was another side to the issue of school entry. Some Winchester parents said they would keep their child in the school. Some parents even proclaimed that they would welcome the attendance of the two HIV infected brothers at the school. One parent, Cindy McGinnis, also a part-time librarian at the school, said, "Of course I'm worried about AIDS. But I'm not only comfortable, I am also grateful that Winchester is the school where they are going. I'm glad this happened now. If I were to pull my children out of elementary school, they are going to come across the virus later, in high school or in adult living. Presently, my kids are still at the age when they will listen to their parents. If they learn the facts about AIDS now, it will prepare them well for adult life." She said she thinks the amount of opposition for admission to the school has been exaggerated. "The people I have talked with," she confided, "have been concerned about AIDS; however, they are sympathetic and not in favor of exclusion of the two HIV infected brothers."

Another parent, Kim Blenk, offered, "People who want to pull their kids out of school are overreacting. I don't believe the danger is great. The Winchester school personnel and the Roseburg School District are doing a great job safeguarding the children's health and their rights. I have a lot of confidence in the school."

"We would all like to run away from this virus," said Kay Russell, a parent who works in a doctor's office. "All of us are angry toward this virus, just like we are angry about the fear of cancer." She believed parents and children must learn to face the reality of HIV; they must learn to live in its presence. "The more that I thought about it, the more I was convinced that I could not yank my son out of school and think that he would be safe. Everyone knows that wherever we go, we will be unknowingly rubbing elbows with persons who are infected with the virus that causes AIDS. The way I see it, my son will learn the facts about HIV and AIDS sooner or later. The sooner, the better."

Her husband, Bruce Russell, the pastor at the First Christian Church in Roseburg, supported enrollment of the two boys in Winchester. He also expressed understanding for the parents who wished to pull their children out of the school. "There is a risk," he said, "even though the risk is small. We must learn to live with the risk of HIV just like learning to live with the risk of becoming ill with cancer." Pastor Russell said they would send their child to Winchester with a feeling of confidence, knowing that their child was being well prepared by his teachers for understanding how to cope with the ubiquitous presence of the AIDS virus.

Another pastor family, Sue and Phil Evans, from the Roseburg Christian Fellowship Church, who attended the presentations by the health experts, commented that they were impressed with the way the school board had handled the HIV infected boys' application for enrollment in Winchester. "We commend the school, the school board, and the staff for the way they have handled everything," they announced. The Evans parents believed that only a minority of parents would respond to the admission of the HIV infected boys by withdrawing their children from school. "We have been given an opportunity to put feet to our faith and to show love and compassion for those who are suffering. Here is a chance to be a good example for all of America."

No one could estimate how many parents opposed school attendance of the HIV infected boys. No one knew how many parents were undecided, watching and listening before making up their minds.

Origin of the Fear of HIV and AIDS

A question arose after consideration of the public response to the entry of the two boys to Winchester. Why was their presence such a threat in Winchester compared to their previous attendance in the Glide school? Bruce Daily discussed the difference in the comfort level of the

Roseburg parents compared to the families with schoolchildren in Glide in the Roseburg Sunday paper of September 13, 1987.[116]

The paper said that HIV-AIDS is a new disease with a stigma attached because typical victims have been homosexual men and intravenous drug users. The scene of the late stages of the disease, emaciation, weakness, feebleness, is accompanied by death without dignity. The disease is relegated to a fatal outcome without a cure. The stigma of the disease, coupled with the mortality, evokes a frightening response in parents of innocent children. Those may be parents who have heard about obscure cover-ups by government officials. They have ignored the records of public health concerns of the past, when government officials developed programs to immunize children in the schools, eliminate polio and small pox, and remove the fear of tetanus. Why do they harbor the suspicion that school and public health officials are not telling them the truth when they proclaim that the chances a child will become HIV infected from contact with another child on the school playground are almost zero?

They dwell on the scene of two boys on the playground exchanging red blood between open cuts, allowing the deadly virus to seep into their child's bloodstream, followed by subsequent destruction of his immune system.

Perhaps the fears did not arise in the school of the small town of Glide because the boys lived there. They weren't newcomers, and the community knew them. They had already been in the school when HIV infection was announced during the middle of the school year. The boys did not appear to be any different after the discovery of HIV; nothing had changed. In contrast, the newcomers in the Winchester school elicited fear in the minds of the parents. Fear of the unknown is not unprecedented. Those fearful parents take their kids to the pediatrician for checkups, bake cakes for the school carnival, buckle up

---

116 Permission received from Vicki Menard, editor of the *News-Review*, January 16, 2009, to cite and quote the news articles that appeared in the Roseburg newspaper discussing AIDS in the school.

their seat belts, help out in the school library, and avoid cigarette smoke. They want someone to calm their fears although they may not believe them when they are confronted with an ugly unknown threat to their children. Some of these parents had already decided the danger to their children was real and concluded the persons who have devoted their careers to the education and health of children are not concerned with what happens at Winchester school. Bruce Daily pointed out that all the daily risks in the entire world cannot be eliminated but that should not eradicate basic human compassion and cause persons to become paralyzed with imaginary fears.

Return to Glide

David and Peter were enrolled in Winchester Elementary School in Roseburg but did not begin attending classes on Monday, September 14, while the school board completed their infectious disease policy, which was intended to spell out protective measures for the boys and their classmates. They were expected to begin attending classes by Wednesday, September 16. As many as one hundred parents of Winchester schoolchildren threatened to withdraw their children from school on the day of Peter and David's arrival to attend classes.

Unexpectedly, Monday morning, September 14, 1987, Superintendent Eisenhauer announced at a press conference that the two HIV infected boys would not be enrolled in Winchester, as had been planned. They had moved out of the school district. The destination of their move was not to be revealed (Schnell 1987). The superintendent announced that the school board would continue its planned meeting the next day to review policies for dealing with AIDS in the Roseburg schools. He said that the recent controversy had been a positive event. He indicated that the school district's residents had become better educated, and they had been allowed to express their concerns. The school district's policy was not a personal thing. It is the responsibility of any school district to handle problems the best way they can, with professional competence. He hoped they wouldn't forget all they had accomplished. He went on to say that although the law protects the confidentiality of the individual who is infected with HIV, their identity will be revealed to teachers or persons who may be in close contact on a "need-to-know" basis.

The boys returned to Glide to attend the same school where they had been students the previous year, without alarm in the Glide school (Martin September 15, 1987). Their return caused a reaction by parents who had not reacted to their presence the previous year. On the first day of school, Monday, the Glide school board was convened and presided over by Scott Mutchie, superintendent of the Glide School District. He described the mood of several parents as concerned but not angry. The boy's return to the Glide school spurred eight parents of Glide students to attend the school board meeting. Four of the parents spoke about their concerns. One of the parents, whose young son sat beside him at the meeting, told the board he wanted a policy that would require children who are HIV infected to be segregated from other children until the federal government announced definitive answers about AIDS. He said he was determined to change the situation. He was prepared to go great lengths to see that change occurred.

In 1987, AIDS was a reportable disease, but name-based reporting of HIV was not in place in Oregon until 1992. (Oregon Department of Human Services 1997). All four parents who addressed the school board disagreed with state and federal rules for reporting HIV. They believed all cases of HIV should be reported. The public has the right to know when HIV is present, they maintained. One parent asked the board how the laws could be changed. The board advised her to contact state and national legislators. Superintendent Mutchie agreed with the parents, suggesting that HIV infection should be designated as reportable. But in the case of the two brothers in the Glide school, he said that the school district had acted properly and covered all aspects that had risen from their HIV infection. He had confidence in the school district's policy of examining each case separately and developing a plan that would prevent danger to any other students.

Another parent emphasized that their hearts went out to these two kids. Then he asked school board member Sandy Hendy, an obstetrical nurse, if she was comfortable with the Glide School District's policy on handling the AIDS virus. She replied that she was more than comfortable. Her biggest concern was not the children who are known to be HIV infected. She said that her concern was with the people who do not know they are HIV infected. The problem is not with the people who have the virus. Naturally, we are going to be more cautious with them. Sandy Hendy emphasized the importance of preventative measures in all infectious diseases. The parents, the school teachers, the staff, and the children must become familiar with health precautions. Such measures include washing hands and cleaning up whenever there is a bleeding wound. A father responded to Sandy Hendy's comments by saying he was not convinced that the HIV infected children should be attending school with the rest of the children. Another parent asked questions about sharing the restrooms and drinking fountains. She asked if their kids were being used as guinea pigs by the federal government.

Both school districts, Roseburg and Glide, had carefully protected the identity of the parents and their two HIV infected children. Mr. Mutchie proclaimed that the kids at the school knew who they were. It's not because the school released their names. School authorities recognized the right of every child to attend school. A proposed education plan would help ensure the safety of the two boys and the other schoolchildren.

Back in Roseburg, the school board continued its scheduled meeting even though the two HIV infected students were gone; they had moved away. The Tuesday noon board meeting, September 14, 1987, had originally intended to clarify and solidify the plans for the two boys. That item was stricken from the agenda; the board instead discussed a communicable and infectious disease policy that included

AIDS as well as other diseases. The members of the school board, in the wake of the controversy over HIV in schools, resolved to formulate a clearer policy for diseases and proclaimed that they would engage in a more active role in meeting the education requirements for HIV infected students' education. The AIDS issue would come back, school board member Keith Cubic acknowledged, referring to David and Peter Witbeck (Martin September 16, 1987). The board had approved the policy the week earlier, on September 9, with the provision that the policy could be reviewed and amended.

During the weekend, when the two brothers were waiting for entry to the Winchester classrooms in Roseburg, the board was besieged with telephone calls. The parents, who were concerned and anxious over the prospect of two HIV infected boys in the midst of their children in the same school, demanded a more clear and comprehensive school district policy. They wanted to know how an IEP was formulated. One member of the school board said she believed board members should be in closer touch with the planning of the IEP. Several board members favored appointment of a board member to the IEP committee, who could report back to the school board. Board chairman John Stenbeck suggested that board member Dr. Larry Hall, a pediatrician, serve on IEP teams whenever an IEP was formulated for an HIV infected student. All the board members agreed that such an appointment to the IEP committee should be at the discretion of the board chairman, and the participating board member should serve as an observer. Dr. Hall replied that he did not want to be tagged as an "AIDS expert," but he would serve on an IEP team if asked. Another board member, also a physician, Dr. William Roady, offered that they should have had the policy in effect ten years ago. He said the board should remember that other diseases in addition to AIDS, such as hepatitis, affect the school districts.

As the board meeting continued, reports were received revealing that nearly all the teachers, support staff, and school bus drivers within the school district had received in-service training in managing AIDS issues.

First-aid kits were in place in schools and in school buses, containing plastic gloves and necessary materials for sanitizing after blood spills or bleeding from wounds. The curriculum committee continued to update and refine teaching materials used for discussing HIV and AIDS in all grade levels.

Carmelita had moved from Glide to Roseburg on August 25. Her sons, David and Peter, enrolled in Winchester Elementary School of the Roseburg School District. After it was announced last spring in Glide Elementary School that the two brothers were infected with HIV, one of the parents of a Glide student pulled his son from the school and moved him to another school district, to Winchester Elementary School in Roseburg (Martin September 20, 1987), the same school the Witbeck brothers intended to attend. Since then, the father of the child moved his son back to the Glide School. After three weeks of turmoil, the two brothers also returned to the Glide school.

The teacher who was assigned to teach HIV prevention at Winchester, Claudia Vangstad, said that most of the children attending the school were great. Of the students in the school, 95 percent were prepared to welcome the brothers if they would have begun attending classes. In contrast, parents who attended the school board meetings loudly voiced their objection to the presence of the boys in the classrooms. No parent attending the board meetings spoke in favor of the boys' entry into the school. Two hundred signatures were affixed to a circulated petition requesting that the boys be prevented from attending the school. One hundred parents, it was rumored, had agreed that if the boys were admitted to the school, their children would be withdrawn from the school.

One week later, after the confusion surrounding the entry of the boys into the school was nullified by the sudden last-minute announcement that the boys would not enter the school, time had allowed reflection about HIV threat in the school. Comparing parents who would have welcomed the HIV infected brothers in the school with those who threatened to pull their children from the school in protest if the boys entered the classrooms revealed differences. One of the mothers of a child at Winchester, who is also a health worker, said that there is no guarantee anywhere. We are rubbing elbows with people who are HIV infected. This mother maintained that the boys would have been welcomed, for their presence would have created an opportunity for her son to learn compassion and proper hygiene.

Another couple believed the same for the lesson in compassion, but they were concerned, not with the known HIV infected boys but rather the unknown. They didn't know who could be HIV infected. They took the lesson so seriously that they discontinued sending their children to any school. Instead, they decided to teach their two children at home, homeschooling, until the state and federal laws were improved to truly protect their children from HIV infection.

They said that it didn't make a whole lot of difference that the HIV infected brothers left their children's school. What truly mattered was that there was a state law that was not protecting the health of its people. They were referring to the laws requiring reporting of infectious diseases. Doctors and health departments were required to inform a school if a student had AIDS. HIV infected cases were not required to be reported. That regulation seemed absurd to the parents. It is the same virus that affects a child at all levels of HIV infection and disease. The virus is as infectious at all stages, whether the child has HIV infection without signs of AIDS or whether the child has the sickness of AIDS. The parents wanted the presence of the virus to be reportable at all stages of infection (Oregon Department of Human Services 1997).[117]

The same parents were frustrated by insinuations that they didn't care about the two HIV infected boys and by parents who were boasting "We won'" after the two brothers moved away. They were not against the brothers who were victims of the AIDS virus. It's the virus they were against.

---

117 AIDS case reporting began nationally in 1989. Oregon has kept records of the number of new HIV infections in Oregonians over the age of thirteen years since 1992. By 1997, HIV case reporting by name was performed in twenty-seven states, including Oregon.

Robert McAlister, speaking as the AIDS program manager for the State of Oregon Health Division countered those parents who were protesting the state regulation and policies: "AIDS virus does not spread by casual contact. State, federal, and school regulations protect the rights of HIV infected children as well as the other schoolchildren."

Dr. William Roady and Dr. Larry Hall, two physicians who were school board members, and Sharon Thrall, Douglas County health officer, echoed McAlister's message. "Risk management" had become a buzzword. Dr. Roady stated that people were not interested in hearing about AIDS. They wanted absolute guarantees about HIV protection. But no one could give them absolute guarantees in any area of life. The school board couldn't guarantee a kid a safe ride on the school bus. If the parents wanted an absolute foolproof guarantee, school buses would be shut down.

Dr. Hall reinforced Dr. Roady's comments. He emphasized that the school board could not make any guarantees. Nobody could. What could be said is that there are no known cases of HIV infection, from one person to another, from casual contact, such as on the school playground. Health professionals such as Robert McAlister hoped that a lesson had been learned by the school parents—simple health precautions, such as hand washing, can help people who are in contact with HIV infected persons avoid becoming infected with the AIDS virus.

Impact of HIV in the School Controversy

The impact of the controversy from the proposed entry of David and Peter into the Winchester school lasted after their departure. Kathy Crenshaw, the school principal, announced that the yellow nylon bags containing towels, plastic gloves, disinfectant, and gauze in the Roseburg District schools were there to stay. They were permanent. In addition, other changes had been implemented, including lists of precautionary measures hanging on doors and walls in all the district's schools. There was placement of plastic liners in the trash cans that were gathered at the end of each day, sealed, and disposed of. She announced that the school district was going to continue the safety precautions at all levels.

Although the boys did not actually attend the Winchester Elementary School, the Roseburg School District had learned a lot from their proposed move. Reaction had been a mixture of caution, anger, fear, and concern. Some parents welcomed the brothers. Others were willing to accept the school district's hygiene programs even though they had doubts about the minimized risk to their children. They were reminded of the necessary vigilance to prevent HIV infection, symbolized by the bright yellow plastic first aid bags marked ROSEBURG SCHOOL EMERGENCY KIT—placed around the school.

The training of teachers and school personnel was being put to good use. They were making certain the schoolchildren used the precautions, whether they were six, eight, or twelve years of age. Thrall added that parents and schools must protect children by knowing *how* to protect. Parents must teach their children the basics at home. The most basic rule is to treat all blood as though it is infectious. School Superintendent Eisenhauer reported to the school board that teachers had completed precautionary training, students were being trained, and the yellow emergency kits were in every school in the district. Reflecting about the two boys who had intended to enter Winchester but ended up returning to the Glide School, he said that we were wrong if we thought the problem would go away just because those two boys had gone away. But he said that something positive had come from this experience—even if we had only explored the problems and if we had learned something. He hoped things went well for the two innocent boys.

Bob Allen, who was appointed chairman of the Douglas County AIDS Council, said he was certain there would be additional cases of HIV infection in the future in Roseburg Schools. The Winchester Elementary School experience with HIV infection had helped the school board refine policies and set goals. He regretted that there was so much fear response. He was sorry for the distress imposed on the family of the two boys. He stated that communities must learn to directly face their fears. Now and in the future, the issues must be faced up front. It would not be easy. The HIV experience with the two brothers made them see themselves as they were, not the way they thought they would like to be.

In addition to increasing preparedness for infectious diseases in the schools, the intended entry of the two HIV infected brothers provoked discussion of another principle: Why are the rights of the minority more important than the rights of the majority? Over and over again, the question was asked by many parents of schoolchildren where the brothers were scheduled to begin classes. At the Roseburg Unitarian Church, twenty-seven of twenty-nine parishioners attending a church meeting signed a petition requesting that Winchester welcome the brothers without harassment and without instilling fear in them. One of the church members who signed the petition, Larry Flanagan, a psychologist, was bothered by the concept of the majority ruling over the minority. He proclaimed that some people think democracy means the majority rules override the rights of the minority. Instead, he said that democracy represents the protection of the right of the minority. Larry Flanagan was concerned about the effect of a rumor that had been circulated, maintaining that a wealthy gay rights lobby was behind an attempt to protect the rights of HIV-positive persons. It reminded him of McCarthyism in the civil rights struggle of the 1960s. But this time it was the gay rights people, not the communists, who were characterized as the villains. He hoped the community's goal would be to protect the rights of everyone. Larry Flanagan said that the best solution to this conflict would be a "win-win situation," but it's difficult to say what that would be.

One of the parents of a Winchester schoolchild expressed a different opinion. She said she was sick and tired of hearing about equal rights stuff after she attended a school board hearing. She made it clear that she bore no ill will toward the two young brothers. In fact, she had invested many years, as a foster parent, providing care for scores of children who had become victims of life's tragedies. She had thought about those two little boys a lot. She said she worried about the cost of their medical care and wondered if they were able to get the medical treatment they need. But the question is one of medical common sense, not individual rights. She said she believed it was not only best for the entire school but also best for those two boys to be schooled at home. She further said that as boys with hemophilia, and as children with lowered immune systems, they were at risk in school from other children. It went both ways. She continued, noting that she didn't believe the two boys were run out of town. Instead, she maintained that parents were only requesting that they be educated at home. She said she was proud of the way dissenting parents behaved during the turmoil after the issue of the AIDS virus arose. They were nonviolent and kept cool heads. She suggested that the people be recognized as a town that cared and as a town that educated itself.

School board member Dr. William Roady worried that many parents may have miseducated themselves. He said there had been an enormous volume of research assembled characterizing the virus, enough for the Centers for Disease Control, CDC, and state health departments to use with assurance in deciding questions of rights and risks. Dr. Roady worried that parents had been reading uncommon literature written by irresponsible authors with axes to grind. He predicted that the questions of rights would come into play more often as schools continued to deal with AIDS issues. The state attorney general's office, Dr. Roady confirmed, had their antennae out for victims of rights violations. He offered an example in Portland, where a dentist was recently penalized for charging AIDS victims higher prices than other patients for dental treatment. The attorney general's office would be on the lookout for violations of human rights for a long time.

In the fall, one month after school opened, although the two brothers who were HIV infected had moved away, their impact continued to affect the Roseburg School Board. Wednesday evening, October 14, 1987, the school district's patrons watched closely as the board adopted two amendments to its infectious and communicable disease policy (Martin October 15, 1987). The amendments unanimously approved the method used for informing the school board when a student had a communicable disease. The first amendment allowed a school board member to be appointed to the team that developed the IEP for a student who was HIV infected. This plan would include the extent of contact allowed between an HIV infected student with other students. The second amendment directed the school board to meet and review the IEP for an HIV infected student before the plan was put into action. These amendments helped answer the school board members' desires to become better informed of the plans for educating an HIV infected student. Parents continued to be concerned about protecting their schoolchildren from becoming HIV infected.

At Wednesday's board meeting, Joyce Parsons, a school parent who had been active in the AIDS-school controversy, said she recommended the different stages of HIV infection be considered as one entity. Whether an HIV infected child was without symptoms or had symptoms of AIDS—it was the same disease. She also believed that the first priority of the school board should be the health of the children who were not HIV infected rather than the individual rights of an HIV infected child. Another school patron at the Wednesday board meeting, Vicki Linderman, praised the teachers at the Winchester Elementary School for their outstanding efforts teaching HIV preventative measures to students. She suggested a supplemental policy for grades one through three. Younger children, she said, are more susceptible to cuts and scrapes and are more likely to lack "common sense" when a blood-borne virus might be transmitted following an open wound of a young schoolchild.

The "Top Ten Stories of 1987," which appeared in the Roseburg Sunday newspaper[118] as the year ended, listed the Douglas County schoolboys infected with the virus that causes AIDS as number two, after the number one story, "Forest Fires."

---

118 *News-Review* December 27, 1987

Federal Response to HIV

On Monday, September 21, 1987, the Associated Press released from Washington, D.C., a report stating that the Reagan administration opposed most provisions of a bill before Congress to expand AIDS testing, including sections that would insure confidentiality and bar discrimination against people who are infected with HIV.[119] The secretary of Health and Human Services, Otis R. Bowen, testified before a House subcommittee, saying that the states were working on the confidentiality problem and that they (the states) should have the primary role in determining whether additional protection is needed to prevent discrimination. The secretary said he supported expanding HIV testing, as called for in the bill, but opposed the $400 million authorized by the measure to pay for the testing. He said that the Reagan administration had requested more than $90 million for AIDS testing in fiscal year 1985 and the individual states were contributing funds of their own. "It is not clear at this time that such substantial funding beyond that amount is needed," Bowen said in his testimony before the House Energy and Commerce Subcommittee on Health. The antidiscrimination section of the bill, sponsored by subcommittee chairman Henry Waxman, Bowen contended, "would create a burdensome new federal administrative enforcement bureaucracy which is not used to protect the rights of persons with any other diseases or handicaps." He continued, saying that HHS[120] was reviewing its own programs to discover how current laws could be used to prevent

119 *News-Review*, September 21, 1987
120 Health and Human Services

discrimination against AIDS victims. He noted that the Supreme Court recently ruled that the law protecting handicapped citizens against discrimination may be applied to AIDS victims.

Secretary Bowen said he would not necessarily oppose all new legislation on the discrimination issue, but he added, "At this time, I believe it is preferable to defer action on specific proposals for new substantive rights or new enforcement procedures until we have the information needed to make a more informed decision." Similarly, he argued against the confidentiality provisions of the Waxman bill, which was introduced into the Senate by Senator Edward Kennedy, Democrat of Massachusetts, a bill that was supported by most of the country's medical groups. When Martin Fitzwater, the White House spokesman was asked about the Reagan administration's stand on the Waxman bill, he replied, "We oppose discrimination, but we do believe the states probably have preemptive responsibility in this area." He added, "When you have a contagious disease, there may be some special situation that would call for controls that need to be accounted for in the legislation."

On Friday, September 25, the Associated Press released an announcement that the Reagan administration had decided to disregard the congressional recommendation to mail an AIDS information pamphlet to every household in the USA.[121] Instead, the government planned to distribute the printed eight-page brochure through private and public outlets. Congress criticized the administration for failing to allow a national mailer, similar to what was done in Great Britain. Ann E. McFarren, executive director of the AIDS Action Council reacted: "This doesn't fit the bill of making sure every household gets information, which I think is the goal we need to work toward." She added, "I don't believe Congress is going to be pleased with this at all." Her group lobbied Congress on behalf of three hundred different AIDS organizations and the treatment providers.

---

121 *News-Review*, September 25, 1987

A spokesman for the Department of Health and Human Services, Campbell Gardett, announced that twenty-five million copies of the pamphlet would become available for distribution on September 30, in conjunction with National AIDS Awareness and Prevention during the month of October. He said that health department officials questioned the appropriateness and the effectiveness of mailing the brochure to every postal address in the United States. A more explicit and more lengthy brochure had been developed by C. Everett Koop that stated that condoms should be used during sex by persons who do not follow his advice that sexual abstinence or limiting sex to only a monogamous relationship with a partner who does not have HIV is the surest way to avoid infection from the fatal disease. Two million copies of the brochure were scheduled to be distributed to Defense Department personnel and military servicemen and servicewomen, Gardett announced. The remainder of the pamphlets was to be distributed, determined by the printing schedule, he said.

U.S. Congressman Ron Wyden, a Democrat from Oregon, accused the White House of delays in mailing AIDS information to the public. However, President Reagan's assistant for domestic policy, Gary Bauer, rebuffed Representative Wyden's criticism, maintaining that if Congress appropriated funds for mailing, the Department of Health and Human Services was obligated to do the mailing. A few days earlier, September 22, HHS Secretary Otis R. Bowen addressed a letter to Senator Lawton Charles, Democrat of Florida, stating that his agency had planned a national mailing, but it would not be ready by October, explaining, "The time required to develop the materials and to arrange logistical support was not adequate." In his letter to Senator Lawton, Bowen continued, "The White House Domestic Policy Council suggested that President Reagan's AIDS Commission should be involved in discussions concerning a mailing to American households." Bowen also stated in the letter that "$30 million allocated by Congress in a supplemental AIDS appropriation is used for a variety of purposes other than mailings." He cited advertising for an AIDS hotline, an AIDS clearinghouse, wider distribution of Koop's AIDS pamphlet, and education grants to state and local health departments, businesses, and nonprofit groups. Representative Henry Waxman, Democrat from California and chairman of the House Energy and Commerce Subcommittee, was skeptical of the Reagan administration's intent to combat AIDS with public information.

The Roseburg Sunday paper[122] published the Associated Press report of Dr. Gary Noble, the highest-ranking full-time official assigned to fight AIDS. He stated, "A person who has a belief will have the belief forever, regardless of any facts you marshal." After a year of observing a society in the first stages of grappling with an epidemic, Dr. Noble was worried about the damage when beliefs and facts collide. He was worried that a cure for AIDS would be illusive, and that frustration, fueled by fear and lack of information, would exhaust the patience of the people of a usually compassionate nation. Many people were familiar with the name of the surgeon general, C. Everett Koop, but unfamiliar with the name of Dr. Gary Noble. He is a graduate of Harvard Medical School, a Rhodes Scholar who has had a unique perspective as the coordinator of the AIDS activities of the huge Public Health Service. Included are the Centers for Disease Control, the Food and Drug Administration, and the National Institute of Health. He had become somewhat of a philosopher after twenty-two years of evolution from a laboratory researcher to an administrator. Dr. Noble was convinced that the social impact of AIDS overshadowed the medical concerns. After his first year as AIDS coordinator, he professed, "Americans have always risen to the pressures of the times in an admirable way, and I am optimistic that we will again." He continued, "Unless drugs are developed to prevent those 1.5 million persons who are already HIV infected from developing signs of illness, we are going to see more and more persons progressing to AIDS."

---

122 *News-Review*, Sunday, September 27, 1987

"A question that remains unanswered in my mind is whether we, as a society, will retain our traditional compassion as an example of the American way. What I have witnessed during the past year has brought home to me direct concerns about our ways." He soberly continued, "As a society we have had to cope with the increasing number of people who have developed AIDS, cope with the burden demanded from our medical resources, on the number of hospital beds, on physicians' and nurses' times, and the spiraling cost of medications. I am worried that we will be stretched beyond our limits of compassion and tolerance."

Dr. Noble paused, attempting to be optimistic. He said that he subscribed to Abraham Lincoln's assessment for human tolerance: "If given the truth, the people can be counted upon to meet any crisis." He reminded all of us that we are not without blemishes on our history. We did hang witches at Salem in 1692 after nineteen were sentenced to die for the felony of witchcraft (Linder 2009). We removed many Japanese families from their homes in the 1940s and forced them into camps during World War II. We cannot guarantee that our society will act rationally when confronted with fear. Although there are promising signs, such as leaders in the executive branch of government and in Congress publicly making stands that are not mere quick political fixes, it's too early to say how society will react to AIDS.

In Atlanta, Dr. Noble continued addressing the AIDS issue as deputy director of the CDC in charge of AIDS activities. In September of 1986, one year earlier, he had been recruited from CDC, with only a twenty-four-hour notice, for the one-year assignment as coordinator of the federal government's AIDS efforts. The role of coordinator had not always been translated into policymaking, especially with some Reagan administration figures not in accord with recommendations of professionals in the Department of Health and Human Services, but he had considerable influence. He was highly regarded among many members of Congress who had been critical of the Reagan administration's AIDS policies. Although Dr. Noble declined to discuss specific policy issues where his council did not prevail, and he was reluctant to discuss successes, it was obvious that a high point was the tone that President Reagan attempted to set in his only full-length speech devoted entirely to AIDS. Although much of what President Reagan said in May 1987 on that Sunday evening was overshadowed by the hostile reaction by the listeners to his request for expanded testing for the AIDS virus, Dr. Noble regarded the Reagan speech as the highlight of his one-year assignment to a no-win job. "Whenever you read some of the words included in the speech, which I have used in other speeches of my own, I believe they are very positive—his calls for urgency rather than panic, compassion not blame, understanding instead of ignorance. It is important that Americans not reject persons who have AIDS, but instead, care for them with dignity and kindness. Regardless of what else President Reagan said, those were important phrases."

Dr. Noble explained that for the most part, he was pleased that AIDS was not looked upon from a "partisan view." The time he was most frustrated was when some persons looked at AIDS as a political issue. He stated that he had also been frustrated with the amount of time and energy that health officials had been required to spend countering blatant misunderstandings of the ways in which AIDS is spread from one individual to another. One false rumor that popped up over and over again is that AIDS is spread by mosquito bites, a notion that health officials said they had disproved. "It is frustrating to have to quaff myths. But if myths exist, they exist. And if they are of sufficient concerns, I'm willing to continue answering questions. What is most frustrating is when people have concerns based more upon prejudice rather than fear. But I am trained as a research scientist, and I expect it is necessary to defend intellectual ideas. If you don't have the facts to convince another intelligent person, you must get the facts.

"It's arguing beliefs or values where there is no victory because a person who has a belief will retain that belief forever, regardless of the facts you marshal," Dr. Noble explained.

Carmelita's Response to the Community's Reaction to Her Sons' HIV Infections

———————

On Wednesday, September 23, 1987, Bruce Daily of the *News-Review* met with Carmelita at the Colliding Rivers Park in Glide to review her thoughts about the experience she had when she moved with her sons and her younger daughter, Maria, to Roseburg from Glide, August 25, for personal reasons and then moved back again to Glide, where Peter was enrolled in the third grade and David in the sixth grade of the Glide school. Their sister, Maria, age six years, did not have hemophilia, nor was she HIV infected, in contrast with her two brothers. Despite close daily contact, living in the same household as her two HIV infected brothers did not result in infection.

The public opposition to entry into Winchester had been strong. "There are some people, no matter how you try to help them with their fears and misbeliefs, you can't," Carmelita professed. "Not until they are ready." She continued after thinking cautiously for a moment. "The Roseburg school officials did a wonderful job of working with my family and me, and the schoolteachers and staff. They were determined to assure that Peter and David would receive the education they needed and deserved."

She reflected and suggested that there were two critical meetings at the beginning of the Winchester school year that had made the difference in the way her sons were received in the school. At the first meeting, when the school board met September 9 to consider a communicable disease policy, a group of parents spoke out against her sons. They had prepared a petition against their entry. The next night, a public information meeting revealed that the boys' entry was regarded with fear by parents of schoolchildren, despite information presented by authorities that they were not a threat for infecting other children with HIV. Carmelita did not attend the meetings. After the first meeting, Superintendent Eisenhauer met with her the following morning, informing her of the proceedings of the meeting and the petitions. "He gave me both positive and negative feedback from the comments of the meeting," Carmelita reported. "You know, I wasn't sure. There was a sizable group of negative people, which concerned me. I said to Eisenhauer, 'I'm just going to wait and see what happens tonight at the second meeting, the public meeting.' I wondered what the parents would do in a larger group meeting. How would they respond when more people were listening to them? Would their opinions be the same?" She discovered that the numbers were the same. Parents opposed the entry of her sons into Winchester.

"My children, in the end, would have taken the greatest brunt of the turmoil," she continued. "I was afraid that parents would show up in protest at the school. My boys were already suffering from too much stress. They were developing feelings that were not welcome. Finally, they asked me, 'Is there any way we can go back home, Mom?' The parents of the children at the school could not take their eyes off their fears long enough to listen."

Carmelita was aware of other events in the hemophilia-AIDS world beyond Roseburg. A year earlier, in 1986, three brothers of the Ray family—Ricky, Robert, and Randy—who lived in Arcadia, Florida, and were affected with hemophilia, were discovered to be HIV infected from the concentrate they used for infusions to treat their bleeds. With their parents, they petitioned the De Soto County School Board for entry to the school classrooms after they were denied admission to the Arcadia school. Later, they sued the school board. The case was referred to the federal courts, which ruled in favor of the Rays for the three brothers' admission to the Arcadia school. Following the legal decision in favor of school admission, the Ray's home was burned to the ground on September 4, 1987. "I was not fearful that someone would torch my house and burn us out," Carmelita responded. "More than anything else, I was concerned about the other children at the school as well as my children. It's an example of an extreme. I really hope that stops. You can never tell how far people will go because of their fears.

"I'm a stubborn lady," she proudly said. "If we had not had Glide to return to, I wouldn't have left Roseburg. I know my sons are strong. They have courage. They would have stuck it out."

Carmelita was not required to inform the school that her sons were HIV infected. HIV reporting was not a name-based reportable disease in Oregon in 1987. Retrospectively, would she have been better off by just not saying anything? "I don't work that way," she emphasized. "Honesty when dealing with people is a quality that is ingrained in me; it's my nature. I do not want to risk any chances with my children when their entire lives lay ahead of them. It's much better to be aware of a problem and know what precautions exist for avoiding its threat than attempting to cover it up and hide it."

If similar instances arise confronting other families, Carmelita advises them to "look at all sides of the big picture. There is a price to pay for secrecy. And there is also a price to pay for honesty. Neither one is an easy choice to pay. I imagine there have been people in the same situation who have made the choice to say nothing and deal with HIV privately." She continued, "I have learned honesty is the best policy. Even those people who were expressing their fears were being honest. They were afraid. They were honest saying so. It's beneficial to say 'I am worried. I am afraid.' It's far better than holding it inside yourself, withholding your feelings. If we discover what we fear, we can learn ways to handle our fears."

Carmelita went on to say, "If people want to have the privilege of knowing what causes their fears, they must take responsible action. In many cases, their reaction must change. The reaction to my sons'

HIV infection back in Glide was different compared to Roseburg. My husband was attending a softball game in Glide in the first part of September, where people talked to him about David and Peter after hearing about the reaction in Roseburg. They told him we should bring the boys back home to Glide. Our church in Glide was with us all the way, even though we had moved away. They helped us so much.

"What I hoped for," she said, "was that those people who were still afraid would, in the near future, set aside their fears and learn to listen. The numbers of HIV infected persons will increase. They cannot all be confined. Not everyone who is infected will be quarantined. It is up to all of us to become compassionate and caring in whatever capacity we are able to be. Hopefully, some learning about HIV has taken place. You can say 'Here's something we must deal with.' People, by nature, procrastinate and put things off for another day. Then, when they must deal with it, it's like a sudden, unexpected slap in the face. But even though they do not realize it, they have learned something. Whether it's a schoolchild or someone at their work, they will be better prepared next time."

Carmelita maintained that one of the problems is "people receive information from many different resources. It's important to check out the source and get information from correct, reputable origins." Carmelita acknowledged that there were many people in Roseburg who accepted her sons in school. They were willing for their children to share classrooms with Peter and David. Opposition to their school entry was not unanimous.

In the park on a glorious September day, as the clear water from the two small rivers rushed to be joined together, Peter was playing without any signs of illness, no suggestion of AIDS from HIV infection. He emphasized that he was glad to be back home. "It's good to be back in school with my friends," he said with a big smile. There were no signs of the fear that a few days earlier had pushed him and his brother, David, into moving back to Glide.

David's and Peter's Last Days

During the last months of their lives, Peter and David became ill, weaker. Cheerfully, David maintained that there were three goals he would have liked to have attained in his life.[123] His first choice was to become a pastor of a church. His next choice was to become a sports announcer. Third, he would have liked to become a musician.

Weakness overtook the two brothers by Christmas 1992, necessitating hospitalization in Mercy Hospital in Roseburg, where the family shared their last Christmas together. The Roseburg Fire Department came to visit them, bringing teddy bears to be distributed in their names to other hospitalized children at Christmastime. On Christmas night, December 25, Peter wanted to play a game of checkers with his mother. However, he was so weak she had to take his hand, holding a red checker in hers, a black checker in his, and help him move his hand. Carmelita left his bedside in the late evening and was called at 2:00 AM, receiving word from the hospital that her son was gone.

In the next hospital room, David was weakening. He told his mother, with a faint smile on his face, "I took all that medicine, and AIDS still beat me."

David looked up at his mother from his hospital bed, his dark eyes looking into hers, and softly said "I know you love me." He was aware that his brother had died in the room next to his.

The doctor took Carmelita aside and told her that he recommended assisting David's breathing with a ventilator. She explained to David

---

123 Conversation with Carmelita Witbeck on June 23, 2008 in her home in Roseburg, Oregon

that going on the ventilator included insertion of a small tube down his throat. David was too weak to talk, but he responded with a thumbs-up. David was wheeled into the ICU and sedated and then intubated with the ventilator to maintain his respirations.

Later in the afternoon, David's color was blue. The pulmonary specialist located Carmelita in the parking lot, where she was talking with Dale, her ex-husband, the boys' father.

"I must talk to you," the doctor said in a grave tone. "There has been no improvement of your son's condition on the ventilator. I am requesting your permission to take him off the ventilator."

Dale and the boys' sister, Maria, were there with Carmelita when David died at 4:00 PM on a Sunday afternoon, December 27 1992, the day after his younger brother died.

"David didn't die first because he knew he must remain alive for his younger brother. They loved one another so much," Carmelita offered. "Loving his brother and serving God was the meaning of life for David."

The next day, sad people, including persons from the mortuary, were in tears as David and Peter were prepared for their burial side by side in the Roseburg Cemetery.

Carmelita, softly weeping, recalled, "Both boys knew they were dying. Their minds were clear until the moment they died; they never lapsed into unconsciousness. My boys loved each other dearly. They did everything together. And now they are together in heaven."[124]

She explained their premature deaths, saying, "The two boys believed they had been called upon by God to educate others about AIDS. They answered God's call by coming to the forefront with bravery and inspiration to educate and to challenge people about AIDS. Through their lives with AIDS and hemophilia, they showed extraordinary bravery and demonstrated their faith in God, which revealed the meaning of life for them."

---

124 *News-Review,* January 3, 1993

"We received extensive support, for me and my family, from the community and the schools," Carmelita said. "Scott Mutchie, the superintendent of the Glide school telephoned to express his condolences. The classmates of the boys, the teachers, and the church family were wonderful to us. David and Peter did a lot of living in just a few years. Their faith in God helped guide them through the suffering caused by the illness." Referring to her oldest son, David, who was seventeen when he died, she revealed, "David intended to become a minister if he survived the disease. He wanted people to know what God had done for him. He wanted them to know Jesus."

Isabella Wallick, health and AIDS educator for the Douglas County Health Department, compassionately offered, "The health department, the schools, and the entire community were saddened by the deaths of those two courageous boys."

Obituaries of Two Brothers Who Died of AIDS

The obituaries of David and Peter were printed in the Monday edition, December 28, 1992, of Roseburg's the *News-Review*, announcing the death of Peter, one day after Christmas, December 26, 1992, and David, one day later, December 27, 1992.

Also in the newspaper, the next day, it was cited that schoolchildren in the state of Oregon were beginning to be identified with AIDS. The two brothers were the first schoolchildren to die of AIDS in Douglas County.[125] Isabella Wallick recalled that the controversy surrounding their entry into the Roseburg School District five years earlier brought AIDS out into the open. "Presentation of their situation to the community was a learning experience and revealed how schools would react to the presence of an HIV infected schoolchild. People began to understand that it wasn't just one segment of the population that must face the dreadful disease. AIDS could affect any part of our community. The

---

125 Swan, B: *News-Review*, December 29, 1992

boys were the catalyst for the Glide school's AIDS policy, which became a model document for the other school districts," she announced. "The policy addresses infection control, confidentiality, and the rights of all schoolchildren, including those who are HIV infected."

The newspaper proclaimed the two brothers heroes, for they touched the lives of all they knew. The opinion section of the Sunday *News-Review* of January 3, 1993, proclaimed, "Glides teens' lives an example in courage," referring to the death of David and Peter Witbeck the previous weekend. The newspaper extended its sympathy to their family and friends and noted that their battle with AIDS helped increase community awareness of the threat of HIV infection. The newspaper acknowledged and commended the entire Glide community for accepting and rallying around the boys and for protecting them from outside pressures, including the media. The publication made an important point by noting that during the recent election season, some politicians sought to capitalize on antihomosexual sentiments by saying that AIDS should be treated like any other disease. "These people need to understand that AIDS is not a gay disease. Rather, it is an epidemic with a potential to devastate the world like few other diseases ever have." The newspaper continued, explaining, "It often requires a tragedy to remind people that the AIDS crisis is not going to go away. Like most epidemics, it will only get worse until breakthroughs occur in treatment and prevention."

After all the years of treating many bleeds in her sons—seventeen years for David, fourteen for Peter—Carmelita has put aside the needles, syringes, alcohol wipes, and bottles of saline that cluttered her small kitchen. Her sons no longer need them. Her daughter, Maria, was tested and discovered to be a carrier of the hemophilia trait, like her mother. Maria has since married an air force man, with whom she has had two children, Lilly and a little boy, Brandon. Brandon does not have hemophilia.

The young Protestant pastor of the Glide Full Gospel Assembly, Mick Owings, officiated during the memorial services for David and Peter Witbeck, where more than two hundred persons crammed into the Glide Community Hall on Monday, December 28, 1987. Those attending to pay their last respects to the two brothers were teachers, classmates, doctors, nurses, neighbors, and residents of the community.

"The two brothers never lamented their fate," Pastor Owings remarked. "I never saw them angry or upset about what happened to them. They led their lives without letting anything hinder them. That is how they attacked the AIDS virus. In the end, they were the victors."

One of the teenagers who spoke at the memorial service said that David, who was attending the eleventh grade at Glide High School until his death, had been his best friend since the fifth grade. "The two brothers had a great influence on my life," he proclaimed. "No matter how bad things were, David and Peter could always look on the bright side of things. They knew their time was limited, their time was coming up, but they did what they could. They carried on. David was a good friend."

A longtime Glide neighbor and family friend, Susie McReady, said that memories of love of the two brothers would forever remain with everyone that they had known. "Their faith in God helped them cope with their illness. Each time they came to a bridge in their lives, they crossed over it with faith and courage. They urged youths to gather strength among themselves, for the days pass too quickly."

Several Sunday school teachers recounted the boys' love and devotion to God. One of the teachers described David as "an angel on earth."

Another woman attending the memorial service recalled that when the church members first learned of the boys' illness, people withdrew from them, held back, because of fear of the unknown disease. But the boys were full of love, she said, which eased all the fears. "I am a better person because of David and Peter," she said, "for they showed all of us how to have strength, courage, and to love one another."

One of the women observed, "The two young brothers were confronted with a hopeless fate, but their suffering ceased to be suffering, for they found a meaning for it through love for one another and for love of God. They did not believe their existence, their relegation to a life burdened with illness, which ended prematurely, had no meaning. All of us were affected by their love for each other, which promoted the development of our love for our neighbor, which enriched the meaning of life for all of us."

Pastor Owings said that David, who longed to become a preacher, "drew great comfort from his faith. We are all proud of the way the community, the school, and the church supported the boys. The way this community responded by placing a protective barrier around the boys is something to be proud of. The community responded, doing something that no other community in this nation has done."

The pastor served a small, rural community, regardless of denomination, without a substantial personal income from his parishioners. He met their spiritual needs, including giving the last rites of two brothers who'd died from AIDS after receiving concentrate contaminated with HIV that was intended to treat their hemophilia. All the while, executives of the pharmaceutical manufacturers who made the medicine that brought death to the brothers lived in luxury compared to the lives of these two boys. Expenses to pay for the executives' luxury was derived from selling concentrates used by the brothers and many others like them. The executives and the stockholders of the pharmaceutical manufacturers benefited; the boys died. The humble minister, a pauper compared to the drug company executives, rose to his calling to provide relief from grief for the family and the community. When talking with the attendees after the memorial service, the minister, when asked, said he was happy serving this small community. His actions were not accompanied with unsuspected consequences that led to grief. This was in contrast with the doctors who intended to bring relief to suffering from hemophilia with a wonderful medicine that unsuspectingly brought more harm and grief than existed from the condition it was intended to overcome.

On June 23, 2008, Carmelita was interviewed at age fifty-four, sixteen years after the death of her two sons, in her home in Roseburg. She has remarried and has a large family who surround her with love. She professes that everyone has a story. She believes David's and Peter's lives had to be as they were. Their lives would never be forgotten because of the change they brought about. She said they did so much good despite their medical problems. "We must learn to be patient for change to come about," Carmelita said. "Abraham had to wait one hundred years to become a father. After Abraham and his wife, Sarah, had Isaac, God ordered Abraham to sacrifice his only son. Abraham did not realize this order was a test of his obedience to God. After Abraham demonstrated his willingness to sacrifice his son, Isaac, God intervened, saving Isaac, who lived to become a very old man. In the same way," Carmelita explained, "I do not know God's meaning in the loss of my sons. But I have faith and know there is a meaning of life in their loss, a message."

Confusion permeated the hemophilia treatment center as well as the homes of the families where a son, or brother, or husband with hemophilia lived. Doctors and families were restless, frustrated by unanswered questions that emanated from the new disease, which was a threat but not understood. Who would be next? Why were some persons who were infused with concentrate dying from AIDS while others were spared? Why did the Witbeck brothers die of AIDS in contrast to the Singer brothers, who had been infused many times without becoming ill, without becoming HIV-positive, after they were infused with contaminated concentrate, avoiding infection with the threatening virus?

Part VIII

Conclusion

Brent's Final Days

B rent became ill as the later stages of AIDS overcame him during the last six months of 1992, when he was sixteen. A grief counselor helped him accept his approaching death. He was known for his honesty and directness, and he expected the same honesty and directness from others.

"My son was the most honest person I have ever known" Gwyn remarked. "He detested sweet talk from well-meaning persons just to make him feel better."

Emile Vidal, a man of small stature but not of small character, recognized that Brent needed to socialize rather than shut himself off from others. He was not a religious man, but he was spiritual. He did not give out easy answers to difficult questions. Emile became a steadfast source for Brent as his medical condition deteriorated. Brent did not seem bitter. He didn't rail against his fate, although at times he was deeply sad. As the days of January 1993 slowly passed, one day at a time, He became weaker and weaker.

"When I recall those last days of my son's life" Gwyn said, "I am reminded of the beautiful sound made by fine crystal when it is tapped."

At 3:00 AM on January 25, 1993, Brent went to sleep, and he never woke up. He was tired of struggling. His struggles of seventeen years finally ended. His mother and father and his two sisters were beside him when he sighed, eyes closed, and breathed his last deep breath.

Gwyn said that even though they grieved, his death also brought relief. "He was peaceful at the end; he was ready to go."

But why did Brent have to die at such a young age? Could his death have been prevented?

Emile Vidal was present in the home the night Brent died. "Where will he go?" Gwyn asked Emile.

"I do not know where he will go, but wherever he goes, he will be received," he replied.

Three happenings marked the end of Brent's life of seventeen years: his birthday party, his death three months later, and the memorial service for him.

Many of his family and friends who'd helped him celebrate his seventeenth birthday, some of whom were in his home when he sighed his last breath, assembled for the final time at Menucha Lodge, set high up on a rocky ledge on the south side of the Columbia River. The mighty Columbia flowed gently westward toward the Pacific, far below the retreat lodge. The mountains of Southern Washington were visible to the north. The snow-covered Cascades of Oregon rose in the east and south.

Eulogies and remembrances were shared as the guests sat on the floor close to one another, holding hands, before the fireplace of the stone and timber lodge. Perhaps the legends of the Indians who had lived there were accurate. They recalled their forefathers telling stories passed down through many generations, recounting how the mountains guarded the people in the area of the Columbia River, assuring them a place in heaven. Mount Rainier, Mount St. Helens, Mount Adams, Mount Hood, and Mount Jefferson speak to one another and watch over the creatures, including humans, who live in their midst.

The events of Brent's seventeenth birthday party in October 1992, his death in January 1993, and the gathering at his memorial in February were sad as well as joyful, part of the broad spectrum of human emotion from sharing the experiences with the family and friends who were part of his life.

Who Was Responsible?

> - Brent's life was filled with suffering and pain caused by hemophilia.
> - The quality of his life was improved with infusions of concentrate.
> - Infusions with infected concentrate caused his illness and death.

The doctors who provided care for Brent were wrong. But were they guilty? "Take this medicine," they said, "and your life will be nearly normal. You will not suffer from hemophilia. You will be safe and not die from hemophilia." That proclamation was partially correct. Hemophilia was not the cause of Brent's death.

But the medicine was not safe. The doctors were wrong. The medicine subdued his hemophilia but caused his death. Was the doctor guilty? Or was the doctor only wrong? Doctors are not usually malicious; however, in some instances, they are wrong or even negligent. Maybe irresponsible. Shouldn't the doctors, the hemophilia treaters, have demanded increased efforts to improve the safety of the medicine for treatment of hemophilia, to purify the concentrate? They accepted the premise that the medicine, contaminated with a virus, was better than no medicine, the lesser evil. They didn't speak out and demand accelerated vigilance from the pharmaceutical manufacturers, who were profit oriented. The government surveillance—the United Sates Public

Health Service and the Centers for Disease Control—was ineffective in preventing disaster in hemophilia caused by polluted medicine. Why didn't the doctors speak out? Were the doctors misdirected by the confusion surrounding the appearance of a new disease that had surfaced within their lifetimes, a disease unfamiliar to them during their medical careers and medical training?

Dr. Taillefer recalled his early days in medicine, when he was a medical student. One of the first patients he cared for after beginning his clinical years of training at the University of Minnesota Medical School impressed him for the remainder of his medical career. He never forgot the experience of being a member of a medical team caring for the man's medical problem. The middle-aged man was a gentle, innocent, humble man. For his working life in rural Minnesota, the man operated a county road grading machine. He lived in the countryside with his wife and children, a good life. He was admitted to the university hospital when he became jaundiced at fifty-six years of age. Quickly, the evaluation revealed that the man had lung cancer that had spread to his liver and bones. Before the man died shortly after admission to the hospital, he revealed that he had smoked cigarettes for forty years.

At that moment, in 1957, while still a medical student, Dr. Taillefer wondered why the medical profession didn't acknowledge that smoking cigarettes caused lung cancer. The attitude of the doctors was that although smoking might not be desirable, it was a personal matter. Doctors didn't caution their patients about the danger of smoking. The American Medical Association made no proclamation about the harm of smoking. And yet, Dr. Taillefer recalls, all of those in the medical profession recognized the harm of smoking and its association with lung cancer. However, doctors put their heads in the sand and didn't speak out. Finally, in 1982, the surgeon general of the United States Health Service, C. Everett Koop, proclaimed that smoking is harmful and one of the causes of lung cancer. Koop announced that cigarette smoking is the major single cause of cancer mortality in the United States. A public health awareness program became effective in educating the youth of

America, informing them of the harm of smoking. Until then, many persons, like Dr. Taillefer's innocent first medical patient, unnecessarily died. The tobacco companies who manufactured cigarettes resembled the pharmaceutical manufacturers who produced concentrate. Both were motivated by profit. According to the philosophy of capitalism, CEOs and directors of private corporations are responsible only to their shareholders for generating profits on their investments, not to the consumers of their products (Magnuson 2008). The medical community did not speak out until many lives were unnecessarily lost from tobacco smoke. A difference between pharmaceutical and cigarette manufacturers compared with medical doctors is the motive. The motive of the drug and tobacco companies was profit. The doctors' motive was to relieve illness. The pharmaceutical manufacturers, in the production of concentrate, were reckless, greedy. The doctors were not malicious, but they were wrong.

An outstanding example of doctors being wrong in treatment of patients, cited by Magnuson (2008), was the management of illness of President George Washington, which resulted in his death at age sixty-eight on December 14, 1799 (Vadakakan 2005). After the president rode horseback, inspecting his Mount Vernon estate on December 12, in snow, hail, and rain, from ten in the morning until three in the afternoon, he became ill. Although inclement weather does not cause sickness, President Washington's exposure was not beneficial at the onset of a sore throat. His developing illness was followed by laryngitis and pneumonia. After summoning his doctors, various remedies were applied. Over the next day, five separate bloodlettings were completed, of 12 ounces, 20 ounces, 20 ounces, 40 ounces and finally 32 ounces of drained blood, totaling 124 ounces of blood, or eight pints. A typical adult male has a blood volume of five liters, or ten pints of blood. The medical doctors attending President Washington depleted 80 percent of his blood volume to make him well—they were wrong.

Doctors can be wrong. They told Gwyn that she was not a carrier of hemophilia. They said her mother and sisters were not hemophilia carriers. The birth of her son eventually revealed that Gwyn is a carrier. Her mother is a carrier. Her sisters are carriers of hemophilia.

The doctors told Gwyn to give her son medicine to help treat his medical disorder. They said the new medicine would allow him to live a normal life. The medicine was infected, and Brent died when he was seventeen. The doctors were wrong.

Doctors are human. They have good intentions, but they are not infallible. They can be wrong, but are they guilty?

When a young doctor graduates from medical school, he swears by the Hippocratic oath. Part of that ancient Greek document, believed to have been written by Hippocrates during the fourth century BC, includes guidelines intended to assist Doctors of Medicine as they tread along an ethical path in their practice of medicine, which Dr. Taillefer recalled:

I will prescribe regimens for the good of my patients according to my ability and my judgment and never do harm to anyone.

To practice and prescribe to the best of my ability for the good of my patients, and try to avoid harming them.

Have I violated the oath I swore to abide by when I graduated from medical school in 1959? Dr. Taillefer wrestled with that question when he recalled the number of individuals for whom he'd prescribed medicine that was contaminated, leading to their deaths. *Am I guilty of harming my patients, even unintentionally? Am I guilty or was I just wrong?*

Table 3. Years of Events in Brent's Life

1964 Cryoprecipitate produced by Dr. Judith Pool

1971 Antihemophilia concentrate available for infusions

1975 Birth of Brent

1976 First bleed, age six months

1976 First infusion with concentrate

1976 Move from Spokane to Oregon

1979 Parents learn home infusion for recurrent bleeds

1982 First report of new mysterious disease

1983 Move to California, age eight

1983 Discovery of HIV (named HTLV in 1983) by Dr. Luc Montagnier

1984 Mother learns about new disease

1984 Return to Oregon from California

1984 Recalls of concentrates

1984 First person with AIDS seen by Oregon Hemophilia Center

1984 HIV antibody test available

1984 Brent learned self-infusion

1985 Heat-treated concentrate available

1986 Western Blot test for HIV

1987 First death from AIDS at Oregon Hemophilia Treatment Center

1987 HTLV name changed to HIV

1987 Brent tested for HIV, age twelve

1991 Enrolled in AZT study group

1991 Pentamidine inhalation

1992 Symptoms of AIDS appeared in Brent

1992 Pneumocystis pneumonia develops

1993 AIDS claims Brent's life at age seventeen

Table 4. Hemophilia and HIV/AIDS

Heat treatment of plasma	1950
Plasma identified as source of homologous serum jaundice	1962
Cryoprecipitate produced for treatment of hemophilia	1964
Humafac Concentrate marketed for treatment of hemophilia	1971
Federal funding of Hemophilia Treatment Centers	1976
First report of a mysterious disease (AIDS) in hemophilia	1982
Term AIDS introduced	1982
Cause of AIDS discovered, named HTLV	1983
Heat-treated concentrate produced in USA	1983
Heat-treated concentrate available for treatment	1985
Cutter discontinued shipping non-heat-treated concentrate overseas	1985
Solvent-detergent method of producing concentrates	1985
Antibody test for HTLV	1986
Western Blot test for HTLV	1986
HTLV renamed HIV, the cause of AIDS	1987
AZT approved for treatment of AIDS	1987
rFVIII recombinant antihemophilia factor concentrate	1990
AZT approved for prevention of AIDS	1990
Oral Polio Vaccine (OPV) theory for origin of AIDS (Tom Curtis)	1992
HAART combination of drugs for treatment of AIDS	1996
The River; Research on the source of HIV and AIDS by Edward Hooper	1999
Hepatitis B vaccine origin of AIDS	2001

Afterword

I mprovement in the treatment of hemophilia has brought relief from suffering and improved the lives of thousands of affected persons throughout the world. The agony experienced during previous centuries has been overcome with modern medicines. Arrival at the level of treatment available today is an example of the effect of research and development in science, medicine, and marketing. A medicine has been produced that allows persons affected with hemophilia to attain near-normal lives. Attainment of this goal is the result of the energy of free enterprise and capitalism.

Development of a medicine to treat hemophilia was not by the way of an easy road. Along the way, unpredictable hazards were encountered, resulting in harm and loss of life. A new disease, AIDS, appeared, and the effects of a recognized disease, hepatitis, exerted its toll. Thousands of persons affected with hemophilia became infected with HIV and hepatitis. Whenever new medical treatments emerge, it is necessary to balance the trade-offs between advantages and hazards of the medical advancements. The entrepreneurship of capitalism has been of great benefit to the treatment of medical disorders, including hemophilia. Because of human nature, the free spirit of capitalistic enterprise requires regulation to avoid profiteering and greed.

The concentrates for treatment of hemophilia were developed by drug companies from human plasma procured from persons of high risk. Donors received payment for selling their blood, which was used as the source for the manufacture of a profitable product with worldwide distribution. Doctors knowingly gave medicine containing the hepatitis virus to their patients. They assumed that the risk of hepatitis was acceptable compared to the hazards of hemophilia. They accepted the proclamation of the drug companies, who maintained that the method for viral depletion of hepatitis virus was not known. That proclamation was incorrect. The method for depletion of hepatitis virus from human plasma has been known since World War II. The drug companies were deficient in knowledge. If hepatitis virus had been eliminated, HIV would also have been eradicated.

Unknown factors exerted unpredictable impacts on the path of development of concentrates. This was the case of the development of hepatitis B vaccine. Intention to relieve disease with a vaccine to prevent hepatitis B resulted in transfer of a simian virus to humans and the appearance of AIDS in humans, a new disease. Scientists assumed simians didn't harbor viruses harmful to humans. They were wrong.

Who is responsible for the tragedy that occurred in hemophilia when persons who were infused with concentrates became infected with hepatitis and HIV? Three tiers of responsibility were involved:

First were the drug companies that manufactured concentrate. They devoted energy toward marketing and sacrificed safety.

The second tier of responsibility was the government and public agencies. The agencies should have required the drug companies to produce a safer concentrate.

The third tier of responsibility, closest to the patients, was the doctors. They were not as critical of the medicine they prescribed as they should have been.

Development of medicine for the treatment of hemophilia materialized as a result of free marketing and the spirit of capitalism that prevailed in the United States. The federal government did not produce a concentrate. Concentrate became a reality because of profitability.

Unfortunately, profitability was influenced by greed. Agencies and foundations were influenced by the drug companies. Meetings and research were supported by drug company funds. Medical doctors who treated hemophilia patients were too close to the pharmaceutical manufacturers of concentrate.

The story of the development of concentrates to treat hemophilia successfully has not been all negative. The drive for financial gains by the pharmaceutical manufacturers has led to production of a recombinant medicine, rFVIII. The experience and methods are applicable to other genetic disorders, which will promote longevity.

The ultimate responsibility for treatment of medical disorders rests with the doctors, not the drug companies. Doctors are entrusted with their patients' lives. They cannot look the other way when confronted with imposing risks. In hemophilia, they made a judgment that the benefits of a new treatment outweighed the risks. The doctors were wrong.

References Cited and Sources of Information

Agence francaise de sécurité sanitaire des produits de santé, (afssps), "Long-term National Surveillance of Coagulation Factors Supply in France 2003." http://agmed.sante.gouv.fr/pdf/5/poster/cpagfac.pdf, retrieved 2008-04-08.

Bayer AG Annual Report, 2005, http://www.annualreport 2005id0602/financial report/keydata2005.php, retrieved 2008-04-23.

Bayer AG Annual Report, 2007, http://www.annualreport.bayer.com, retrieved 2008-04-12.

Bayer AG, Bayer health Care Products. Our Best selling Products in 2009. http://www.bayerhealthcare.com, retrieved 2010-03-14.

Billings, M., "The Influenza Pandemic of 1918," 1997, http://virus.stanford.edu/uda/, retrieved 2008-04-13.

BLTC, "Archbishop of Canterbury, John Bird Sumner, 1780–1862." http://www.general-anaesthesia.com/images/john bird-sumner.html, retrieved 2005-10-05.

Bogdanich, W., and E. Koli, "2 Paths of Bayer Drug in 80's: Riskier One Steered Overseas." *New York Times*, May 22, 2003.

British Royal History – "Queen Victoria and her Family", http://www.royalty.nu/Europe/England/Victoria.html, retrieved 2008-04-10.

Brown, D. "Changes Cited in Bird Flu Virus." *Washington Post*, October 6, 2005, A03.

Brown, L. W. "A Private War Escalates; The Dana Kuhn Story." Style Weekly, October 5, 1993, http://members.aol.com/LoveIsHome/DanaKuhn.html, retrieved 2008-02-14.

Burr, T., J. M. Hyman, and G. Meyers, "The origin of acquired immune deficiency syndrome: Darwinian or Lamarckian?" Philosophical Transactions of the Royal Society of London B 356 (2001): 877–887.

Centers for Disease Control and Prevention (CDC), "Deaths among Persons with AIDS through December 2000." http://www.cdc.gov/hiv/topics/surveillance/resources/reports/2002supp_vol8no1/table4.html, retrieved 2008-9-15.

Centers for Disease Control and Prevention (CDC), "Report on the Universal Data Collection Program." (2004): 1–13.

Central Connecticut State University, Africa Update Newsletter, Vol. IX, Issue 1, "Conversation on AIDS." Part 2, http://www.ccsu.edu/afstudy/upd9-1, retrieved 2008-04-07.

Chehab, N., "A Review of Coagulation Products Used in the Treatment of Hemophilia." *Cleveland Clinic*, V, No. IV, (Jul/Aug 2002).

Chen, Christine, "Pharmaceutical Cost Containment. The Potential and Challenges of Reference Pricing. Insure the Uninsured Project." April 2007. http://www.iyup.org/workgroups/CostContainmentReferencePricing, retrieved 2008-11-18.

Chorba, T. L., R. C. Holman, M. J. Clarke, and B. L. Evatt, "Effects of HIV infection on Age and Cause of Death for Persons with Hemophilia A in the United States." American Journal of Hematology 66 (2001): 229–240

Curtis, T., "The Origin of AIDS. A Startling New Theory Attempts to Answer The Question 'Was it an Act of God or an Act of Man?'" *Rolling Stone*, Issue 626 (Mar. 19, 1992): 54–59, 61, 106, 108.

Cramer, P., and Martinet, J., "Factor VIII for haemophilia A patients," *Bioimpact*, http://www.france-biotech.org.monographie FVIII_ENG_.pdf.2004, retrieved 2008-04-26.

Crowley, R., *What If?* New York: Berkley, 2001.

Daily, B. "AIDS response borders on hysteria." *News-Review*, September 13, 1987.

Daily, B. "Mother of infected boys doesn't regret making situation public." *News Review*, September 23, 1987.

Darby, S. C., D. W. Ewart, P.L.F. Giangrande, P. J. Dolin, R. J. D. Spooner, and C. R. Rizza, "Mortality before and after HIV infection in the complete U K population of Haemophiliacs." *Nature* 377 (1995): 79–82.

Darby, S., Wan Kan Sau, R. J. Spooner, et al., "Mortality rates, life expectancy, and causes of death in people with Hemophilia A or B in the United Kingdom who were not infected with HIV." *Blood* 110 (2007):815–825.

Del Amo, J., S. Perez-Hoyos, A. Moreno, et al., "Trends in AIDS and mortality in HIV infected subjects with Hemophilia from 1985 to 2003: The competing risks for death between AIDS and liver disease." *Journal of Acquired Immunodeficiency Syndrome 41,* 5 (2006): 624–631.

Devean, C., and D. Bucquet, "Natural history of HIV disease among a cohort of hemophiliacs in France after three years of follow-up. HEMOCO Study Group." International Conference on AIDS, 9 (June 6–11, 1993): 664.

Diamond, J., *Guns, Germs, and Steel, The Fates of Human Societies.* New York: Norton, 1999.

Direvo, 2008, http://www.direvo.com/page2.asp?PageID+666.

DollarTimes.com, http://www.dollartimes.com/calculators/inflation, retrieved 2009-08-03.

ELISA/Western Blot Test, 2009, http://www.nlm.gov/medlineplus/ency/article/003538, retrieved 2009-07-30.

Enge, M. "Doctor, Supplier Win AIDS Verdict." *Anchorage Daily News,* June 8, 1991.

Evatt, B. L. "The tragic history of AIDS in the Hemophilia population, 1982–1984." Journal of Thrombosis Haemostasis, 4(2006): 2295–2301.

Frankl, V. E., *Man's Search for Meaning.* New York: Washington Square Press, 1984.

Gene Therapy in: *Wikipedia,* http://en.wikipedia.org/wiki/Gene_therapy, 8 May, 2008, retrieved 2008-05-11.

Gilbert, M. T., A. Rambaut, G. Wlasiuk, T. J. Spira, A. E. Pitchenik, and M. Worobey, "The emergence of HIV/AIDS in the Americas and beyond." http://www.pnas.org/cgi/doi/10.1073/pnas.0705329104, retrieved 2008-04-15.

Graw, J., H. H. Brackmann, J. Oldenburg, R. Schneppenheim, M. Spannagl, and R. Schwaab, "Haemophilia: from mutation analysis to new therapies." *Nature Reviews Genetics* 6 (2005): 488–501.

Guirguis, H. S., and E. G. Rogoff, "Strategies and impacts of new drug introduction: Hemophilia treatment." *J. Health Care Finance* 30 (2004):14–25.

HAART, "Highly Active Antiretroviral Therapy," http://www.haart.com/, retrieved 2009-01-12.

Healthcare Sales & Marketing Network, http://salesandmarketingnetwork.com/news_release.php?ID=201634, February 1, 2007, retrieved 2008-04-21.

Higgins, A., E U Conference on Pharmaceutical Innovation, Keynote Address, Nov 19, 2007, http://bayer.com, retrieved 2008-04-11.

Hill, H. M., S. Deam, B. Gordon, and G. Dolan, "Mutation analysis in 51 patients with haemophilia A: report of 10 novel mutations and correlations between genotype and clinical phenotype." *Haemophilia* 11 (2005): 133–41.

Hooge, O., "The chances of you existing." http://www.members.shaw.ca/frisen/chances_of_you_existing, retrieved 2008-05-10.

Hooper, E. *The River, a Journey to the Source of HIV and AIDS*. Boston: Little, Brown and Company, 1999.

Horowitz, L. G. "Early Hepatitis B Vaccines and the "Man-Made" Origin of HIV/AIDS." http://originofaids.com/articels/early.htm, retrieved 2008-04-06.

Human Ovulation Process, http://www.syl.com/hb/humanovulationprocess.html, retrieved 2008-05-10.

Institute of Medicine, U.S. Department of Health and Human Services, Washington, D.C., National Academy Press, Jul 13 1995.

Kay, M. A., J. C. Glorioso, and L. Naldini, L., "Viral vectors for gene therapy: the art of turning infectious agents into vehicles of therapeutics." *Nature Medicine* 7 (2000): 33–40.

Kroner, B. L., et al. "HIV-1 infection incidence among persons with hemophilia in the United States and Western Europe, 1978–1990." *Journal of Acquired Immunodeficiency Syndrome,* 7 (1994): 279–286.

Linder, D. O. "Salem Witchcraft Trials 1692," http://www.law.umk. edu/faculty/projects,ftrials/salem, retrieved 2009-12-10.

Lozier, J. N., A. Dutra, E. Pak, et al. "The Chapel Hill hemophilia A dog colony exhibits a factor VIII gene inversion." *Proceedings of the National Academy of Sciences* 99, 2 (2002): 12,991–12,996.

Magnuson, J. *Mindful Economics.* New York: Seven Stories Press, 2008.

Mannucci, P. M. "Hemophilia and Related Disorders: Looking Back, Looking Forward." 2002 Thomas Ham/Lois Wasserman Memorial lecture, http://www.medscape.com/viewarticle/446881, retrieved 2008-04-26.

Marriott, S. J., T. H. Lee, B. Slagle, and J. S. Butel, "Activation of the HTLV-1 long terminal repeat by the hepatitis B virus X protein." *Virology* 224 (1996): 206–213.

Martin, M. "Glide students transfer to Roseburg, are infected with AIDS-related virus." *News-Review,* August 25, 1987.

——— "Parents object to AIDS students." *News-Review,* September 10, 1987.

——— "Health experts try to calm Winchester nerves." *News-Review,* September 11, 1987.

——— "Tiny HIV virus causing large commotion, Winchester school parents continue soul-search over two 'AIDS' students." *News-Review,* September 13, 1987.

——— "Concern in Glide over return of two infected brothers." *News-Review,* September 15, 1987.

——— "School board calls for clearer disease policy." *News-Review,* September16, 1987.

——— "AIDS — What we have learned." *News-Review,* September 20, 1987.

———— "Board approves two changes in AIDS policy." *News-Review*, October 15, 1987.

Measuring Worth, 2009, http://www.measuringworth.com/indicator, retrieved 2009-08-03.

Miller, R. H., and W. S. Robinson, "Common Evolutionary Origin of Hepatitis B Virus and Retroviruses." Proceedings of the National Academy of Sciences 83 (1986): 2,531–2,535.

Oregon Department of Human Services, 1997, "Confidential HIV Case Reporting – Oregon." http://www.oregon.gov./DHS/ph/hiv/data/reporting/name.shtml, retrieved 2009-03-22.

Origin of AIDS, "The origin of AIDS and HIV May Not Be What You Have Learned." http://originofaids.com/, retrieved 2008-04-06.

Money Central News 2007, "GTC Biotherapeutics Obtains License to Factor IX, Factor VIII, and Fibrinogen." http://www.news.moneycentral.msn.com, retrieved 2008-04-25.

Nachman, M. W., and S. L. Crowell. "Estimate of the Mutation Rate per Nucleotide in Humans." *Genetics* 156 (2000): 297–304.

News-Review, "Roseburg School Board approves disease policy." September 11, 1987, p. 3.

News-Review (AP), "AIDS bill opposed at hearing." September 21, 1987, p. 1.

News-Review (AP), "AIDS brochure to be distributed." September 25, 1987, p. 24.

News-Review (AP), "AIDS social implication overshadow medical." September 27, 1987, p. C-7.

News-Review, "Top 10 stories of 1987." AIDS # 2, December 27, 1987, p. D-1.

News-Review, Obituaries, "David Christopher Witbeck." "Peter J. Witbeck." December 28, 1992.

News-Review, Opinion, "Glide teens' lives an example in courage." January 3, 1993, p. C-4.

Nuss, R., J. M. Soucie, and B. Evatt, "Changes in the occurrence of and risk factors for hemophilia-associated intracranial hemorrhage." *American Journal of Hematology* 68 (2001): 37–42.

Oxford, J.S., "The so-called Great Spanish Influenza Pandemic of 1918 may have originated in France." Philosophical Transactions Royal Society London B 356 (2001): 1857–1859.

Philipp, C. S. and the Monoclate-P Study Group. "Viral safety of a pasteurized, monoclonal antibody-purified factor VIII concentrate in previously untreated haemophilia A patients." *Haemophilia* 7 (2001): 146–152.

Pollack, A., "Wyeth Deal May Slow Pfizer Biotech Acquisitions." *New York Times*, January 26, 2009.

――――― "Is Money Tainting the Plasma Supply?" *New York Times*, December 6, 2009.

Qunintana, M., J. del Amo, A. Barrasa, S. Perez-Hoyos, I. Ferreros, et al. "Progression of HIV infection and mortality by hepatitis C infection in patients with haemophilia over 20 years." *Hemophilia* 9 (2003):605–612.

Resnik, S., *Blood Saga. Hemophilia, AIDS, and the Survival of a Community.* Berkley: University of California Press, 1999.

Reuters, 2008, "Norse Receives Milestone Payment from Novo Nordisk on Factor VIII Program." http://www.reuters.com/article/pressRelease/idUS163360+06-Feb-2008+BW20080206, retrieved 2009-07-24.

Revel-Vilk, S., M. R. Golomb, C. Achonu, et al. "Effect of intracranial bleeds on the health and quality of life of boys with hemophilia." *Journal of Pediatrics* 144, 4 (2004): 490–495.

Rogoff, E. G., H. S. Guirguis, et al. "The upward spiral of drug costs: a time series analysis of drugs used in the treatment of Hemophilia." *Thrombosis and Haemostasis* 88 (2002):545–553.

Sabin, C.A., A.N. Phillips, T.T. Yee, A. Griffoen, and C.A. Lee, "Twenty-five years of HIV infection in haemophilic men in Britain: an observational study." *British Medical Journal* 331 (2005): 997–998, retrieved 2008-04-23 from: bmj.com.

Schnell, L. "Aids brothers moving out of district." *News-Review,* September 14,1987

Serwadda, D., R. D. Mugerwa, N. K. Sewankambo, et al., "Slim disease: a new disease in Uganda and its association with HTLV-III infection." *Lancet* 2 (8460), (October 19, 1985): 849–852.

Sharp, P. M., E. Bailes, R. R. Chaudhuri, M. Rodenburg, M. O. Santiago, and B. H. Hahn, "The origins of acquired immune deficiency syndrome viruses: where and when?" *Philosophical Transactions Royal Society London B* 356 (2001):867–876.

Shaw, D. "On the Trail of Tainted Blood – Hemophiliacs Say U.S. Could Have Prevented Their Contracting AIDS." *The Philadelphia Inquirer,* Editorial Review and Opinion (Sunday, April 16, 1995).

Shilts, R., "Portland doctor withholding new version of clotting factor." *San Francisco Chronicle* (Tuesday, December 5, 1989).

Simmonds, P., "The Origin and Evolution of Hepatitis Viruses in Humans." 2000 Fleming Lecture, *Journal of General Virology* 82 (2001): 693–712.

Smith, D. B., S. Pathirana, P. Davidson, E. Lawler, J. Power, P. L. Yap, and P. Simmonds, "The Origin of Hepatitis C Virus Genotypes." *Journal of General Virology* 78 (1997): 321–328.

Smith, J. L., and M. L. Tamplin, "Pigs, People and Hepatitis E. The Organism, Its Disease and Habitat," USDA, http://www.ars.usda.gov/News/docs.htm?docid=6813, retrieved 2008-04-06.

Sobesky, R., P. Lebray, B. Nalpas, A. Vallet-Pichard, H. Fontaine, J. L. Lagneau, and S. Pol, "Pathological evolution of hepatitis C virus – 'Healthy Carriers.'" World Journal of Gastroenterology 14, 24 (2008): 3861–3865.

Stafford, R. S., M. Hegewald, C. Haag, L. Wolff, and E. Lovrien, "Life Expectancy in Hemophilia." *Clinical Research* 28 (1980): 103A.

Starke, Amy Martinez, "Stretching beyond limitations." *Oregonian,* Obituaries and Life Stories, Sunday, December 5, 2004, B5.

Swan, B. "Brothers with AIDS remembered for their courage." *News-Review,* December 28, 1992, p. 3.

———— "Young AIDS victims called heroes, Memorial service honors Glide teens exposed to virus through tainted blood." *News-Review,* December 29, 1992, p. 1.

T Helper Cells, http://en.wikipedia.org/wiki/T_helper_cell, retrieved 2009-01-22.

Taubenberger, J. K., A. H. Reid, R. M. Lourens, R. Wang, G. Jin, and T. G. Fanning, "Characterization of the 1918 influenza polymerase genes." *Nature* 437 (2005):889-893.

Tencer, T., H. S. Friedman, J. Li-Mcleod, and K. Johnson. "Medical Costs and Resource Utilization for Hemophilia Patients with and without HIV or HCV Infection." *Journal Managed Care Pharmacy* 13 (2007): 790–798.

Theophilus, B.D., M.S. Eynayat, M.D. Williams, and F.G. Hill, "Site and type of mutations in the factor VIII gene in patients and carriers of haemophilia A." *Haemophilia* 7 (2001): 381–391.

UCLA School of Public Health, "Anesthesia and Queen Victoria," http://www.ph.UCLA.edu/epi/snow/Victoria.html, retrieved 2005-11-05.

Vadakakan, V. V. "A Physician Looks at the Death of Washington." *Early America Review*, Winter/Spring 2005, http://www.earlyamerica.com/review/2005_winter_spring/washington_death.htm, retrieved 2009-01-17.

Verbeeck, J. et al. "Investigating the Origin and Spread of Hepatitis C Virus Genotype 5a." *Journal of Virology* 80 (2006):4220–4226.

Vogel, F., and Motulsky, A. G. *Human Genetics, second edition.* Berlin: Springer Verlag, 1986, chapter 5, p. 334.

White, A. "Reagan's AIDS Legacy." *San Francisco Chronicle*, June 8, 2004, p. B 9.

Worldwide AIDS & HIV Statistics Including Deaths, "Global HIV/AIDS estimates, end of 2007." http://www.avert.org/worldstats.htm, retrieved 2008-04-20.

Appendix I: To Be Remembered

Listed in table 5 are names of some of the persons who had hemophilia, whose bleeding episodes were treated with concentrate prescribed by the Oregon Hemophilia Treatment Center. They died from AIDS caused by HIV infection, or liver failure or cancer of the liver from hepatitis infection. They were instructed to infuse concentrate and their suffering from hemophilia would be lessened; they would experience near normal lives.[126] The medicine was discovered to be contaminated with HIV and hepatitis viruses, which led to AIDS and liver disease. Although the doctors did not intend for these persons to develop AIDS and liver failure, if they were not guilty of prescribing harmful medicine, they were certainly wrong.

I wish to say to the survivors of these persons, their parents, children, spouses, brothers and sisters, and families, *I am sorry.* I apologize for the fatal results of my actions and on behalf of all the doctors, nurses, and all the Oregon Hemophilia Treatment Center staff that unknowingly caused harm.

E. W. Lovrien, MD
2010

---

126 Infusions of concentrates were recommended by the medical and nursing staff at the hemophilia treatment center, proclaiming benefits, at the time of clinic evaluations during the 1970s and 1980s.

Table 5. To be remembered

Vance Adney	Mark Gillespie	Carl Ross
Paul Aina	Claudius Groves	Kevin Royer
John Alread	Tom Guerara	Bill Ruff
Jerry Angel	Steve Hatch	Ben Sherry
Donald Austin	Michael Hollub	Joe Singler
Richard Austin	David Jarrard	Tim Singler
Eric Benz	David Jones	Curtis Stevens
Jim Berry	Joe Kennedy	David Utecht
John Berry	Joe Krostag	Dick Wagner
Dale Branham	Barry Kurath	John Warren
Granville Boynton	Nathaniel Kurillo	Don Weil
Chris Cairns	Mark Laam	Curtis Whitley
Sean Cairns	Jeff Lawson	David Witbeck
Donald Calahan	Jeff Leppaluatto	Peter Witbeck
Cary Carlstrom	Doug McAllister	James Worthy
Mike Charles	John McAnulty	
Seth Cline	Terry McConnel	
Gary Clinton	David Midkiff	
Jason Cobb	Leonard Moffit	
Frankie Cornelius	Gary Morgan	
Tom Dameron	Terry Nelson	
Larkey DeNeff	Roger Norman	
Bruce Dessellier	Wayne Palmer	
Russell Dickman	Jack Peterson	
Jeff Dinsdale	Gerald Peterson	
Michael Durr	Phillip Peterson	
Eric Dutson	Sally Phillips	
Danny Fitzgerald	Steve Phillips	
Randy Gibson	David Reardon	
Cindy Gibson	Tim Reeves	

Appendix II: Hemophilia in Queen Victoria's Family

B rent was critical of information presented to him. He was almost skeptical. When his mother explained the first appearance of hemophilia in his family, he questioned the discovery of hemophilia in the royal family, the appearance in Leopold. Results of tests indicate that the mutation for hemophilia appeared for the first time in Brent's family in individual 2000, Prudence (figure 1). Considerable information is available for assessing the appearance of hemophilia in the family of Queen Victoria; the royal family was well chronicled. Review of records suggests that she was the first person to posses the mutation in the royal family (figures 3 and 4).

Leopold was Queen Victoria's fourth son, her eighth of nine children, born to her and Prince Albert at one fifteen in the afternoon on April 7, 1853. He was the first person in the royal family to have hemophilia. His birth event was a first for Queen Victoria in two respects: first was his painless delivery utilizing chloroform. The introduction of ether in 1846, and chloroform in 1847, only six years before Leopold's birth, as anesthetics, offered patients merciful relief from suffering during childbirth and surgery (British Royal History 2007). Prior to the advent of anesthesia, surgery was a terrifying prospect, resulting in indescribable agony for its victims. The utopian prospect of surgery without pain was a nameless fantasy, as fanciful as life without suffering seems in our present world. General anesthesia, putting a patient to sleep, in the delivery rooms and during surgery, offered hope and great relief to patients. Surgeons were grateful, for they could perform surgical operations over longer time spans and complete delicate procedures on anesthetized persons who weren't thrashing about. Although we might suppose adoption of painless surgery would be uniformly welcomed, such was not the case. A debate whether anesthesia should be used in dentistry, obstetrics, and surgery during the 1800s rose from the voices of a minority of churchmen and laity, even from some physicians, who believed in the psychic healing power of pain. Also, critics rightfully questioned the safety of anesthetics when it became apparent that one in fifteen thousand persons died as the direct result of ether, and one in twenty-five hundred persons given chloroform anesthetic died.

John Bird Sumner, the archbishop of Canterbury from 1848 until his death in 1862, endorsed the use of anesthetics, rebuffing ministers who condemned obstetric anesthetics, claiming their use mocked the curse of "primal sin." London physician Dr. John Snow, age forty, moved to the affluent Sackville Street. He administered chloroform to the queen at the birth of Leopold. Five weeks following his birth, the influential medical journal *The Lancet*, May 14, 1853, criticized the queen's physicians for giving chloroform to the queen during Leopold's birth. The next year, in 1954, after Queen Victoria received chloroform for Leopold's delivery, Sumner's daughter received chloroform obstetric anesthesia (BLTC 2005). The prominence of Queen Victoria's obstetric anesthesia and the advocacy of the archbishop of Canterbury combined to add a significant endorsement, promoting relief from pain during childbirth for many women.

The second remarkable aspect of Leopold's birth in 1853 was the discovery of hemophilia, the first appearance of the medical condition in Queen Victoria's family. No males who were affected with hemophilia had been born in the royal family prior to Leopold. He was two years of age before his affection was recognized. Of all of Queen Victoria's nine children, Leopold was the smallest, the most frail. He appeared to be delicate from birth. He suckled poorly from a wet nurse, which was attributed to a problem of digestion resulting in a change of wet nurses (UCLA School of Public Health 2005). Leopold was named after the queen's uncle, Leopold I, the king of Belgium, and christened when he was two months of age on June 28, 1853, the anniversary of the queen's coronation, sixteen years previously.

In early infancy, bruises began to appear on the little boy's body that became severe by age two, when he was said to have lameness of the legs. Queen Victoria and her husband, Prince Albert, who was one of her first cousins, did not recognize their son's malady. They believed he was clumsy and badly behaved. His stumbling, they reasoned, resulted in the bruises they discovered on his arms and legs. Most doctors were unaware of the medical condition, hemophilia.

In 1803, Dr. John Otto in Philadelphia described a hemorrhagic disposition existing in some families. The first use of the word "hemophilia" was published by Hopff in 1828, twenty-five years before Leopold was born. In 1858, at age five years, while on a walk with the family, Leopold fell, cutting his knee. His parents became alarmed when they could not stop the bleeding. Queen Victoria, in a letter to King Leopold, wrote that his poor little namesake was laid up again from a bad knee after an inconsequential fall. She confessed that her son was very sad and would never be fit for military service. She said no medicine or remedy brought relief from his suffering. Leopold dreaded being alone when he was bedridden with a bleed.

One hundred years separated the births of Brent Perry and Dick Wagner compared to Leopold's birth. They differed in respect in their family history—Brent had a cousin, and Dick had a grandfather who had hemophilia; Leopold was the first known instance in the royal family. Leopold was born into royalty; individuals in Brent's and Dick's family were commoners. Queen Victoria became aware of her son's bleeding problem, but she was not aware that his problem was inherited and that she was a carrier. Although he was the first instance of hemophilia in the royal family, he was not the last. The mutant hemophilia gene can alight in any family, rich or poor, nobility or average. Regardless of the family, the victims shared the same effect of agonizing pain and loneliness. Similar to Brent, Leopold suffered the pain from joint bleeds. And like Dick Wagner, Leopold recorded in his journal his dread of loneliness while he endured endless days alone in bed, motionless, suffering.

Doctor Guilt?

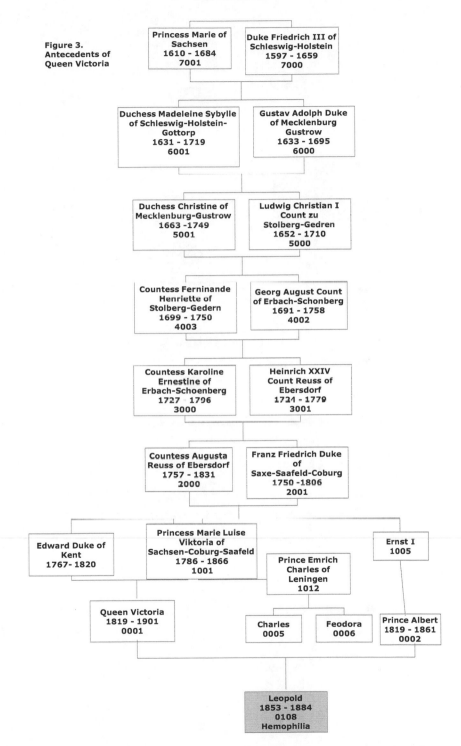

Figure 3.
Antecedents of
Queen Victoria

Princess Marie of
Sachsen
1610 - 1684
7001

Duke Friedrich III of
Schleswig-Holstein
1597 - 1659
7000

Duchess Madeleine Sybylle
of Schleswig-Holstein-
Gottorp
1631 - 1719
6001

Gustav Adolph Duke
of Mecklenburg
Gustrow
1633 - 1695
6000

Duchess Christine of
Mecklenburg-Gustrow
1663 -1749
5001

Ludwig Christian I
Count zu
Stolberg-Gedren
1652 - 1710
5000

Countess Ferninande
Henriette of
Stolberg-Gedern
1699 - 1750
4003

Georg August Count
of Erbach-Schonberg
1691 - 1758
4002

Countess Karoline
Ernestine of
Erbach-Schoenberg
1727 - 1796
3000

Heinrich XXIV
Count Reuss of
Ebersdorf
1724 - 1779
3001

Countess Augusta
Reuss of Ebersdorf
1757 - 1831
2000

Franz Friedrich Duke
of
Saxe-Saafeld-Coburg
1750 -1806
2001

Edward Duke of
Kent
1767- 1820

Princess Marie Luise
Viktoria of
Sachsen-Coburg-Saafeld
1786 - 1866
1001

Prince Emrich
Charles of
Leningen
1012

Ernst I
1005

Queen Victoria
1819 - 1901
0001

Charles
0005

Feodora
0006

Prince Albert
1819 - 1861
0002

Leopold
1853 - 1884
0108
Hemophilia

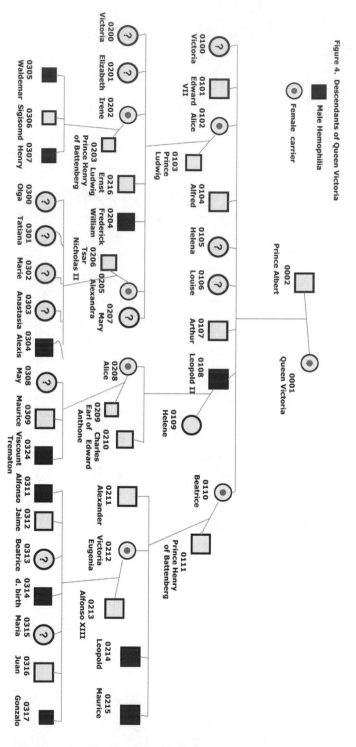

Figure 4. Descendants of Queen Victoria

Eleven male descendents of Queen Victoria who were affected with hemophilia were born into the royal family (table 7, figure 4). The possibility that a mutation occurred in the hemophilia gene in one of Queen Victoria's ova to be fertilized with her husband's sperm, which developed into a male affected with hemophilia, Leopold, can be dismissed since there were multiple male descendents who were affected with hemophilia. Not just one ovum contained the mutant hemophilia gene that could have been present if the queen were a gonadal mosaic. Instead, all the cells in her body contained the mutant hemophilia gene; she was made that way from the beginning, from the time she was an embryo. She was created from the union of a sperm or an egg that contained the mutant gene.

The origin of the mutation of the hemophilia gene within Queen Victoria's family has been debated. No living male descendents are available for modern molecular testing to search for the mutant gene. The last living affected person in the queen's family, Waldemar (0305, table 6), died in 1945 at age fifty-six. Is it possible that the hemophilia recessive mutant gene was inherited through the females, in generations preceding Queen Victoria, silently passed down from generation to generation without any signs of the disorder? The likelihood, the chances the gene would not appear, if it were inherited from previous generations of females, depends upon the number of males born to the females, females who might be carriers of the mutant gene.

Table 6. Hemophilia in descendents of Queen Victoria

Pedigree Number	Name	Hemophilia	birth	death	age
0001	Queen Victoria	hemophilia carrier	1819	1901	82 y
0002	Prince Albert, spouse 0001, died of typhoid fever		1819	1861	42 y
0100	Victoria, Princess Royal		1840	1901	61 y
0101	King Edward VI, Prince of Wales		1841	1910	69 y
0102	Josephine, Grand Duchess of Hesse, died typhoid fever	hemophilia carrier	1843	1878	35 y
0103	Louis IV, Prince Ludwig IV Grand Duke of Hesse spouse 0102		1837	1892	55 y
0104	Alfred, Duke of Saxe-Coburg died of throat cancer		1844	1900	55 y
0105	Helena, Princess Christian of Schleswig-Holstein		1846	1923	77 y
0106	Louise, Marques of Lorne		1848	0939	91 y
0107	Arthur, Duke of Connaught		1850	1942	91 y
0108	Leopold, died from claret and morphine for knee hemorrhage*	hemophilia	1853	1884	31 y
0109	Helena, spouse 0108		1861	1922	61 y
0110	Beatrice	hemophilia carrier	1857	1917	87 y
0111	Henry of Battenburg, spouse 0110		1858	1896	38 y
0200	Victoria, Marchioness of Milford Haven		1863	1950	87 y
0201	Elizabeth, Grand Duchess Feodorovna murdered		1864	1918	54 y
0202	Princess Irene	hemophilia carrier	1866	1953	87 y
0203	Heinrich, spouse 0202		1862	1929	66 y
0216	Ernst Ludwig		1868	1937	68 y
0204	Frederik, died of brain hemorrhage	hemophilia	1870	1873	2 y
0205	Alexandria, Tsarista of Russia murdered	hemophilia carrier	1872	1918	46 y
0206	Tsar Nicholas II murdered		1868	1918	50 y
0207	Marie, died of diphtheria		1874	1878	4 y
0208	Princess Alice	hemophilia carrier	1883	1981	97 y
0209	Earl of Athlone, spouse 0208		1874	1957	82 y
0210	Charles Edward		1884	1954	69 y
0211	Alexander		1886	1960	73 y
0212	Victoria Eugenie	hemophilia carrier	1887	1969	81 y
0213	Alfonso XIII, King of Spain, spouse 0212		1886	1941	54 y
0214	Leopold, died during knee surgery from hemorrhage	hemophilia	1889	1922	32 y

Doctor Guilt?

Pedigree Number	Name	Hemophilia	birth	death	age
0215	Maurice, died in military, Kings Royal Rifle Corps	hemophilia	1891	1914	23 y
0305	Waldemar, died fleeing the Russians	hemophilia	1889	1945	56 y
0306	Sigismund		1896	1978	82 y
0307	Heinrich, died from hemorrhage after bumping head	hemophilia	1900	1904	4 y
0318	Olga, murdered		1895	1918	22 y
0319	Tatiana, murdered		1897	1918	21 y
0320	Maria, murdered		1899	1918	19 y
0321	Anastasia, murdered		1901	1918	17 y
0304	Alexis, murdered	hemophilia	1904	1918	13 y
0322	Lady May of Cambridge		1906	1994	88 y
0323	Prince Maurice of Tek		1910	1910	6 mo
0324	Rupert, Viscount Trematon died head bleed (car crash)	hemophilia	1907	1928	21 y
0311	Alfonso, bled at circumcision; died bleeding (car crash)	hemophilia	1907	1938	31 y
0312	Jaimie		1908	1975	67 y
0313	Beatriz		1909	2002	93 y
0314	Infante Ferdinando Borbon y Battenburg	?	1910	1910	birth
0315	Maria		1911	1996	85 y
0316	Juan		1913	1993	80 y
0317	Gonzalo, died bleeding (car crashed into a wall)	hemophilia	1914	1934	20 y

* Sources conflict on the cause of Leopold's death: Excess morphine and claret for a knee bleed vs. a head bleed after falling in Club Villa Nevada in Cannes, or both.

Table 7. Eleven males in the royal family with hemophilia

Pedigree No.	Name	born	died	age at death
0108	Leopold	1853	1884	31 y
0204	Frederick	1870	1873	3 y
0305	Waldemar	1889	1945	56 y
0214	Leopold	1889	1922	33 y
0215	Maurice	1891	1914	23 y
0307	Henry	1900	1904	4 y
0304	Alexis	1904	1918	14 y
0311	Alfonso	1907	1938	31 y
0314	stillborn	1910	1910	birth
0317	Ganzalo	1914	1934	20 y
0324	Trematon	1907	1928	21 y

Average age at death, not including 0314: 23 years

Queen Victoria was the only child born of the union of her father, Edward, Duke of Kent, and her mother, Princess Marie of Sachsen-Coburg-Saafeld, 1001 (figure 3). Her mother was a widow after her first husband, Prince Emich Charles of Liningen, 1012, died before she married Queen Victoria's father. With her first husband, Princess Marie bore two children, a son Charles, 0005, and a daughter Feodora, 0006. If Queen Victoria inherited the hemophilia gene from her mother, the chances that Charles, 0005, would have had hemophilia was one half.

Similarly, if Queen Victoria's mother, Princess Marie, 1001, inherited the mutant hemophilia gene from her mother (Queen Victoria's grandmother), Countess Augusta, 2000, (figure 3) who had nine children, including four sons and five daughters, the chances that hemophilia would not have appeared, if the mutant gene had been present, in one of her four sons are $\frac{1}{2} \times \frac{1}{2} \times \frac{1}{2} \times \frac{1}{2}$, or 1/16. If all the children born to Queen Victoria's maternal antecedents—during seven generations back to Princess Maria, 7001, of Sachsen, born in 1610, who gave birth to sixteen children, including eight daughters and eight sons—were counted, thirty-nine daughters and twenty-three sons were born. If Princess Maria, 7001, was a carrier of hemophilia and passed the mutant gene down to Queen Victoria during seven generations, without hemophilia appearing in one or more males before the birth of Leopold, if hemophilia was inherited, the chances the family tree would have been observed without hemophilia is $(\frac{1}{2})^{23}$ or $\frac{1}{2}$ to the square of the number of males born, which equals 0.00000135, or 1 in 769,230 chances that hemophilia would not have appeared in one of the male offspring if Queen Victoria inherited the mutation from Princess Maria. However, this reasoning is not completely valid unless the age of death of all the males is considered. If the males died early, hemophilia could have been present without discovery. Of the sixteen children born to Princess Maria of Sachsen, 7001, and Duke Friedrich III of Schleswig-Holstein, 7000, during nineteen years, six died before the end of their first year, including two daughters and four sons. Of the ten male descendents of Queen Victoria affected by hemophilia, the average age at death was twenty-three years. Only one person affected with hemophilia, Waldemar, 0305, lived past his fortieth birthday (table 7).

Considering the possibility that hemophilia may have been present but not detected in earlier generations of Queen Victoria's family, it is unlikely that the family tree would have been as it has been recorded if hemophilia was inherited. Instead, another explanation for the appearance of hemophilia within the royal family is offered. It is likely that the mutation occurred in a sperm of Victoria's father, Edward, Duke of Kent, who was fifty-two years of age when Victoria was born. If his sperm contributed the mutation when the ovum of her mother was fertilized, all the cells in her body would contain the mutant hemophilia gene on the X chromosome that she received from her father to pair with the maternal X chromosome she received from her mother. As a result, Queen Victoria would have produced two kinds of ova: half her ova would bear the hemophilia mutant; half would be without the hemophilia mutant. Her children who received her X chromosome without the hemophilia mutant would not be female carriers or sons with hemophilia. Half her offspring would be expected to receive the hemophilia mutant gene. For females, they would be hemophilia carriers; for males, they would have hemophilia.

Review of the royal family tree reveals that of the nine children born to Queen Victoria, three females were not known to be carriers; two females were carriers of hemophilia. Three of her sons did not have hemophilia; one son was affected with hemophilia (figure 4).

Queen Victoria's nine children

Five daughters
- three non-hemophilia carriers: Victoria, Helena, Louise
- two female hemophilia carriers: Alice, Beatrice

Four sons
- three non-hemophilia sons: Edward, Alfred, Arthur
- one hemophilia son: Leopold II

Index

Bold page numbers indicate photos.
t indicates tables. *n* indicates notes.

A

accountability
  of drug companies, 8
  of patients' families, 51, 52, 60,
    226
Acquired Immunodeficiency Disease
  (AIDS). *See* AIDS (Acquired
  Immunodeficiency Disease)
Adney, Vance, 442*t*
adrenalin, 21
"AFRAIDS," 378
Africa
  children of HIV-infected
    mothers, 217
  deaths from AIDS, 298
  emergence of HIV/AIDS in, 305,
    307
  plasma collection centers in, 321
AHF (antihemophilia factor)
  amount of, per infusion, 50
  as clotting factor, 37, 85, 201n70
  replacement treatment, history of,
    55–56
  testing, 16
AHF (antihemophilia factor)
  concentrate
  availability of, 6
  costs of, 87, 236, 326n109
  discovery of, 55–56, 66

heat-treated (HT) concentrate.
  See heat-treated (HT)
  concentrate
HIV-contaminated, 153, 209
Humafac. *See* Humafac
immunization by, 75
Koate. *See* Koate (concentrate)
Kogenate. *See* Kogenate
  (concentrate)
Konyne. *See* Konyne
  (concentrate)
manufacture of safer concentrate,
  157, 234, 316, 321
as miracle treatment for
  hemophilia, 7
Monoclate. *See* Monoclate
producers of, 122
production of, 6
recalls of. *See* recalls, of
  concentate
recombinant AHF (rFVIII). *See*
  recombinant FVIII (rFVIII)
sales of, 326n109
storage of, at clinic, 121–122
in whole blood, 201n70
Xyntha, 340n111
See also concentrate
AHF (antihemophilia factor) factor
  VIII, deficiency of. *See* factor VIII,
  deficiency
AHF F8 (gene), 22
AHF F9 (gene), 22

AIDS (Acquired Immunodeficiency
Disease)
  association of homosexuality
    with, 100, 110, 209, 292, 297,
    298, 307, 310, 311, 332, 378,
    387, 412
  as a bad word, 153
  "big bang theory" for origin of,
    306, 307
  cause of, 147n54, 151
  as chronic illness, 227
  common cause of death in
    survivors of, 136
  deaths from, 298, 305
  Dr. Taillefer's first case of, 117
  Dr. Taillefer's second case of, 118
  drugs users association with, 298
  first cases in hemophilia in
    United States, 322
  as frightening threat, 374
  government information
    pamphlet on, 400–401
  and hemophilia, 426t
  length of time between HIF
    infection and onset of, 217
  as man-made, 305
  naming of, 244n91
  as new territory for attorneys, 265
  as new territory for doctors, 265
  onset of, 244
  Pat Buchanan on, 297
  in persons treated with blood-
    derived AHF concentrate, 7
  as political issue, 404
  as preventable, 231
  as red flag, 332
  as reportable disease, 389
  reporting of, 393
  Ronald Reagan on, 297–298,
    399, 404
Ronald Reagan's administration
    on, 400, 403
  signs and symptoms of, 117n40,
    120, 168
  social impact compared to
    medical concerns, 402
  society's reaction to, 403
  spread through plasma products,
    322
  stigma associated with, 209, 292,
    298, 387
  teaching materials for, 392
  as universally fatal disease, 207, 227
AIDS Action Council, 400
AIDS clearinghouse, U.S.
  government, 401
AIDS Commission, 401
AIDS Conference (British), 306, 309
AIDS coordinator, U.S.
  government, 402
AIDS for Douglas County
  (Oregon), 373
  See also Douglas County AIDS
    Council
AIDS hotline, U.S. government, 401
AIDS information pamphlet, U.S.
  government, 400–401
AIDS memorial, at Camp
  Tapawingo, 207
AIDS pandemic, potential trigger
  of, 305
AIDS policy, Glide Elementary
  School, 412
AIDS prevention, questions about
  from hemophilia patients, 245
AIDS warning, on concentrate
  package insert, 286
Aina, Paul, 208, 442t
Albert, Prince, 443, 445
albumin, heat-treated, as alternative
  for plasma, 318

- 456 -

hepatitis B (HB) vaccine, as proposed theory for transfer of SIV in chimpanzees to HIV in humans, 304t, 306–307, 308f, 309, 311, 428

hepatitis B virus (HBV). *See* type B hepatitis (HBV)

hepatitis C virus (HCV). *See* type C hepatitis (HCV)

hepatitis E virus (HEV), 303

hepatitis viruses
in blood-derived AHF concentrate, 6
elimination of, 157n62, 158
See also hepatitis E virus (HEV); type A hepatitis (HAV); type B hepatitis (HBV); type C hepatitis (HCV)

hepatoma, 136

heroin addicts, and AIDS, 298, 312

heterochromia, 353

HEV (hepatitis E virus), 303

HFO (Hemophilia Foundation of Oregon), 113, 137, 142

HHS (U.S. Department of Health and Human Services), 238, 399, 401

Higgines, Maxine, 275

Higgins, Donald, 269, 275, 276

highly active antiretroviral therapy (HAART), 179, 227, 228, 434

Hinckley, Abby, 177

hip bleeds, 60

Hippocratic oath, 424

HIV (human immunodeficiency virus)
in blood-derived AHF concentrate, 6–7
community discussion of, in school, 378–381
compared to hepatitis, 230
described, 150–151
in existence since 1970s, 309

and heat-treated (HT) concentrate, 158
and hemophilia, 426t
as infectious substance in blood supply, 114
as new territory for attorneys, 265
as new territory for doctors, 265
origins of, 303
path to from SIV via HBV, 308f
protection against contact with, 383
reaction of inoculation into chimpanzees, 311–312
as reportable infectious disease, 152, 389, 393
from SIV (simian immunodeficiency virus), 303, 304t
teaching materials for, 392
testing for, 147–151, 222

HIV and hepatitis infection in hemophilia, as "an unavoidable tragedy," 231

HIV antibody test, 147

HIV infection
from concentrate. *See* Oregon Hemophilia Treatment Center, patients to be remembered
diarrhea as sign of, 118n41
as displaying no symptoms, 310
as frightening threat, 374
length of time between and onset of AIDS, 217
previously known as HTLV-III infection, 118n41
reporting of, 152, 332, 372, 389, 393, 407
routes of infection, 151n56
stigma associated with, 292

HIV-1 (human AIDS virus), 309, 311

HIV-positive
confirmation with Western Blot
test, 147, 148n55
designation, 150, 151
diagnosis (Bantu person 1959),
305
diagnosis (Brad Craigdon), 261,
263, 272
diagnosis (Brent Perry), 152, 153,
154, 155, 239, 244, 245, 246,
333
diagnosis (Davy Jarrard), 166, 168
diagnosis (Mike Charles), 222–223
diagnosis (persons in Hong
Kong), 324
diagnosis (Sally Phillips), 292
diagnosis (Steve Phillips), 292
Hollub, Michael, 442t
home infusions
advantages of, 51
of cryoprecipitate, 319
of Humafac, 56
and Oregon Hemophilia
Treatment Center, 205
use of (Brent Perry), 46–49
use of (David Whitbeck), 364–365
use of (Doug McAllister), 204
use of (Mike Charles), 219–220
use of (Randy Gibson), 177
use of (Roger Norman), 127
homeless people, as blood donors,
58, 229
homologous serum jaundice, 318
See also type B hepatitis (HBV)
homosexual men
new disease discovered in, 100, 110
as one of the 4Hs, 297, 311, 387
simultaneous emergence of AIDS
in Africa and in, 307
as volunteers to help develop
hepatitis B vaccine, 310

as volunteers to help develop
polio vaccine, 310
homosexuality, association of AIDS
with, 100, 110, 209, 292, 297, 298,
307, 310, 311, 332, 378, 387, 412
Hong Kong, as market for non-HT
concentrate, 314, 324
Hooper, Edward, 299, 304, 307,
434
Hopff, Friedrich, 445
Horowitz, Bernard, 325
HTLV, 147, 425, 426
HTLV-III infection, 118n41
Hudson, Rock, 297, 375
Huge, Clyde, 259
Hugo, Ellen, 259
Humafac, 56, 85, 127, 204, 205,
219
human immunodeficiency
virus (HIV). See HIV (human
immunodeficiency virus)
Hunt, Dr. Stephen, 58
Hunter, Jim, 37
"the Hurricane" (topical anesthetic),
167
Hyland Laboratories, 55, 56
Hyland Pharmaceutical, 85, 122,
204, 313, 318, 319, 320, 323, 326
hyporeflexia, 70

I

ice packs, use of, 39, 59, 97, 126,
218, 219
immune system, 150, 224, 225,
240, 245n93, 325, 368, 387, 397
immunoaffinity chromatography,
234n83, 236
infectious, compared to contagious,
151
infectious diseases, origins of, 300
inflammation of gums, 116, 120

influenza
    epidemic of 1918, compared
        to HIV/AIDS scenario in the
        1980s, 301
    epidemic of 1918, deaths from,
        300
    origins of, 300
infusions
    costs of, 87, 236–237, 326n109
    frequency of, depending upon
        age, 87–88
    home infusions. *See* home infusions
    importance of early, 45
    as preventative, 53–54
    self-infusions. *See* self-infusions
    use of butterfly needle for, 39, 47,
        123, 365
    "when in doubt, infuse!" 159
inherited mutation, 353, 355
insulin, production of, 337–339
intracranial hemorrhage, 24*t*, 32,
    42, 86, 126–127, 156
intrahepatic portosystemic shunt
    procedure, 256
intron 22 inversion, 32, 355–356
Isabella (clinic staff), 36, 68, 80, 170
Italy, and development of safer
    concentrate, 234
IV drug users, 210

J

Jacob (in McCann family), 24*t*, 29*t*,
    33*t*
James, Dr. Harold, 84
Japan, as market for non-HT
    concentrate, 160, 230, 314
Jarrard, David (Davy), 165–170,
    233, 442*t*
Jarrard, Julie, 166, 169
jaundice, homologous serum, 318
    See also type B hepatitis (HBV)

jaw bleeds, 60
Jergens, Dr. Elisabeth, 278
Joe (in Norman family), 124*t*
Johns Hopkins Medical Center,
    carrier testing, 15, 26, 27, 31
Johnson, Hutchinson Kimberly
    (Hutch), 334–342
joint bleeds
    Brent Perry, 44–45, 59
    in child compared to older man, 62
    Dick Wagner, 252, 257
    Doug McAllister, 204, 206
    Leopold, 446
    Norman children, 126
    Phillips children, 292
Jones, David, 241–243, 442*t*
Joseph (in McCann family), 25*t*,
    29*t*, 33*t*
Josephine (office staff), 170
*Journal of the American Medical
    Association*, 317, 320

K

Katrina (office staff), 170
Kennedy, Edward, 400
Kennedy, Joe, 146, **193**, 231, 442*t*
Kerlix bandage, 166
ketoconazole, 166
Kingston, Dr. Aaron, 111, 260, 278
knee bleeds, 60, 78
knee joint replacements, 63, 66–67,
    292
Koate (concentrate), 75n25, 122,
    226, 263, 278, 327
    See also Koate HP (concentrate);
        Koate HT (concentrate)
Koate HP (concentrate), 121, 158,
    160
Koate HT (concentrate), 101, 121,
    158, 160, 226

Kogenate (concentrate), 239,
326n109
Konyne (concentrate), 75n25, 76,
122, 248, 249
Koop, Dr. C. Everett, 298, 401,
402–403, 422
Korean War, and ultraviolet
irradiation of pooled plasma, 319
Krostag, Joe, 123, 124t, 131–132,
442t
Kurath, Barry, 235, 237, 442t
Kurillo, Nathaniel, 442t

L
Laam, Mark, 442t
labial frenum, 175n67
laminectomy, 73–74
The Lancet, 444
Latin America, as market for non-
HT concentrate, 324
Lawson, Jeff, 442t
lawsuits
    Brad Craigdon as plaintiff,
    261–287
    class-action suit 1993, 326
    for contaminated concentrate, 231
    against doctors, 238
    against manufacturers of
    concentrates, 327
    against school board, 406–407
    against using unheated pooled
    plasma, 325
Legg-Calvé-Perthes disease, 204
Leopold, 42, 77–78, 443–446,
447t, 448t, 449, 450t, 452t
Leopold I, King, 445
Leppaluatto, Jeff, 442t
lidocaine, 167
life expectancy, in hemophilia, 42,
55, 57, 83, 204, 351, 358
Lincoln, Abraham, 403

Linderman, Vicki, 398
liver cancer
    in persons infused with HIV
    contaminated concentrate who
    survive AIDS, 136
    in persons treated with blood-
    derived AHF concentrate, 7
    Roger Norman, 136
liver disease, in persons treated with
blood-derived AHF concentrate, 7
liver failure
    Dick Wagner, 255
    Mike Charles, 232
Los Angeles County Hospital, 99, 100
Los Angeles Times, 100
lyonization, 23n9, 31, 290t
lyophilized concentrate, 55, 85
lyse, 61n22

M
Mack, Viktor, 277
malaria
    contraction of, 299–300
    origins of, 300
Manson, Dr. Purcel, 40
Margaret (in McCann family), 24t,
29t, 33t
marketing, of medicines, 95, 159,
210, 237, 326, 335, 336, 338,
339, 427, 428
Martin, Mary, 375, 383, 435–436
MASAC (Medical and Scientific
Advisory Committee of the National
Hemophilia Foundation), 277
Maternal and Child Health Division
of NIH (MCH), 90, 91, 92, 93, 320
    See also Region X Comprehensive
    Hemophilia Treatment Center
    grant
Maternal and Child Health Services
(Alaska), 111

in study program on benefits of
AZT, 245
and Wayne Palmer, 133–134
on withholding infusions because
of fear of becoming stricken
with new disease, 147
Perry, Leland Hubert (Lee)
effect of recalls on, 113
giving Brent shots, 46–49, 52–53
infusions, on withholding of,
because of fear of becoming
stricken with new disease, 147
learning about hemophilia, 43–44
learning about HIV and AIDS,
156
marriage to Gwyn McCann, 13
McCann family history, 29t, 33t
separation from Gwyn, 334
work history, 34, 36, 99, 100, 105
Perry family, mistrust of medical
community, 158–159
Peterson, Gerald, 442t
Peterson, Jack, 62–63, 442t
Peterson, Phillip, 442t
Pfizer, 56n20, 340
pharmaceutical manufacturers. See
drug companies
phenobarbital, 128
Philadelphia Inquirer, 316
Phillips, Sally, 288–293, 363, 442t
Phillips, Steve, 290, 292, 293, 363,
442t
phylogenetic and sequence analysis,
300
Pierrette (friend of Gwyn), 14, 17, 97
Pierrette (wife of Dr. Taillefer), 172,
173
pigs, and HEV, 303
the plague, origins of, 300
plasma
collection centers, 229, 312, 321

and cryoprecipitate (cryo), 319
from donors. *See* blood donors
fractionating industry, 315
freeze-dried, 318
heat treatment of, 317, 325, 326
pooled, as vehicle that caused
homologous serum jaundice, 318
purification of, 316, 317
transfusions of, on battlefields in
World War II, 317
ultraviolet irradiation of pooled
plasma in Korean War, 319
plasma-derived concentrate, 239
platelet plug, 21–22
platelets, 21
Pneumocystis jiroveccii, 245n93
pneumocystis pneumonia (PCP)
and Brent Perry, 331–332, 333,
349, 360, 425
described, 245n93
pneumonia
as later sign of AIDS, 120, 245–
246
prevention of, 245
poems
by Dick Wagner, 250–251
by Linda Charles, 232–233
polio, contraction of, 299
Pool, Dr. Judith, 55, 319, 321
pooled plasma, as vehicle that
caused homologous serum
jaundice, 318
poor appetite, early sign of AIDS, 120
porta vein, 54
Porter, Dr. Don (dentist), 68, 166,
167, 168
Portland Red Cross, 58
Portland Teachers Credit Union, 82
previously un-infused persons
(PUPS), 239n90
Price, Alfred, 325

primates
  and development of polio
    vaccine, 304–305
  and HIV-related retroviral gene,
    307
  and pathway for origin of HIV,
    309, 311
  sequences of genotypes, 302
  viruses in, 303, 305, 310
prophylactic infusions, 101, 226
prophylaxis, compared to demand
  treatment, 54
proteases, 61n22
proteolytic enzymes, 61
prothrombin assay, 176
prothrombin complex, 75n25
pseudotumor, 242
psittacosis, 117n39
psoriasis, 117
public health policies
  on drug pricing, 236
  reporting of HIV-positive
    students, 332
publications, funded by drug
  companies, 209
Puget Sound Blood Center, 90
"punctuated origin event," as origin
  of HIV/AIDS pandemic, 305, 306
PUPS (previously un-infused
  persons), 239n90
purification, of blood supply, 114,
  234, 316, 317

Q
quadriceps atrophy, 64

R
race, and hemophilia, 111n37, 113,
  123
Ramsley, Dr. Hunter, 111, 116

Rappaport, Captain Emanuel, 317,
  318
Rappaport, Dr. Sam, 84–85
Ray, Randy, 406
Ray, Ricky, 406
Ray, Robert, 406
Ray family, 406–407
Reagan, Ronald
  administration on AIDS
    information pamphlet, 400
  administration's AIDS policies, 403
  on AIDS, 297–298
  on AIDS testing, 399
  speech on AIDS, 404
Reardon, David, 442t
recalls, of concentrate, 109, 112,
  158, 160, 206, 293, 313, 367
recombinant FVIII (rFVIII), 134,
  234, 239, 326n109, 355, 429
recombinant technology, 210, 239,
  338
Red Cross. See American Red Cross;
  Portland Red Cross
Redeker, A. G., 319, 320
Reed College, 57
Reeves, Tim, 442t
Region X Comprehensive
  Hemophilia Treatment Center
  grant, 90–93, **184**
Region X Hemophilia Center,
  Oregon Hemophilia Treatment
  Center as, 110
regulations
  governing contagious illnesses
    and school attendance, 376,
    379, 393, 394
  lack of, in United States in
    health-care industry, 8, 229,
    316, 336, 339, 340
  punishment for failure to impose,
    327

Stenbeck, John, 377, 391
Stevens, Curtis, 442*t*
stockholders, interests of, 237
    See also drug companies
string sign, 75
stroke, causes of, 22
Strong, Dr. Ned, 85, 169, 224, 299, 331, 332, 333
suffering, concentrate as relief for, 159
summer camp
    balloon release, **197**
    Brent Perry at, 137–142, **193**
    counselors who died from AIDS, 146
    David Witbeck at, **196**, 369–370
    Doug McAllister at, 207
    funded by drug companies, 209
    Peter Witbeck at, **196**, 369–370
Sumner, John Bird, 444
surgery, for persons with hemophilia, 62–63, 86
swelling, 37, 39, 44, 51, 59, 98, 127, 131, 133, 176, 200, 218, 219, 225, 255, 367
swimming, as therapy for joint problems, 292
Syme's amputation, 130
synchronous epidemics, 306
synovectomy, 366
synovitis, 366
synovium, 61

T
T4-helper cells, 224, 245
    See also T-helper cells
Taillefer, Dr. Anton
    appointed director of Oregon Hemophilia Treatment Center, 84
    background of, 81–84
    and Barry Kurath, 235, 237–239
    and Brent Perry, 36, 39, 40–41, 47–48, 333
    on contact with drug company reps, 234
    Craigdon lawsuit and trial, 258, 261, 265–269, 270–287, 327
    and Davy Jarrard, 165–170
    devastated at tainted concentrate, 119
    and Dick Wagner, 253
    and drug company incentives, 341–342
    and financial concerns of patients and clinic, 87–89
    and Hippocratic oath, 424
    on his early days in medicine, 422
    and Jason Cobb, 114–118
    and John McAnulty, 118–119
    and MCH funding of regional clinic, 90–92
    and Mike Charles, 223, 232
    and Nora Warren, 143–144
    and pharmaceutical competition, 95
    on polluted medicine, 182
    and Randy Gibson, 172–175, 178, 180
    at summer camp, 369–371
    and Wayne Palmer, 133–134
    and Wendell Singer, 69–73, 75
target joints
    Brent Perry, 61, 109
    Mike Charles, 219
    tracking development of, 226, 227
T-cell leukemia, 147n54
Ted (in McCann family), 24*t*, 29*t*, 33*t*
temporomandibular joint (TMJ), 60
tests/testing
    AHF (antihemophilia factor), 16
    carrier testing. *See* carrier testing